W9-AZO-563

Introduction to
Information Systems for Health Information Technology

FOURTH EDITION

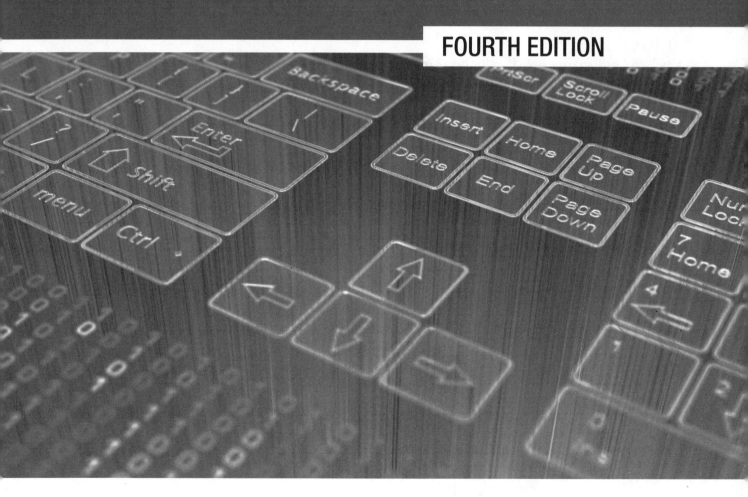

Nanette B. Sayles, EdD, RHIA, CCS, CDIP, CHDA, CHPS, CPHI, CPHIMS, FAHIMA
and Lauralyn Kavanaugh-Burke, DrPH, RHIA, CHES, CHTS-IM

AHIMA
PRESS

Copyright ©2021 by the American Health Information Management Association. All rights reserved. Except as permitted under the Copyright Act of 1976, no part of this publication may be reproduced, stored in a retrieval system, or transmitted, in any form or by any means, electronic, photocopying, recording, or otherwise, without the prior written permission of AHIMA, 233 North Michigan Avenue, 21st Floor, Chicago, Illinois, 60601-5809 (http://www.ahima.org/reprint).

ISBN: 978-1-58426-742-3

AHIMA Product No.: AB103419

AHIMA Staff:
Chelsea Brotherton, MA, Production Development Editor
Megan Grennan, Director, Content Production and AHIMA Press
James Pinnick, Vice President, Content and Product Development and Licensing
Rachel Schratz, MA, Assistant Editor
Cover image: ©iStock

Limit of Liability/Disclaimer of Warranty: This book is sold, as is, without warranty of any kind, either express or implied. While every precaution has been taken in the preparation of this book, the publisher and author assume no responsibility for errors or omissions. Neither is any liability assumed for damages resulting from the use of the information or instructions contained herein. It is further stated that the publisher and author are not responsible for any damage or loss to your data or your equipment that results directly or indirectly from your use of this book.

The websites listed in this book were current and valid as of the date of publication. However, webpage addresses and the information on them may change at any time. The user is encouraged to perform his or her own general web searches to locate any site addresses listed here that are no longer valid.

CPT® is a registered trademark of the American Medical Association. All other copyrights and trademarks mentioned in this book are the possession of their respective owners. AHIMA makes no claim of ownership by mentioning products that contain such marks.

For more information, including updates, about AHIMA Press publications, visit **http://www.ahima.org/education/press**.

American Health Information Management Association
233 North Michigan Avenue, 21st Floor
Chicago, Illinois 60601-5809
ahima.org

Contents

Detailed Contents

Chapter 3   Introduction to Databases and Data Analytics   35

Chapter 6   Computerization in Health Informaticsand Information Management   **113**

About the Authors

Nanette B. Sayles, EdD, RHIA, CCS, CDIP, CHDA, CHPS, CPHI, CPHIMS, FAHIMA

Dr. Sayles has a bachelor of science degree in medical record administration, a master of science in health information management, a master's degree in public administration, and a doctorate in adult education. Dr. Sayles has more than 10 years of experience as a health information management practitioner with roles in hospitals, a consulting firm, and a computer vendor. She has 20 years of health information management education experience. She was the 2005 American Health Information Management Association (AHIMA) Triumph Educator award winner. She has held numerous offices and other volunteer roles for AHIMA, the Georgia Health Information Management Association (GHIMA), the Alabama Association of Health Information Management (AAHIM), the Middle Georgia Health Information Management Association (MGHIMA), and the Birmingham Regional Health Information Management Association (BRHIMA). These positions include: AHIMA Educational Strategies Committee, AHIMA Co-Chair RHIA Workgroup, GHIMA Director, and President of MGHIMA. Dr. Sayles has published a number of health information management textbooks and is currently the professor of health information management at East Central College in Union, Missouri.

Lauralyn Kavanaugh-Burke, DrPH, RHIA, CHES, CHTS-IM

Dr. Burke earned her bachelor of science degree in health record administration with a minor in biology from York College of Pennsylvania, a master of science degree in Community Health Education from West Virginia University, and received her doctor of public health (DrPH) with a concentration in epidemiology from Florida A&M University. She has almost 40 years of management experience in hospital health information departments, coding consulting and DRG analysis, health education programs, and teaching in both health information technology and management programs. Through her extensive experience, Dr. Burke's main areas of interest are hospital disaster preparedness, bioterrorism and infectious diseases, and the implementation of technology in health information management. In addition to her degrees, she also a certified health education specialist (CHES) and certified in implementation management for health information technology (CHTS-IM). She has published in the Journal of the American Health Information Management Association, Perspectives in Health Information Management and Educational Perspectives in Health Information Management and is the author of the medical science chapter of Cengage Learning's Professional Review Guide for the RHIA and RHIT Examinations. Dr. Burke has also held positions and participated in committees within the Northwest Florida Health Information Management Association (NWFHIMA) and the Florida Health Information Management Association (FHIMA). She currently is an associate professor in the Division of Health Informatics and Information Management at Florida A&M University.

Acknowledgments

From Nanette Sayles:

This book is dedicated to my husband, Mark, and my daughter, Rachel, who are my biggest supporters. I love you both. Thanks to AHIMA Press for your vote of confidence in publishing this book. Thanks, Lauralyn, for your partnership on this book. You have made it better. To the students and faculty who use this book, I hope you find it a valuable resource.

From Lauralyn Kavanaugh-Burke:

This book is dedicated to my husband, John K. Burke, Jr. and my late parents, Lieutenant Colonel (Ret.) Richard D. and Cathryn C. Kavanaugh for their unconditional love, unwavering support, and encouragement in my educational journey and achieving this personal goal. A special thank you to Dr. Nanette Sayles for inviting me to coauthor the fourth edition of this great textbook. It has been a challenging and worthwhile experience. To all who use this book, may it provide the stepping stone in a long and productive career.

AHIMA Press and the authors would like to thank Ray Hylock, PhD, and Nathan Taylor, MS, MPH, CHDA for their review and feedback on this book.

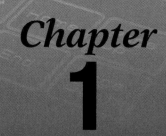

Introduction to Computers in Health Information Management

Learning Objectives

- Identify and discuss the impact of computers on healthcare.
- Discuss the history of computers in healthcare.
- Compare and contrast the similarities and differences among the Internet, intranet, and extranet as used in healthcare.
- Explain data analytics and health informatics and how information systems (ISs) apply.

Key Terms

Certified health data analyst (CHDA)
Clinical pathways
Clinical practice guidelines
Cloud computing
Computer on wheels (COW)
Dashboards
Data
Data analytics
Data mining
Descriptive analytics
Descriptive statistics
Diagnostic analytics

Dumb terminals
Electronic health record (EHR)
Evidence-based medicine
Extranet
Financial applications
Health informatics
Health information exchange (HIE)
Inferential statistics
Information
Information system (IS)
Internet

Intranet
Local area network
Mainframe computers
Patient safety
Personal computer (PC)
Protocol
Point of care (POC)
Predictive analytics
Predictive modelling
Prescriptive analytics
Wireless on wheels (WOW)

Computer use in healthcare and health information management (HIM) is not a new concept. Computers have been used in patient care, public health, and research since the 1960s. Even though the HIM profession has relied on data since the time of the first paper health record, the way that the data—raw facts and figures—are collected, stored, and shared has changed dramatically with the implementation of information systems. An information system (IS) is an automated system that uses computer hardware and software to record, manipulate, store, recover, and disseminate data (that is, a system that receives and processes input and provides output). Input is the data that is entered into the information. Output is the data displays, reports, and other means of pulling data from the information system. These changes range from data interaction among individuals and departments to system-wide networks and hospital information systems that span several states. It is the role of the HIM professional to collect, analyze, use, and maintain data at all levels of ISs and networks in hospitals and other healthcare organizations. This responsibility can be a challenge as technology changes, quickly requiring constant updating of skills and knowledge. Adoption and implementation of the technology in a healthcare organization generally move at a much slower rate. For example, electronic health records, defined in the next section, have been around for decades but have only recently been implemented in many healthcare organizations. ISs now play a major role in healthcare. This chapter covers the history of computers in healthcare, the impact of computers on healthcare, an introduction to health informatics, an introduction to data analytics and the impact on HIM.

History of Computers in Healthcare

The first computers in healthcare used punch-card systems prior to the 1960s. Punch cards were cards with holes punched in them to represent data to be read by the computer. See Figure 1.1 for an example of an unpunched card. At that time, computers were large machines that filled entire rooms and needed extreme cooling controls; these machines used vacuum tubes for circuitry and magnetic drums rather than microchips for memory. Much of the healthcare-related information systems used in those days involved manual data entry.

Figure 1.1. Unpunched punch card

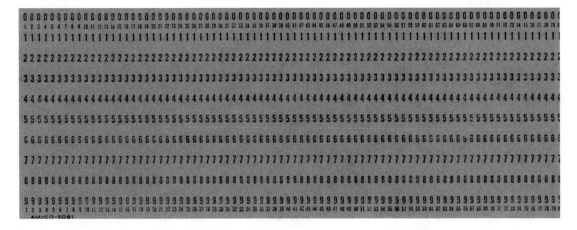

Source: Burchfield, G. *Personal punch card.*

Figure 1.2 is an example of a punch card that has been punched. It provided the computer instructions on what to do. For example, it might provide an instruction on what to do.

Early Information Systems

The first ISs installed in the 1960s were mostly financial applications, which were among the few information systems available and were some of the simplest software packages. **Financial applications** are software applications that handle patient accounts, budgets, and other financial activities of the healthcare organization. With the use of mainframe computers throughout hospitals, the healthcare industry was beginning to experience the benefits computers could provide. **Mainframe computers** are large computers that are used by the government and other organizations that require speed and the ability to process large amounts of data. Although the trend has been to use smaller computers, some mainframe computers are still in use today.

In the 1970s, technology evolved and the memory capability of computers increased. In the late 1970s, the healthcare industry began to use departmental ISs, such as those used in the laboratory, radiology, and HIM departments. See chapters 6–8 for details on ISs.

Figure 1.2. Punched card

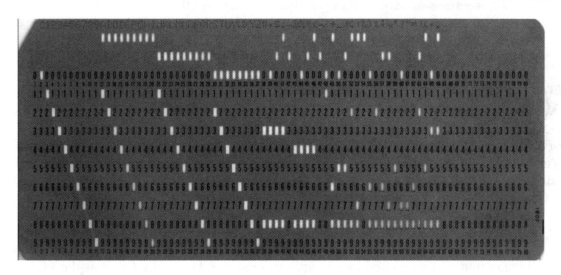

Source: Gwern. *Blue Punch Card Front*.

In HIM departments, computers were used to help the personnel with master patient index (MPI) functions and abstracting, which are further discussed in chapters 6 and 7. Most of the computers used were **dumb terminals**. In dumb terminals, all of the processing is performed at the server or mainframe, whereas with **personal computers (PCs)** some or all of the processing is performed on the PC. The **personal computer** is a computer that has a central processing unit (CPU), computer memory, and data storage devices designed to support a single individual. The CPU is another name for a microprocessor, which is a microchip that processes the information and the code (instructions) used by a computer, the "brains of a computer." Some advanced HIM departments in the 1970s began having employees input patient data into the dumb terminals, capturing various patient or clinical data for reporting and ordering purposes. Previously, all abstracting of data from the health record was done by the HIM technicians on paper abstracts. These abstracts were then mailed to the various reporting agencies for data entry and report creation. The ability to abstract patient data once into an information system and being able to send the abstracts to several agencies or used to generate several reports, was innovative for the time. Using the old paper abstracts for reporting purposes was a time-consuming process for the personnel. The new ISs also decreased the possibility of errors made when transcribing by hand any notes from the primary record to a secondary source. The data from the computerized abstract was used to print reports.

The 1980s and 1990s saw even more advancement in computers' memory capacity and speed. The physical size of the computers and their costs decreased while memory and the amount of storage increased at tremendous rates. Use of computers in business continued to increase, and purchases of home computers multiplied during this period. The PCs for consumers became more affordable, making the computer a machine that home users could enjoy and not just a tool for business and industry.

During the 1980s, wired networking among hospital departments became more common, and computers and other digital devices helped healthcare organizations share data more quickly and with greater ease. These networks, which connect devices in close, physical proximity, are known as a local area network (LAN). In the 1990s, the Internet became mainstream. The Internet comprises thousands of networks with millions of computers linked together to share data and information. The Internet enables physicians, HIM professionals, and others to remotely access patient and other information for patient care, billing, quality improvement, and other purposes. It allows patient information as well as administrative information to be shared outside the healthcare organization with insurers, healthcare providers, health departments and others. The 1990s also saw data entry being performed using technologies such as barcoding of data, speech recognition, touch screens, light pens, and microphones. Hospital departments—such as admissions, business offices, quality improvement offices, and utilization management—that worked closely with the HIM departments were networked so that data were shared and less time was spent rekeying data. This network made these departments more efficient, and data sharing within hospitals increased significantly.

Modern Information Systems

Today wireless devices, such as tablets and cellular phones, are used throughout the healthcare organization. These wireless devices frequently utilize Wi-Fi. Wi-Fi is wireless connectivity protocol (set of communication rules) that uses radio waves to connect computers and other devices to a local area network and the Internet. Many of these wireless devices are small and are easily carried to nursing units for patient care at the bedside by healthcare practitioners. Wireless computers are often seen at the **point of care (POC),** the place or location where the physician administers services to the patient, such as the patient's bedside. POC is used to document the care provided when it is provided. One type of device used at the POC is the **computer on wheels (COW)**—also referred to as **wireless on wheels (WOW)**—which involves a wireless computer mounted on a mobile cart that can be moved from patient to patient. Using the COW at the POC improves documentation because the documentation is completed as soon as the care occurs. Point of care documentation also gives current information to other healthcare professionals involved in the patient's care. One of the downsides to wireless computers is that they are easy targets for both physical (the device itself) and virtual theft (data).

Healthcare organizations have been working toward the **electronic health record (EHR)** for decades as they have implemented other ISs that feed data into the EHR. The EHR is an electronic record of health-related information on an individual that conforms to nationally recognized interoperability standards and that can be created, managed, and consulted by authorized clinicians and staff across more than one healthcare organization. Many healthcare organizations, however, began the transition to the EHR after the American Recovery and Reinvestment Act of 2009. This law enacted an incentive program known at the time as Meaningful Use, which gave healthcare providers who met the requirements financial incentives for implementing the EHR and using it in a meaningful way such as improving the quality of care provided to the patients. For example, the EHR will monitor the medications ordered for the patient to ensure that the combination of drugs is safe. In other words, to ensure there are no negative drug interactions.

Within the healthcare industry, computers helped increase employee productivity. Since the end of the 1990s, most HIM department employees have used PCs at their workstations to better perform their HIM roles within the healthcare organization. Some HIM departmental employees may use laptops, tablets, or other portable devices to perform their work. There are risks in using the portable devices, as they can be easily lost or stolen. See chapter 12 for additional information about these risks.

Today, cloud computing is used to store data and run applications by many healthcare organizations. **Cloud computing** is the delivery of computational services (e.g., analytics, storage, and application sharing) by a vendor over the Internet. The healthcare organization uploads or enters data remotely into the vendor-owned information system. This storage of data at a remote location is often referred to storing data "in the cloud". One of the benefits to cloud computing is the facilitation of information sharing. For example, this allows a healthcare organization with multiple hospitals can share data among the hospitals. The data stored at a remote location can be accessed by all authorized users. When the healthcare organizations need more processing, more data storage, and so forth, the vendor can easily add computers to handle the volume.

Many healthcare organizations have a private network, known as an intranet. The intranet is used by the healthcare organization's own employees and other authorized individuals. The **intranet** is a private information network that is similar to the Internet in that it uses Internet technologies; however, its servers are located inside a firewall or security barrier so that the general public cannot gain access to information housed within the network, distinguishing it from the

Internet. The firewall built around the intranet will prevent unauthorized access to it or restricted parts of the website. (See chapter 12 for a description of a firewall.) A healthcare organization's intranet might give updates on upcoming events, house the bylaws and rules and regulations as well as the policies and procedures of the healthcare organization, provide a repository for forms, and contain an employee directory, map of the healthcare organization, or other items helpful for employees. It can provide links to information systems such as the EHR. The intranet can also provide users with a site search engine for items not found in the contents page.

Healthcare organizations may also have an extranet. An **extranet** uses a system of connections of private Internet networks outside an organization's firewall and uses Internet technology to enable collaborative applications to allow external users to access limited portions of the IS. For example, the extranet, through a patient portal, can be used by healthcare organizations to allow patients to access health information and schedule appointments. For (for more on patient portals refer to chapter 10). Also, suppliers can use the extranet to monitor a hospital's supply levels and make shipments without the healthcare organization having to place an order. Likewise, vendors can allow healthcare organizations access to its extranet so they can track the status of orders.

CHECK YOUR UNDERSTANDING 1.1

1. A patient can access his test results by using the _____.

   a. Intranet
   b. Extranet
   c. COW
   d. Meaningful Use

2. Cloud computing refers to _____.

   a. Data that is inaccurate or incomplete
   b. Computational services provided by a vendor over the Internet
   c. The use of a single information system across the entire healthcare organization
   d. Outdated information that is purged from an IS

3. Documentation at the bedside is known as:

   a. Point of care
   b. Extranet
   c. Intranet
   d. Creation of an intranet

4. The early information systems used in health included _____.

   a. Financial applications
   b. Cloud computing
   c. EHR
   d. POC system

5. Identify where an employee working at the healthcare organization can locate the form required to request reimbursement recent travel within the organization's network.

   a. Internet
   b. Intranet
   c. Extranet
   d. WOW

Impact of Computers on Healthcare

The healthcare industry continues to grow in size and in complexity. Without information systems to aid in the management of patient data, the healthcare industry would not be able to obtain the information needed to function in this complex environment. Technology allows the healthcare industry to use data in ways that enhance patient care, research, business practices, education, and public health. These ways include identifying effective medications or treatments, monitoring for epidemics, improved decision making, and sharing information between healthcare providers at other healthcare organizations. Technology has also enabled significant changes in such areas as patient safety, quality of patient care, and access to information.

Impact of Technology on Patient Care

The impact that ISs have on patient care is seen in multiple ways including

- Actual care provided to the patient
- Patient engagement in healthcare
- Creation of evidence-based medicine
- Creation of practice guidelines
- Patient safety

The care provided to the patient has been improved in multiple ways through the use of technology. The EHR provides immediate access to the patient's past medical history, current test results, allergies, and so forth. It also reminds physicians of tests that should be considered and helps with the quality of documentation. Chapter 9 provides more information about the benefits of EHRs.

Health information exchange (HIE) is the exchange of health information electronically between providers and others with the same level of interoperability. Interoperability is the ability of different information technology systems and software applications to communicate; to exchange data accurately, effectively, and consistently; and to use the information that has been changed. It allows healthcare providers access to patient information even if health records are located at other healthcare organizations, whether local or in other states. Figure 1.3 shows an example of how an HIE links various healthcare providers in the local area. See chapter 11 for more information on HIE.

Today patients are more engaged in their own healthcare than ever before. Patients use the Internet to research their symptoms, diseases, treatments, and medications. They also access the Internet to communicate with their healthcare provider, schedule appointments, check test results, access a summary of their care, and more. These practices will be discussed in chapter 10. One of the most important impacts that technology can have on patient care is supporting patient safety efforts.

Patient Safety

Patient safety is a hot topic in healthcare and has been since the publication of *To Err Is Human: Building a Safer Health System* by the Institute of Medicine (now known as National Academies of Medicine). This report was published in 1999 and related that up to 98,000 people died each year in hospitals as a result of preventable medical errors (IOM 1999). This report prompted the healthcare industry to take steps to improve patient safety.

Patient safety has been enhanced through the use of technology. Examples of these efforts include:

- Use of barcodes to verify patient identification for medication administration (see chapter 9)
- Checking medications ordered against allergies and other medications (see chapter 8)

Figure 1.3. Health information exchange

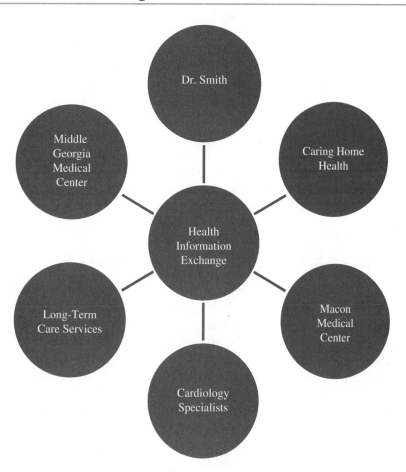

Source: ©AHIMA.

- Improved data quality through edits and standardization (see chapters 2 and 3)
- Clinical provider order entry (see chapter 8)

With the paper health record, the capturing of data on the patient's care and then analyzing the data was very difficult, time-consuming, and costly. Now with the EHR and other technologies research and data analysis can be performed using the existing databases. The EHR along with data mining (discussed later in this chapter) offers healthcare providers valuable knowledge, such as drugs with serious complications, best treatment for a condition or disease, and so forth. See chapter 3 for more information on databases used in healthcare.

Technologies such as the EHR eliminated illegibility issues that were found in the handwritten patient health record and that can lead to errors in medication dosage and other patient safety issues. Technology can also help reduce or even eliminate incomplete information. For example, when a physician orders a medication in the paper health record, the physician may leave off a key piece of information such as the route of administration. The EHR would not allow this.

With the use of clinical provider order entry (CPOE), which is where the physician orders tests, medications, and other procedures (discussed in chapter 8), the physician is prompted to provide all of the required information. Technology cannot solve all patient care issues; there may still be errors in software, issues with usability of an information system, wrong medication ordered, and more. It can, however, improve patient outcomes and give patient confidence in the healthcare system.

Evidence-Based Medicine

Research concerning drugs and other medical treatments is critical to patient care. Physicians and other healthcare providers need to know that the drugs and other treatments used are effective. One of the ways this is accomplished is through evidence-based medicine. **Evidence-based medicine** describes healthcare services based on clinical methods that have been thoroughly tested through controlled, peer-reviewed biomedical studies. Evidence-based medicine uses data analysis from the EHR and other ISs to determine which treatment(s) worked the best. The findings from the review of data in the EHR and other ISs are used to develop clinical pathways. **Clinical pathways** are a tool designed to coordinate multidisciplinary care planning for specific diagnoses and treatments. For example, if a patient has an acute myocardial infarction, the clinical pathways define the best practices for treatment. Another tool is the **clinical practice guidelines,** which provide a detailed, step-by-step guide used by healthcare practitioners to make knowledge-based decisions related to patient care and issued by an authoritative organization such as a medical society.

Introduction to Health Informatics

Health informatics is a "science that defines how health information is technically captured, transmitted, and utilized" (AHIMA 2019). This field of study uses ISs to manipulate and use information to improve healthcare. Health informatics is only possible because the data are stored in the ISs. Improvement of healthcare can include, standards development, clinical pathway development, clinical practice guidelines development, and more. Standards are a scientifically based statement of expected behavior against which structures, processes, and outcomes can be measured. Standards are covered in more detail in chapter 9. In order to get quality information, quality data are needed. See chapter 2 for more about data collection and data quality.

There are a number of specializations in health informatics, including clinical health informatics, nursing informatics, and public health informatics. All of these use data and information systems to improve patient care, but health informatics goes beyond this. It also facilitates the sharing of data, saving money through improved communication and elimination of duplicate testing, monitoring for communicable diseases, involving patients in their care, and improving efficiency (CIS Consulting 2017).

Introduction to Data Analytics

With the data collected through the EHR and other ISs, HIM professionals and others are able to turn data into information through the use of data analytics. **Data analytics** is the science of examining raw data with the purpose of drawing conclusions about that information. This information can then be used to make business decisions concerning which services to provide and how to improve patient care.

Data and information are important terms in data analytics. Data was defined earlier in this chapter. **Information** is data that have been manipulated into something meaningful. Data and information are not interchangeable. An example of data is "33% of the patients have insurance." This is a fact, but it does not provide context or meaning. The statement "33% of the patients had commercial insurance for the month of December 20XX, which is a 2% increase over this point last year" identifies not only the specific number of patients but also how the number has changed and in what period. This makes it information.

Data analytics is becoming more important to healthcare and HIM. The American Health Information Management Association (AHIMA) sponsors the **certified health data analyst (CHDA)** certification. This advanced certification covers business needs assessment, data acquisition and management, data analysis, data interpretation and reporting, and data governance (CCHIIM 2019).

Data analytics can be divided into four categories: descriptive, diagnostic, predictive, and prescriptive:

- Descriptive analytics looks at the past to determine what has already occurred. For example, how has the patient volume changed over the past five years. This type of analytics helps the organization learn from the past. Descriptive analytics uses descriptive statistics such as mean, frequencies, variance, and so forth. The trends identified in the analysis helps the healthcare organization plan for the future.

- Diagnostic analytics helps a healthcare organization determine why something happened. Diagnostic analytics tools such as dashboards and data mining are introduced later in this chapter. For example, if the patient volume has gone down, you can investigate types of patients, age of patient, physician admissions, and other attributes to identify the reason for the decline such as losing a physician practice on your medical staff that admitted a lot of patients.

- Predictive analytics analyzes historical data to make predictions. For example, predictive analytics may determine the expected readmission rate. The prediction may or may come true as many factors can impact future events.

- Prescriptive analytics builds upon predictive analytics by suggesting possible courses of action the healthcare organization may take and what the implications may be for each. For example, the hospital may see a rise in patient volume. (Brinkmann 2019). Prescriptive analytics can help determine the number of nurses required to care for the patients on a nursing unit.

A number of tools are used in data analytics, including data mining, machine learning, statistics, dashboards, and predictive modelling. These tools utilize ISs to manipulate and analyze the data contained in the database. The data are used for research, monitoring the quality of patient care, and much more.

Data mining is the process of extracting and analyzing large volumes of data from a database for the purpose of identifying hidden and sometimes subtle relationships or patterns and using those relationships to predict behaviors. It uses data to determine differences in the way physicians practice medicine, determine changes in the patients being seen, and more. Refer to chapter 3 for additional information.

Dashboards are summarized or aggregated reports of process measures to help leaders follow progress to assist with strategic planning. The dashboard provides the status on key measures. For example, a hospital chief financial officer might want to know the total charges of unbilled claims, accounts receivable, accounts payment, percentage of patients with various insurers, and so forth. These figures would change automatically as payments are received, bills are submitted, and so forth. The ability to continuously update the data allows the user to have the most current information in one location. This information may be displayed in line graphs, pie charts, and other displays. The dashboard would allow the user to monitor these key measures closely. An example of a dashboard is found in Figure 1.4.

Descriptive statistics is a set of statistical techniques used to describe data, such as means, frequency distributions, and standard deviations; statistical information describes the characteristics of a specific group or a population, such as the mean costs for patients who have had an appendectomy.

Inferential statistics is a set of statistical techniques that allows researchers to make generalizations about a population's characteristics on the basis of a sample's characteristics, such as HIM professionals' continuing education efforts.

Predictive modelling is a process used to identify patterns that can be used to predict the odds of a particular outcome based on the observed data. Predictive models use historical data in order to predict what is likely to happen in the future. The predictive model utilizes algorithms through machine learning. Machine learning is an area of computer science that studies algorithms and computer programs that improve employee performance on some task by exposure to a training or learning experience. An example of predictive modelling might be used to predict the number of inpatient beds needed at the healthcare organization.

Figure 1.4. Sample dashboard

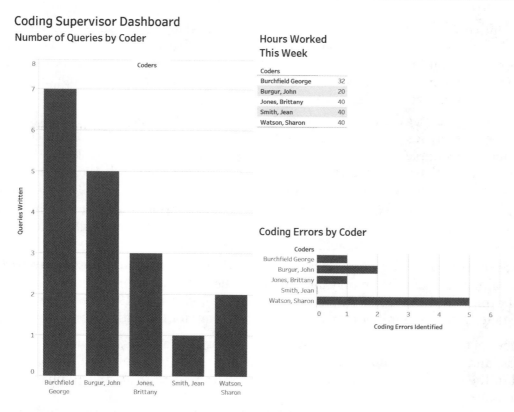

Source: AHIMA Virtual Lab Tableau.

A healthcare organization can use one or more of these tools to perform data analytics. The choice(s) would be based on the objectives of the analyses. For example, a hospital can have a dashboard showing key indicators like hospital census. This census data would be displayed as descriptive statistics.

Impact on the HIM Profession

Technological advancements implemented in healthcare have had a major impact on the HIM profession. For decades, the health record had not changed significantly. With the advent of department ISs such as the laboratory IS (see chapter 8) laboratory reports were computer generated, printed out, and then filed in the health record. This began the slow transition to the EHR. Today many healthcare organizations utilize the EHR to capture, store, and manage patient information. This change in format has enabled the HIM department to use technology to process the health record and manage information to perform many tasks including:

- Assigning diagnosis and procedures codes
- Managing the MPI
- Managing registries
- Transcribing documents such as the discharge summary
- Analyzing the health record
- Documentation of health information activities
- Computer-assisted coding

Before the EHR, these functions were slow, methodical, tedious, and labor-intensive. Using ISs to perform management of information tasks saves time and money and reduces the number of employees needed (thereby saving employers salary costs).

Some healthcare organizations use a virtual HIM department, in which (when the EHR is available) coders, transcriptionists, and other HIM professionals can work remotely, which may be from home. A virtual HIM department benefits both employers and employees. Employees are able to save on transportation costs, they have more flexibility in their job, flexibility, improved job satisfaction, and more.

Employers are able to use the freed up space for revenue producing purposes such as creating additional operating rooms in the space that once housed the HIM department. Allowing employees to work remotely is a great recruiting tool when looking for employees to fill vacant positions. These benefits for the healthcare organization include financial savings, increased productivity, improved recruitment of new employees, and strong retention (Asperian Global 2020).

Another option is providing HIM services at a centralized location rather than having staff at each individual healthcare organization. For example, ABC Hospital System has hospitals in Macon, Atlanta, and Columbus, Georgia. All three of these hospitals utilize the EHR. ABC Hospital System could centralize their HIM services in Atlanta. As a result, most of the HIM services for all three hospitals can be performed in Atlanta, eliminating the need for three HIM directors, coding staff, and work space in all locations.

There are downsides to both the virtual and centralized departments. In both models, there are limited HIM professionals and staff that can support the physicians, committees, and other staff onsite and there are increased security concerns when employees access data remotely.

There are technological tools that allow employees to network, meet virtually, collaborate, and more. Sometimes healthcare organizations require face to face meetings for employees. These onsite meetings allow for training, teambuilding, collaboration, and so forth. These meetings could be monthly, quarterly, annual, or another period.

Employees who work remotely may also experience isolation as the employee does not have the same level of interaction with others. Some employees may have trouble focusing due to children and other distractions (dishes, laundry, and other household chores). They may also have trouble balancing work and home life (Asperian Global 2020). For example, the work environment is always present reminding the employee of work that needs to be done. Alternatively, the household tasks are also ever present.

The skills required by the HIM professional have changed significantly in light of technological advancements. The HIM skills of today include system implementation, databases, data governance, legal health record, data analysis, data mining, healthcare informatics, and much more. The HIM profession has changed from one that is focused on processing health records to one that is focused on data and information that can be used to monitor quality of patient care, patient outcomes, reduce costs, and more. With the paper health record, aggregating health data and turning it into information was difficult because the HIM professional had to review each health record and collect data before it can be turned into information. With the EHR, data can easily be manipulated and turned into information. Many new roles, such as data integrity analyst, data analyst, and mapping specialist, have been created as a result.

CHECK YOUR UNDERSTANDING 1.2

1. AHIMA's certification that addresses data acquisition and management is _____.
   a. CHDA
   b. RHIA
   c. RHIT
   d. CCS

(Continued)

CHECK YOUR UNDERSTANDING 1.2 (*Continued*)

2. _____ is used to assess the status of key indicators.

   a. Predictive modelling
   b. The annual report
   c. Data mining
   d. The dashboard

3. Prescriptive analytics is used to:

   a. Provide possible courses of action
   b. Explain the past
   c. Improve the quality of care provided
   d. Select the best medication for a patient

4. A trend seen in HIM is _____.

   a. The elimination of HIM functions
   b. The ability for staff to be able to work remotely
   c. Bringing staff back into the department to work
   d. To return to the basics of HIM

5. Identify the tool that outlines the best practice to treat a patient.

   a. Prescriptive modelling
   b. Predictive modelling
   c. Clinical practice guidelines
   d. Clinical pathways

Real-World Case 1.1

Sophie is the HIM director at Medical Center of Alabama. The Medical Center of Alabama is part of a five-hospital chain and two health clinics known as Hometown Health. Sophie earned her RHIA five years ago and is excited about the decision to transition to a virtual department. The medical center has an EHR that will support this transition. Sophie and a few other employees will work with patients, physicians, committees, etc. onsite, while everyone else will work remotely. The space currently utilized by the HIM department will be used to expand the operating rooms. As excited as Sophie is, she does have some concerns which are:

- keeping the employees connected with the healthcare organization
- providing training
- ensuring the quality of the work produced by the remote employees
- managing the remote employees

The transition to a virtual workforce will occur in one year and there is much to do to prepare.

Real-World Case 1.2

ABC Hospice is a small inpatient hospice that plans to implement an EHR next year. Since they are small, they do not have a lot of resources to implement and manage the EHR. The management of the EHR includes updates, back-ups, and other maintenance. ABC Hospice has decided to utilize cloud computing so that they do not have to hire a full-time individual just to manage the EHR. They plan to research a number of companies that provide cloud computing services over the next few months and contact the regional extension center and to help them select one in time to get the information system up and operational in time for their desired implementation date. They are looking forward to the use of the EHR not only because of the benefits to patient care, but also for the use of health informatics and data analytics.

REVIEW QUESTIONS

1. To make conclusions about a population, use _____.

   a. Descriptive statistics
   b. Inferential statistics
   c. Predictive modelling
   d. Data modelling

2. The field used to draw conclusions is:

   a. Data analytics
   b. Data modelling
   c. Population health
   d. Health informatics

3. The first ISs used in healthcare were _____.

   a. Financial applications
   b. EHR
   c. Dashboard
   d. Mainframes

4. Identify the true statement about the Intranet.

   a. It is a synonym for Internet.
   b. It is used to communicate with vendors.
   c. It is used to access employee resources.
   d. It is used by patients.

5. The impact of ISs specifically on HIM professionals includes _____.

   a. Improving patient safety
   b. Improving access to health information
   c. The need to assign diagnosis and procedure codes
   d. Skills required

6. Identify the true statement about the EHR.

   a. The EHR allows flexibility by not requiring recognized standards.
   b. The EHR stores information about the population, not individuals.
   c. The EHR utilizes nationally recognized interoperability standards.
   d. The EHR is available only to HIM professionals.

7. The benefit of point of care documentation is that it:

   a. Evidence-based medicine.
   b. Created as soon as the care is provided.
   c. Clinical practice guidelines.
   d. Wireless technology.

(Continued)

8. The technology where the user enters data to a remote system over the Internet is known as:

   a. Intranet
   b. Internet
   c. Cloud computing
   d. Electronic health record

9. The tool used to identify hidden relationships is:

   a. Descriptive statistics
   b. Inferential statistics
   c. Predictive modelling
   d. Data mining

10. Identify the tool used to determine why something happened.

    a. Descriptive analytics
    b. Prescriptive analytics
    c. Predictive analytics
    d. Diagnostic analytics

References

American Health Information Management Association. 2019. *What is Health Information?* https://www.ahima.org/careers/healthinfo.

American Health Information Management Association. 2017. *Pocket Glossary of Health Information Management and Technology*, 5th ed. Chicago: AHIMA.

Asperian Global. 2020. *The Benefits of a Remote Workforce and Virtual Collaboration*. https://www.aperianglobal.com/benefits-remote-workforce-virtual-collaboration/.

Brinkmann, B. 2019. *Comparing Descriptive, Predictive, Prescriptive, and Diagnostic Analytics*. https://www.logianalytics.com/predictive-analytics/comparing-descriptive-predictive-prescriptive-and-diagnostic-analytics/.

Burchfield, G. *Personal punch card*. Scanned 2/2/2020.

CIS Consulting. 2017. *7 Ways Health Informatics Transforms Healthcare*. https://www.cisc-llc.com/7-ways-health-informatics-transforms-health-care/.

Commission on Certification for Health Informatics and Information Management (CCHIIM). 2019. *Candidate Guide*. https://www.ahima.org/media/mhjapwhx/revised-candidate-guide-8-6-2020.pdf

Gwern. *Blue Punch Card Front*. 20 November 2009. Accessed 2/2/20. https://commons.wikimedia.org/wiki/File:Blue-punch-card-front-horiz.png.

Institute of Medicine. 1999. *To Err Is Human: Building a Safer Health System*. https://pubmed.ncbi.nlm.nih.gov/25077248/.

Chapter 2

Information Integrity and Data Quality

Learning Objectives

- Identify the various data sources that populate the electronic health record.
- Apply the American Health Information Management Association data quality management model characteristics to data collection.
- Identify the appropriate field type for a data element.
- Make recommendations to address data quality and data integrity issues.

Key Terms

AHIMA data quality management model
Authorship
Back-end speech recognition (BESR) *p20*
Checkbox *18-19*
Data accessibility
Data accuracy
Data capture
Data cleansing
Data comprehensiveness
Data consistency
Data currency
Data definition
Data granularity
Data integrity
Data mapping

Data precision
Data quality
Data quality management
Data quality measure
Data relevancy
Data timeliness
Date field
Direct data entry
Drop down box
Edit check
Front-end speech recognition (FESR)
Hot spot
Interface
Natural language processing (NLP)
Numeric field

Peer review
Physician advisor (PA)
Primary data source
Qualitative analysis
Quantitative analysis
Radio buttons
Secondary data source
Speech recognition
Structured data
Structured data fields
Template-based data entry
Time field
Unstructured data fields
Version control

Patient history has been recorded on paper for centuries; written records of treating the sick date back to the Middle Ages. Although these documents are not what are currently thought of as quality health records, they show that patient care was recorded through the centuries.

The history of healthcare and the importance of recording written data are a part of the foundation of healthcare. The importance of data quality in healthcare cannot be overstressed or overstated as lives are at stake. For example, failure to document an allergy could result in the patient being given an inappropriate medication that can be life threatening. Every piece of information from the health record is vital to patient care. The healthcare provider must read, review, analyze, and compare the patient's health record to similar cases to make a plan for the patient's care and administer treatment accordingly. Therefore, it is critical that all information is timely, accurate, and complete.

The data contained within the health record by itself would be raw data or figures; however, when these data are organized and presented to produce meaning, resulting in information. Healthcare providers must rely on information so that patient care can be provided at the highest level. A health record containing only raw data is a record full of numbers and other documentation that has little meaning to anyone. These data must have meaning attached to them. Once this occurs, these data become useful information that can be used by the practitioners to treat the patient.

For example, a routine laboratory report contains a list of test results for a patient. The normal range scale for each test is listed next to the results, thus giving it meaning and translating it into information. For example, a complete blood count would have a hematocrit, hemoglobin, white blood cell count, and other blood cell measurements. The hematocrit will have a range such as 34–46. If the normal range scale is not listed and there is no knowledge of where the normal ranges fall, it remains raw data because the numbers have no meaning.

Most health records are documented with the best information available at the time by healthcare providers and personnel who are trained on how to appropriately document within health records and to use electronic health records (EHRs) and databases accordingly. However, errors can still be made when documenting, computer problems can transpire, or other data mishaps can occur. Because of the possibility of errors related to data, the quality of information must be a priority in healthcare. While documentation itself is outside of the scope of this text, information systems play a big role in the quality of that documentation. The content of this chapter includes data sources, screen design, data integrity, data quality management, and data integrity issues which all impact data quality.

Data Sources

Data that populate the EHR come from many sources. Data sources can be categorized into primary and secondary data sources.

Primary Data Sources

Primary data sources come directly from the original source, such as the patient when talking about symptoms or the reason for coming to the healthcare organization. The health record is considered to be a primary source of data as the physicians and other healthcare providers document the treatments, observations, and care provided. The highest quality of data will always come from the primary source, which is the original source of the information.

Secondary Data Sources

Secondary data sources are derived from the primary data sources, such as the health record. Secondary data sources include indices, registries, and other databases. A registry is a collection of care information related to a specific disease, condition, or procedure that makes health record information available for analysis and comparison. Secondary data are typically used to conduct research, address population health issues, and for administrative purposes such as monitoring for possible fraud (Sharp 2020). For example, a cancer registry may identify that a certain region of the state has a higher than average lung cancer rate.

Screen Design

Screen design is an important part of data quality as it influences data capture, which is discussed in the next section of this chapter. Poor screen design can confuse users if instructions are not provided, if the data fields are not in a logical order, and if users are entering data in different ways. An example of an illogical order of the data fields is the placement of the first name at the top of the page and the last name at the bottom. In another example, users might enter data in different ways in response to the data element "state": they could enter the full state name (Georgia) or the abbreviation (GA). This difference in data capture would make data retrieval and analysis difficult as the user cannot be sure that all the appropriate data is retrieved for reporting or display. For more on screen design, refer to chapter 5.

Data Capture

Data capture is the process of recording healthcare-related data in an electronic health record system or clinical database. The healthcare practitioners who input data into the health record are responsible for the quality of data they enter into the EHR or other information system (IS). Poor data capture results in not only poor quality of care but also poor business decisions. For example, if the patient's weight is entered incorrectly, the wrong dosage of a medication may be administered. Also, poor data may result in a healthcare organization closing a profitable service. The adage garbage in, garbage out (GIGO) is applicable to the documentation of healthcare data. There are a number of ways that data are captured to help prevent the "garbage." These methods include direct data entry, template-based data entry, speech recognition, and natural language processing.

Direct Data Entry

Direct data entry includes a number of manual data entry methods such as keyboard, mouse, or other devices for entering data into the information system. A number of data field types are available for use in an IS. Some of these field types can contribute to data quality by limiting the number of choices, by limiting the appropriate entries, and further specifying the data required.

Many vendors use hot spots throughout their software applications to make the data fields as user-friendly as possible. **A hot spot**, also known as a pop-up text, is a type of help message that is triggered when the cursor is placed on top of a data field. The hot spot may indicate the next level of choices, the purpose of an icon, or an explanation of that field including valid entries. The valid entries, number of characters, and other attributes are controlled by the data dictionary, which is discussed further in chapter 3. The field types are selected based on the type of data collected and the flexibility of data entry required. The field type also depends on whether or not structured or unstructured data are needed. More on field types later in this chapter. Figure 2.1 provides an example of a hot spot.

Unstructured Data Fields

Unstructured data fields use data elements that allow for free text entry, which means that the user can type in any data that he or she chooses. Examples of unstructured data include a description of the procedure performed or a patient's explanation of his medical history. Unstructured data complicates data retrieval and analysis, so structured data are preferred. For example, unstructured data would allow different terms with the same meaning to be entered (such as Lou Gehrig's Disease vs. Amyotrophic Lateral Sclerosis)., while structured would present only one option (e.g., Amyotrophic Lateral Sclerosis).

Text box fields allow the user to type free text into the field, so the user is not limited to allowed choices. The data dictionary can limit the characters allowed, such as A through Z or 0 through 9, as well as the number of characters. The type of data collected in the text box will dictate the number of characters allowed. For example, the last name field might be limited to

Figure 2.1. Hotspot example

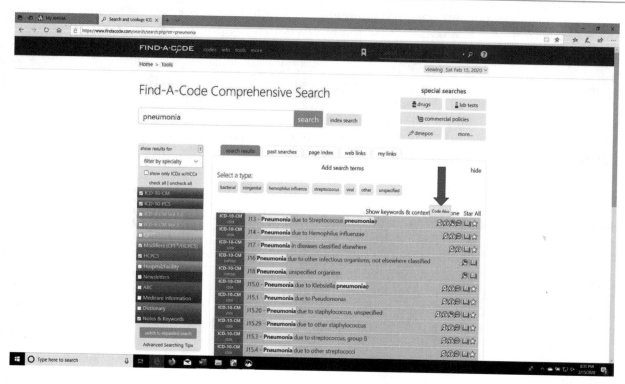

Source: ©AHIMA.

40 alphabetic characters. The address field would accept both numbers and letters. A text field in which the physician enters his or her findings might allow 500 or even 1,000 characters.

Structured Data Fields

Structured data fields guide the user during the data entry process, limiting what a user can enter into the field. A number of different types of structured data fields can be used, including radio buttons, drop-down boxes, check boxes, and more. Some of these fields, such as drop-down boxes and radio buttons, have proved to be an effective and efficient method for capturing data, thus improving productivity and data quality. Other types of user-friendly aids within the health record are examples located near a data field to show the user a suggested response format for a data field. For example, there may be a question mark by the field that when clicked tells the user more about what data should be entered and in what format. For example, the phone number would be in the XXX-XXX-XXXX format. Examples of structured data fields are found in Figure 2.2.

Drop-Down Menus

One type of structured data field frequently found in the EHR is the drop-down menu. The user simply clicks on the arrow to the right (or left) of a data field and a drop-down menu appears with several choices. The choices can be controlled by the healthcare organization based on its needs. For example, a community hospital may populate the drop-down menu choices in the service field as medical, surgical, and obstetrical, while a large teaching hospital may list medical, surgical, transplant, cardiology, nephrology, and many more. Another use for a drop-down menu is patient type such as inpatient, outpatient, and emergency.

Once selected, the data field is automatically populated with the user's selection. A drop-down menu can be used for countless data fields within the EHR. It can be found in the admission record also known as the face sheet, the financial record, the history and physical examination and many more. Drop-down menus save time because the entire data field item does not have to be typed in

Figure 2.2. Examples of structured data fields

Dropdown Box	Checkbox	Radio Button
All states ▼	☐ Living Wheel	○ Male
		○ Female

the data field. They improve consistency because everyone enters data the same way. For example, the state of Georgia is selected from the drop-down box consistently as "Georgia" rather than being entered by some users as GA and others as Georgia.

Check Box

The check box is a type of data field that displays a comprehensive list of approved answers for the data element. The user can choose zero, one, or many of the options. For example, if the check box field is part of the cardiac section of the history, the options may be murmurs, gallops, and rubs. The user can then choose all the options that apply to the patient. As with the drop-down field, the choice of options must be comprehensive.

Radio Buttons

Radio buttons are a type of data field that also identifies a comprehensive list of choices, much like the check box. The difference is that the user can choose only one of the options. This type of field is for data for which only one option should be chosen among a small number of options. An example of this is gender. In this data field, the choices are generally male and female.

Numeric Field

A numeric field allows for the entry of numbers. The number of characters and range can be controlled through the data dictionary. It could control the format, such as decimal points and currency. The values in the numeric fields must be able to be added and subtracted, as with age, weight, and so forth. Lab values, even though they are often entered as numbers, would not be considered numeric because they are not added, subtracted, or otherwise mathematically manipulated.

Date Field

A date field allows for the entry of valid dates. "Valid" does not mean that the date is correct as the date can be entered incorrectly but rather it means that an invalid date (for example, February 30) cannot be entered.

Time Field

A time field allows for the entry of valid times. It would prevent 26 hours in a day or 70 minutes in an hour. This does not mean that the time is correct but rather means an invalid time cannot be entered.

Autonumbering

Autonumbering means that the IS assigns a number in numeric order. This type of field is used for the health record number and the patient account number. For example, the health record numbers would be assigned in numeric order, such as 12-34-56, 12-34-57, and 12-34-58. The use of autonumbering prevents two patients from being assigned the same health record number.

Template-Based Data Entry

Template-based data entry is a cross between unstructured and structured data entry. The user can pick and choose data that are entered frequently, thus requiring the entry of data that change from patient to patient. It assists the healthcare provider by providing direction in what is to be documented. For example, if a physician is documenting a history and physical examination, the template will instruct the physician to document a review of system, history of present illness, physical examination, impression, plan, and other required components. The template helps ensure that all required categories of data are collected. Other examples of templates include those used in pediatrics, surgical consults, and obstetrics.

Speech Recognition

Speech recognition, which also may be known as voice recognition, is technology that translates speech to text. The text must be edited, as speech recognition software may misunderstand words and therefore translate speech into text incorrectly. There are two strategies to editing documents created by speech recognition: front-end speech recognition and back-end speech recognition. Dictation with **front-end speech recognition (FESR)** occurs when the physician or the dictator is the editor of the document that is dictated. The advantage to FESR is that the authenticated document is available in the EHR quickly. The downside is that the physicians and other healthcare providers must be trained in how to edit documents. This takes away from the time available to see patients or read radiology reports.

The strategy known as **back-end speech recognition (BESR)** is the specific use of speech recognition technology in which the physician dictates in the traditional manner and an editor listens to the audio and reviews the document created to ensure it was created correctly. Because the dictated documents do not have to be transcribed, the role of transcriptionist is evolving to the role of an editor, who will edit the document to correct any errors created by speech recognition. The document is sent to the dictating physician for approval following the editing process. The advantage of BESR is that the physician is not required to take the time to perform the editing.

Natural Language Processing

Natural language processing (NLP) is the technology that converts human language (structured or unstructured) into data that can be translated then manipulated by information systems. It is sophisticated enough to be able to identify key words needed to perform specific tasks such as computer-assisted coding (see chapter 6). This technology basically teaches the meaning of a word or phrase to a software application after several uses. For example, the system would learn how to assign the appropriate procedure code for a new procedure. This is done by a statistical algorithm, as the applications can then compare and code these similar expressions accurately and quickly.

Data Integrity vs. Data Quality

Data quality is the reliability and effectiveness of data for its intended uses in operations, decision making, and planning. Thus, data quality focuses on the usability of data, whereas data integrity is about its trustworthiness. When designing an IS, steps should be taken to build in data quality. There are a number of tools that can help accomplish this, including required fields, edit checks, user-friendly data field, and field type. To ensure data integrity within the patient's health record, there are many methods that users can build into their paper-based or electronic systems. Because most health records are electronic, they will be the focus of discussion in the sections that follow.

Data integrity is the extent to which healthcare data are complete, accurate, consistent, and timely. It goes beyond data quality as it includes the validity of the data throughout its lifecycle which makes it usable for reports, decisions, patient care, and so forth (Ortega 2017). This is critical for the health record as life and death situations occur and healthcare providers must trust the data they are using to make decisions on patient care.

There are a number of tools used to help with data quality. These are data dictionary, metadata, required fields, and edit checks.

Data Dictionary

The data dictionary is descriptive list of the names, definitions, and attributes of data elements to be collected in an information system or database whose purpose is to standardize definitions and ensure consistent use. In other words, it defines each data element used in the information system. In this section we will address the data dictionary as it relates to quality which includes metadata. For additional information on the data dictionary, refer to chapter 3.

Metadata

Metadata is defined as descriptive data that characterize other data to create a clearer understanding of their meaning and to achieve greater reliability and quality of information. Metadata tags are used to describe the data. Metadata provides information such as the creator of the data, the date of creation, keywords, and more (MerlinOne 2019).

There are three different types of metadata: descriptive metadata, structural metadata, and administrative metadata. Descriptive metadata is recording descriptive information about the patient in a way that the data can be shared with other healthcare providers. This descriptive information includes demographics, diagnosis, physician and much more. This metadata is used to retrieve data from a database. Structural metadata provides insight into how the data is organized. Administrative metadata tracks the file type, date it was created, permissions and more (MerlinOne 2019). Administrative data includes the data dictionary described earlier in this chapter. Metadata also includes the audit trail which identifies who logged into an information system, what the user did, what the users viewed, and so forth. For more on the audit trail, refer to chapter 12.

Required Fields

The data fields within an IS for capturing data are individual blank fields required to be populated with patient data. A required field is a field in which data must be entered before the IS will allow the user to proceed. If these data fields were on paper, the user would interview the patient for data and write the data into the blanks on the paper to complete the data fields. The paper form would not alert the user that a data field was skipped or omitted, or if wrong data were entered into a field during entry. With an IS, the user may not be able to skip ahead on the screen, although some ISs may allow the user to override the required field to enter other data, and then come back to enter data in this field later. The existence of required fields is one of many reasons why the EHR is the preferred method for capturing data.

The healthcare organization, working with the IS vendor, determines which data fields should be set as required, if any. It is good practice to set fields as required for information that is essential for patient care, a healthcare organization's needs, or other reporting purposes. The healthcare organization must weigh the benefits and disadvantages of required fields to determine what essential information is needed because the user can get frustrated by an excessive number of required fields or when the required data is not available at that time.

Edit Check

Many ISs have functionality within the software to minimize errors and aid in data accuracy. An edit check is a standard feature in many applications' data entry and data collection software packages. Edit checks are preprogrammed definitions of each data field set up within the application. So, as data are entered, if any data are different from what has been preprogrammed, an edit message appears on the screen. For example, an edit message would prevent a user from entering a body temperature of 254 degrees. This edit message is sometimes called a flag because it signals that the user needs to verify the data being entered to ensure that the criteria of the field are met. This flag serves as a quality verification of data being entered into the IS as part of the data collection process.

Edit checks can check for illogical data, such as when a patient's gender does not match patient gender-specific procedure documented. For example, a flag would appear on the screen indicating that a hysterectomy cannot be performed on a male patient. The user would then check the health record for a correct diagnosis and procedure as well as check the patient's gender and determine which information is correct and which needs to be edited. Another example of an illogical data check is a blood pressure of 543/87.

Edits also can make sure that the type of data entered and its format is valid for that data element. For example, the discharge date should be a valid date. For example, the date could not be 02/30/20XX. The discharge data would also be entered in MMDDYYYY or DDMMYYYY format such as 10152020 or 15102020. Even though the information system stores it in MMDDYYYY format, the system may display it in a more user-friendly view, such as 10/15/2020. When data is stored in one format and displayed in another, like in the example given, it does this through the use of a mask. A mask takes the data and displays it in user friend manner without having to save dashes slash marks or other characters. In addition to dates, it can be used for social security numbers, phone numbers, credit card numbers, and more.

CHECK YOUR UNDERSTANDING 2.1

1. Identify a data integrity tool.
   a. Cloning copy/paste
   b. Natural language processing
   c. Speech recognition
   d. Required field

2. Identify the data integrity tool used to assist the users in data entry.
   a. Data dictionary
   b. Primary data source
   c. Hot spot
   d. Automatic save

3. Identify the field type that is BEST for entering gender.
   a. Drop-down menu
   b. Check box
   c. Radio buttons
   d. Text box

4. Identify the primary data source.
   a. Data set
   b. Health record
   c. Registry
   d. Index

5. Identify the BEST field type for service.
   a. Drop-down menu
   b. Check box
   c. Radio button
   d. Text box

Collection
Application
Warehousing
Analysis

Data Quality Management

Data quality management is defined as "the business processes that ensure the integrity of an organization's data during collection, application (including aggregation), warehousing, and analysis" (Davoudi et al. 2015). Collection in data quality management refers to the way that data elements are gathered. Application is the reason for collecting the data. Warehousing involves the methods used to store the data. Analysis entails converting data into information (Davoudi et al. 2015). The American Health Information Management Association (AHIMA) data quality management model (figure 2.3) displays the components of data quality management and the characteristics of data quality.

Data Accessibility

Data accessibility means that data items are easily obtainable by authorized users. Data can be accurate and relevant, but if it is not accessible to the healthcare providers when needed, then it is of no use. With the paper health record, the accessibility is limited because the health record may be in use by another provider, or may be in transit between patient care areas. In the EHR, the health records are immediately accessible to multiple users at the same time unless the IS is down. In case of IS downtime, data must still be accessible; a business continuity plan must be in place to address what happens during downtime. For more information on the business continuity plan, see chapter 12.

Data Accuracy

The patient's health record must be accurate and complete. **Data accuracy** means that data are free of identifiable errors. There are a number of different types of errors that impact data accuracy. Quantitative and qualitative analyses are two methods used to help prevent inaccurate data from occurring frequently within a health record.

Quantitative analysis is a review of the health record to determine its completeness and accuracy. It is used by health information management (HIM) professionals as a method to detect whether elements of the patient's health record are missing. In quantitative analysis, the reviewer determines whether or not the reports are present or absent from the health record.

Figure 2.3. AHIMA data quality management model functions and characteristics

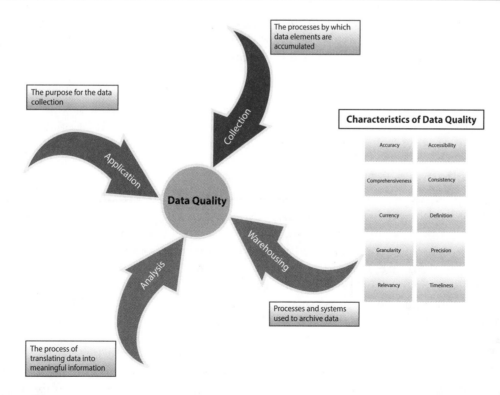

Source: Davoudi et al. 2015.

A **qualitative analysis** is a review of the health record to ensure that standards are met and to determine the adequacy of entries documenting the quality of care. While reviewing a health record, the reviewer considers whether the health record appropriately documents the care provided. A nurse should review the quality of nursing documentation, a physician, the physician documentation, and so forth. This would include ensuring that all required components are in the discharge summary or other document. HIM professionals look at legibility, use of abbreviations, patient identification, and so forth. Physicians, nurses, and others review the actual quality of the documentation.

When qualitative and quantitative reviews are performed retrospectively, it is difficult to make changes when problems are found. Concurrent reviews allow deficiencies to be identified during the course of the patient's care and therefore the documentation can be addressed in the health record. When documentation issues are found, the problem documentation can be used as teaching points to show the medical staff and other practitioners who document within health records what should be written, so that future documentation can improve.

Inaccurate data are useless, are expensive, and can be harmful to patients. Data form much of the body of knowledge used by medical professionals, epidemiologists, policymakers, and public health officials in decision making. These decisions affect patient lives, policies on healthcare reform, and other major issues regarding health. Resources are allocated at local, state, and national levels based on data collected and entrusted to be accurate. Accurate data are needed to evaluate patient outcomes and quality of life, and to determine satisfaction issues and implement procedures for improvement.

Some errors in the accuracy of the health record are obvious. Spelling errors are the most common obvious errors and often occur in paper-based health records. As more healthcare organizations, including hospitals, clinics, and physician offices, become computerized, fewer spelling errors are seen thanks to spell check. Spell check does not catch all spelling errors as the error may spell a legitimate word – just not the correct one. Data errors are often made by carelessness, such as transposition of digits when typing a string of numbers. For example:

- Physician order: Penicillin 250 mg
- Transposed physician order: Penicillin 520 mg

If the physician was hurriedly typing in the order for the patient, it is easy to see how the numbers could be transposed. It is also easy to see how this type of error can be missed when proofing the data entry because the same numbers are there but out of order. Depending on the transposition, there could be serious consequences.

Another data accuracy issue arises when many patients have the same last name or the same first name, raising the possibility that duplicate health record numbers could be assigned to more than one patient. During the admission process, the patient must be questioned to make sure that two different patients with the same or similar name have a different health record number.

Data Comprehensiveness

Data comprehensiveness means that the patient's health record must be complete, meaning that all required data are included. Many governmental agencies, accreditation organizations and medical staffs have standards that mandate what data must be collected to be considered a complete health record. Incomplete health records (missing documents or missing data, or even missing entries or signatures) would not serve any purpose as it would not contain all the needed data to make decisions or otherwise use the data. Any item or element that is not in the patient's health record that should be there is considered missing and qualifies as incomplete data, making the record incomplete.

The HIM profession has been monitoring incomplete patient records since the beginning of record keeping because it is a sound practice of good documentation. Not only is this legally advisable but the primary reason is for the quality of the continuity of patient care. Without accurate and complete data in the health record, practitioners cannot accurately treat the patient.

It is in the best interest of the patient and the healthcare organization as well as all practitioners to ensure that all clinical data on the patient's care are contained in the health record. This is again why HIM professionals perform a detailed review of health records, with a quantitative and qualitative review to ensure that records are comprehensive. Reviews help ensure that the healthcare organization meets legal and regulatory requirements and that the documentation within the health records will reinforce this if ever questioned. Complete documentation also is needed for billing and reimbursement. If there are data missing, there is good reason for the claim to be rejected or denied by a third-party payer.

HIM professionals are trained to conduct quantitative analysis and qualitative analysis within a health record. If during a qualitative review of a record there appears to be documentation that does not reflect best practice, if the notes appear to have a lapse in time covered, or if something does not look right, the HIM technician will submit the health record for review by a **physician advisor (PA)**. The PA is hired by the healthcare organization to act as a liaison between the HIM department or others and the patient's physician. The PA reviews health records for various reasons, including qualitative reviews, utilization reviews, quality reviews, surgical case and tissue reviews, other pathological reviews, and a host of blood and laboratory reviews for various medical staff and hospital committees. Typically, several physicians serve as PAs on an annual basis and are usually from diverse backgrounds, such as pathology, surgery, medicine, and other disciplines so that reviews can be a true peer review.

Peer review is a review by like professionals, or peers, established according to a healthcare organization's medical staff bylaws, organizational policy and procedure, or the requirements of state law. The peer review system allows medical professionals to candidly critique and criticize the work of their colleagues without fear of reprisal, as the feedback comes from the committee, not a specific individual. An example of a true peer review would be a cardiologist reviewing a health record that was documented by another cardiologist and not a physician from any other discipline. Peer review is at its best whenever physicians of the same discipline review each other. However, this is not always possible, especially in small healthcare organizations. These qualitative, quantitative, and peer reviews are more easily performed with the EHR as data are more readily accessible to authorized reviewers. Additionally, the data in EHRs are complete since the EHR can prevent the user from moving forward if required information is missing. In the paper environment, data elements on forms are frequently left blank, so the review process has greatly benefited from the conversion from a paper-based record to the EHR.

Whether data are entered into fields located as entries on a page in a paper-based record or as entries in an EHR, all data must be entered to be considered comprehensive. If data do not apply, a field usually has several options for the user to choose (such as Not Applicable, Not Given, or Not Known) so there are no blank fields in the health record. Using one of the aforementioned options signals that the user has read the option, but there is not a designation that applies from the choices given, and the field was not skipped or left blank unintentionally.

Data Consistency

Data consistency ensures that like data are the same on each document or computer screen. For example, in the paper health record, the patient's date of birth is listed on many different documents. It is easy for someone to write the wrong age on a document, which would create different ages on different documents. With the EHR, the date of birth is entered once and is displayed on multiple screens.

Data Currency

Data currency ensures that data are up to date. A data value is up to date if it is current for a specific point in time, and it is outdated if it was current at a preceding time but incorrect at a later time. Patient care must be provided based on current information. For example, a patient's chest x-ray study from six weeks ago has little to no value when a physician is treating the patient's pneumonia. The physician needs a current chest x-ray study to evaluate the patient's current condition.

Data Definition

The **data definition** is the specific meaning of a healthcare-related data element. Defining each data element provides the foundation that allows everyone to interpret and collect the data in the same way. Meanings can vary by department, healthcare organization, or another factor, supporting the need for a standard definition to avoid confusion. For example, "admission time" can be the time the patient arrived at the hospital, the time the patient's information was entered into the IS, or the time the patient arrived in their room. In addition, if the patient is first seen in the emergency room or when the IS is down, the time of admission would be impacted. Therefore, "admission time" should be defined, and the definition should be made available to all users.

Data Granularity

Data granularity describes the level of detail at which the attributes and values of healthcare data are defined. The required level of detail depends on the circumstances of the patient's care. For example, the documentation in the health record for a patient who is being treated for cardiac disease will describe the patient's cardiac condition much more detail than if the patient had a disease in another body system.

Data Precision

Data precision ensures that all data necessary to support and action. These actions can be, patient care, data analysis, billing, and more. Each task requires different data to be collected in acceptable values. For example, ICD-10-CM codes must be valid so they can be submitted as part of the healthcare claim.

Data Relevancy

Data relevancy is the extent to which healthcare-related data are useful for the purposes for which they were collected. Thus, only data that are needed or are expected to be needed in the future are collected. The type of data is determined by the needs of the healthcare organization. In the case of the health record, relevant data should include demographic data, administrative data, and clinical data. Demographic data are basic information about the patient, such as name, address, and date of birth. Administrative data include consent forms, insurance information, and authorizations to release health information. Clinical data includes information about the patient's care, such as symptoms, test results, physician observations, and treatment performed. The data needed in the health record vary by setting (hospital, emergency department) and service (surgical, medical, obstetrical). The data collected should support the patient's care; for example, one would generally not collect data such as patient's eye color or shoe size.

Data Timeliness

Data timeliness means that data should be recorded in an appropriate period of time after the event and should be available to the user when needed. The healthcare organization determines the appropriate period of time for each data element based on accreditation, state licensure, and other requirements. The timeliness of data entry is of utmost importance and represents one aspect of data quality. Healthcare providers should document the care of the patient at or near the time that the care is provided; however, there is no established standard timeframe for documentation. Timeliness ensures that the information is available to the other care providers and improves the accuracy of the information in the health record as well. The care provider will better remember the details of the care provided when it is documented immediately. This way, the information will not be forgotten or confused with that of another patient. Best practice is to complete documentation of the care provided to one patient before moving on to the next. The documentation must reflect the exact time and date when care was performed. Inaccurate accounting of the treatment may reflect poor quality of care as well as poor documentation of care. Users of the patient's health record depend on accurate and timely data, so it is important that the actual time of care is recorded.

It also helps to meet accreditation standards that list requirements on the timeliness of documents such as the history and physical examination.

The signatures or initials of the healthcare practitioners who oversee each event during a patient's stay, such as verbal and written orders, should be recorded. This verifies that the practitioner has overseen the treatment or plans for treatment and that these plans have been carried out. The timeliness of authentication (a provider's signature or initials) is just as important as the patient's treatment because it represents proof of care, not to mention satisfying medicolegal requirements and billing and claims reimbursement after the patient's discharge.

Data Integrity Issues

Efforts should be made to prevent data integrity issues in order to have the best data available for decision making. Failure to do so can result in poor quality patient care and bad business decisions. These efforts include data collection, data cleansing, data mapping, version control, security, organization, culture of the healthcare organization, and documentation integrity errors.

Data Collection

Data collection is the process by which data are gathered. Data collected by information systems may be entered manually or automatically through interfaces and medical devices (e.g., blood pressure cuffs). Manually collected data can be entered by a user via the keyboard, barcode, mouse, or other data entry tool. Both structured and unstructured data is collected as discussed earlier in this chapter. An interface is the zone between different computer systems across which users want to pass information (for example, a computer program written to exchange information between information systems or the graphic display of an application program designed to make the program easier to use). In other words, it takes data from one information system and shares it with another. For example, demographic data collected in the master patient index (covered in chapter 7) can be shared with other IS so that the data does not have to be entered manually again. This assists in ensuring data quality as the data is collected and entered once thus reducing the chances for errors.

Data is collected not only by the physician and other healthcare professionals but the patient too. The patient adds to the data collection when he or she provides his or her current medications, completes forms, and signs consent forms.

Data Cleansing

Data cleansing is the process of checking internal consistency and duplication as well as identifying outliers and missing data, and correcting any issues. In other words, data cleansing means looking for errors or problems with the data, such as duplicate patients and addressing the discrepancy so that the errors can be corrected. There may be outliers, which is an extreme statistical value that falls far outside the normal range. For example, if a research study has captured the number of continuing education hours that registered health information technicians report and most reported somewhere in the range of 20 and 250 hours but one reported 1,500 hours, then the 1,500 hours would be an outlier. An outlier is not necessarily an error, but it should be evaluated for accuracy because of the impact that it has on the mean and other statistical analysis of the data. Another consideration when performing data cleansing is missing data, such as when the number of continuing education hours is not reported. Efforts should be taken to complete any missing data that is identified. Failure to perform cleansing may lead to poor data integrity.

Data Mapping

Data mapping allows for connections between two systems. For example, the *International Classification of Diseases, Ninth Revision, Clinical Modification* and *International Classification of Diseases, Tenth Revision, Clinical Modification* have similar concepts but are not identical. If the concepts in the two systems are not linked appropriately, there will be problems with data integrity. For example, a link has been established when the codes for an open appendectomy in each coding system are identified as equivalent codes for each other. For additional information on data mapping, refer to chapter 9.

Version Control

The process whereby a healthcare organization ensures that only the most current version of a patient's health record is available for viewing, updating, additions, and so forth. Why is this necessary? While health record data should never be deleted, there are times when the data needs to be altered either to correct (amend) data or to add an addendum (more information). This can occur if data is entered in the wrong patient's health record, erroneous data is entered, addendums to the existing data, and must be made, or through other errors. In the EHR, an unsigned, dictated document such as a history and physical and a signed one are two different versions.

The EHR must notify the user that there is a different version of a document available but not all users need to have access to the original version. There should be a process to provide access to authorized users and those who need access for some reason such as going to court.

Security

The intent of this section is not to provide an overview of security as that topic will be covered in chapter 12, but rather to address the importance of security with regards to data integrity. There is always the possibility of crackers accessing and altering data in a database. Even internal users can intentionally or unintentionally alter data. Data can also be altered as it is being transmitted from one point to another – whether over the internet or a private network. Malware (malicious software that damages computers, ISs, and/or data) can prevent access to data, destroy data, or otherwise cause data quality and integrity issues. For more on security, refer to chapter 12.

Organizational Culture of the Healthcare Organization

The healthcare organization must have a culture that focuses on data quality. Employees make mistakes. Those mistakes can result from carelessness, typographical errors, apathy, lack of training or accountability, or other reasons. It is up to the leadership to create this culture. Methods to create this culture include monitoring the quality of data, training employees on data quality policies and best practices, counseling employees who create data quality errors, and more. This cannot be a one-time initiative but ongoing so that data quality stays at the forefront of everyone's mind.

Documentation Integrity Errors

Data integrity of documentation can be compromised in many ways in ISs like the EHR, such as when a revision is made to an operative report and it is unclear which is the most current version. These integrity errors affect patient identification, authorship, dictation, amendments, cloning, and copying and pasting. These errors not only harm the integrity of the data but can lead to poor quality of care and allegations of fraud and abuse. Potential threats to documentation integrity errors include: patient identification, authorship, dictation errors, copy and pasting, and amendments to the health information.

Patient Identification

Patient identification is identifying the proper patient. For example, there may be several John Smith's who have been treated at the healthcare organization. The proper one must be selected to prevent patient identification errors. Patient identification errors occur when patient A's health information is documented in patient B's health record. This mistake can lead to serious patient care errors for both patients. For example, patient A may have had an appendectomy. If patient B shows symptoms of appendicitis, then appendicitis may not be considered as a diagnosis since the health record states that the patient's appendix has been removed. There may also be issues with billing as the wrong patient may be billed. Healthcare organization should use methods that help ensure the identity of patients, such as algorithms, biometrics, and photography to ensure the correct patient is identified. The EHR should flag users when there are patients with the same name or similar names exist to encourage users to ensure they have the correct patient (AHIMA 2019).

Authorship

Authorship is the origination or creation of recorded information attributed to a specific individual or entity acting at a particular time. In other words, documentation in the EHR or other health record must be credited to the individual who created it. This is typically done through the use of a unique user identifier and a password although other measures may be used. When a digital signature is created, it indicates that the data has been reviewed and approved by the physician or other care provider signing the entry in the health record. A digital signature is an electronic signature that binds a message to a particular individual and can be used by the receiver to authenticate the identity of the sender. Failure to link the documentation to the proper author makes it difficult to determine who actually recorded it when multiple healthcare providers are involved in the patient's care (AHIMA Work Group 2013). It is important to identify the author because the documentation is used for legal reasons to prove what the healthcare professional did or did not do. Authorship is important in other areas, too, including coding, because generally only the patient's physician documentation is used in coding.

Dictation Errors

If speech recognition is utilized, and the documents are not edited after their creation to ensure accuracy, then there may be problems with data integrity. The speech recognition software may misinterpret something that the dictator said which would result in the health record containing incorrect medications and other incorrect words. One study showed that the speech recognition error rate was 7.4% before the documentation was reviewed and edited. Once edited by the transcriptionist, the error rate dropped to 0.4% and when the physician reviewed before signing, it dropped slightly more to 0.3% (Zhou, et al. 2018). The final error rate may be small but depending on what the error is, it could have a serious impact on the patient. Speech recognition is covered in more detail later in this chapter.

Copying and Pasting

One of the ways to speed data entry is through copy and paste functions. Data from one patient's health record can be copied and pasted into another patient's health record or data from the same patient's previous hospitalization may be moved to their current hospitalization. Copying and pasting is commonly done for routine procedures, radiology results, and other conventional entries for which the same information is used repeatedly. The most frequently cited benefit to copy and pasting is consistent in the patient's health history (AHIMA 2019). However, there are risks associated with this, so this practice is not always recommended. For example, the physician may copy and paste a preoperative order from one patient's health record to another's. In the order copied from the first patient's health record, there may be a medication inappropriate for the second patient. If not caught, the patient may be given this medication in error. Copying can also be used in moving data, such as diagnoses and medication, between different visits of the same patient. For example, data can be moved from a patient's October 1 visit to their December 30 visit. Although this function speeds data entry, it raises data quality and integrity concerns as the information copied may not completely apply to the patient's care. When this happens, the patient's health record contains erroneous information that can impact the quality of care. In spite of the risk, copy and paste is widely used. One study found that 46% of a note written by a healthcare professional was copied (Wang, Khanna, and Najafi 2017). This is a huge amount of copied data. This figure shows just how frequently the opportunities for copying outdated or incorrect information truly is.

Amendments to the Health Record

The data contained in the health record must be amended when changes are necessary, such as correcting mistakes, attaching addendums, making late entries, and replacing a draft (unsigned) copy of a document with a final (signed) copy. For example, if the patient's blood type is entered in the EHR as A+ but it is actually B−, then the blood type must be corrected.

Once a health record entry is signed, the document should be locked to prevent further alterations. The IS should also lock the entire record from edits at a predetermined point, such as 30 days after discharge. To amend the health record, it would have to be unlocked by an authorized user so that the necessary changes can be made by the author of the document. There should also be policies in place regarding who has the ability to amend. For example, the HIM professional may be able to correct the spelling of the patient's name or a transposition in the social security number, but only the physician would be able to correct his clinical documentation. The deleted information should not be permanently deleted so that it can be retrieved if needed. Late entries and addendums should be clearly labeled so that it is clear when the documentation was created (Davoudi et al. 2015).

The erroneous information should not be completely deleted; rather, there should be a way to identify that the health record was altered. The best practice is to create a second version of the document. As discussed earlier in this chapter, version control is necessary to manage the various documents. Access to this previous version is necessary in court cases and other legal circumstances.

Data Quality Measure

Data quality measure is a "mechanism to assign a quantitative figure to quality of care by comparison to a criterion. Quality measurements typically focus on structures or processes of care that have a demonstrated relationship to positive health outcomes" (Davoudi et al. 2015). For example, when steps are taken to reduce postoperative infections, the data quality measure would address issues, such as use of antibiotics and wound care. These are used to compare actual patient information to a standard created by an accreditation organization, government agency, or other group to determine the quality of care provided. The data can be aggregated (compiled) and be used to compare healthcare organizations against state or national scores.

Policies and Procedures

Policies and procedures are a critical part of data quality as they set the stage for the steps employees take to ensure the quality of data. Governing principles that describe how a department or an organization is supposed to handle a specific situation or execute a specific process defines a policy. In other words, it is a broad statement of how something is done. A procedure is a document that describes the steps involved in performing a specific function. It gives step by step instructions needed to accomplish the policy.

There needs to be policies and procedures on data collection, data retention, monitoring the quality of data and so much more. Following these policies and procedures provide consistency in how things are done such as the collection of data. For example, a policy and procedure may help an employee confirm that they have identified the correct John Smith.

Ensuring Data Integrity During the Sharing of Data

With the EHR, healthcare organizations have more data available than ever before. This data can also easily be shared with patients, other healthcare organizations, and other authorized users. Many healthcare organizations share data through a health information exchange (HIE). A HIE exchanges health information electronically between providers and others with the same level of interoperability, such as labs and pharmacies. To be able to share data between organizations, all organizations much utilize standards so that they are able to compare not just "apples to apples" but Gala apples to Gala apples. This means that data is stored in the same format, data fields have the same definition, same diagnosis and procedure coding systems, and more. Application programming interfaces (APIs) enables one information system to access another information system. The APIs are being used to facilitate the sharing of health information. APIs are used by HIE but they are also used to share information with patients, with other healthcare providers, and with registries (HealthIT 2020). For additional information on HIE, refer to chapter 11.

Data integrity issues can be impacted by poor data collection and other practices within a healthcare organization but can also occur through data sharing. For example, data can be altered or seized during electronic transit between two healthcare organizations.

Patients may be seen at multiple healthcare organizations. When health information is shared via a HIE, there is the risk of patient duplication in the HIE's database (i.e., one patient with two unlinked records), fragmenting the patient's record resulting in incomplete health information available to healthcare providers. Data integrity issues also result from overlays in the HIE's database (Butler 2018, 15). An overlay is when two patients' health information are commingled under one patient. This could be two people with the same name, siblings born on the same day, or other patients.

CHECK YOUR UNDERSTANDING 2.2

1. The identification of the individual who recorded a progress note in the health record is known as _____.

   a. Edit check
   b. Data integrity
   c. Version control
   d. Authorship

2. Addressing missing information and outliers is known as _____.

   a. Edit check
   b. Qualitative analysis
   c. Data cleansing
   d. Quantitative analysis

3. Documentation integrity issues include _____.

   a. Amendments
   b. Data precision
   c. Edit check
   d. Data capture

4. Identify the characteristic of data quality that addresses the usefulness of the data collected.

   a. Data relevancy
   b. Data precision
   c. Data accuracy
   d. Data granularity

5. Identify the attribute of data quality that addresses data being displayed in the same format on different screens in the EHR.

   a. Data relevancy
   b. Data consistency
   c. Data accessibility
   d. Data granularity

Real-World Case 2.1

In order to improve patient safety and efficiency, XYZ Hospital recently implemented a clinical provider order entry (CPOE) system. One of the functions of the CPOE system is to notify physicians of any problems at the time that an order is entered. Days after the CPOE system was implemented, Dr. Smith ordered medication X for a patient named Mary Johnson. Immediately, the CPOE came back with a message stating that medication X was contraindicated (not recommended) for patients on medication Y and that Mary was taking medication Y. Dr. Smith realized that he had almost ordered a medication that could have significantly harmed Mary. The immediate availability of this information via the CPOE allowed him to cancel the order of medication X and order medication Z instead. Mary received the appropriate medication in a timely manner, quickly improved, and was discharged from the hospital in two days.

Real-World Case 2.2

A patient was admitted to XYZ Medical Center with abdominal pain. He had been at the medical center several times over the years for various conditions and treatment. The patient's health record was reviewed and showed that the patient's appendix had been removed five years ago. Because of this entry, the diagnosis of appendicitis was ruled out. Other conditions were considered but were ultimately ruled out. In talking further with the patient, the physician learned that the patient never had an appendectomy. The patient was then diagnosed with appendicitis and had surgery to remove the appendix. This erroneous entry in the health record was corrected, the patient improved, and was discharged home.

REVIEW QUESTIONS

1. Identify the type of data field that is most appropriate for the health record number.

    a. Numeric field
    b. Autonumbering field
    c. Text box field
    d. Radio button field

2. Identify the benefit of front-end speech recognition.

    a. It does not impact the physician.
    b. The document is available immediately upon completion of the dictation.
    c. It speeds availability of the document.
    d. It eliminates data quality issues.

3. The data quality characteristic that includes a missing document would fall under data _____.

    a. Comprehensiveness
    b. Accuracy
    c. Consistency
    d. Definition

(Continued)

REVIEW QUESTIONS (*Continued*)

4. The data quality characteristic that identifies the need for the data element is data _____.

   a. Precision
   b. Currency
   c. Constancy
   d. Definition

5. The fact that there is missing data would be identified in _____.

   a. Authorship
   b. Data consistency
   c. Data mapping
   d. Data cleansing

6. Linking two systems is known as _____.

   a. Patient identification
   b. Authorship
   c. Data mapping
   d. Validation

7. Identify the statement that is true about amending a health record.

   a. Anyone should be able to alter the health record at any time.
   b. The author is the only one who should alter the health record.
   c. Any documentation deleted should be retrievable if needed.
   d. Health records cannot be amended.

8. Ensuring that only the most recent report is available for viewing is known as _____.

   a. Documentation integrity
   b. Authorship
   c. Validation
   d. Version control

9. Edit checks ensure that _____.

   a. The format is appropriate for the data element
   b. The data entered is accurate for that patient
   c. The health record is complete
   d. The data entered is at the level appropriate for the situation

   preprogrammed definition

10. Qualitative analysis reviews the quality of _____.
    a. Forms in the health record
    b. Screen design
    c. Documentation in the health record
    d. The data dictionary

References

American Health Information Management Association (AHIMA). 2019. Ensuring the Integrity of the EHR. Journal of AHIMA 90(1) 34-37.

American Health Information Management Association. 2017. *Pocket Glossary of Health Information Management and Technology*, 5th ed. Chicago: AHIMA.

AHIMA Work Group. 2013. Integrity of the Healthcare Record: Best Practices for EHR Documentation (2013 update). http://bok.ahima.org/doc?oid=300257#.WjxsKeRy5jo.

Butler, M. 2018. Ensuring Data Integrity during Health Information Exchange. Journal of AHIMA 89(10) 14-17.

Davoudi, S., J. A. Dooling, B. Glondys, T. D. Jones, L. Kadlec, S. M. Overgaard, K. Ruben, and A. Wendicke. 2015. Data Quality Management Model (2015 update). http://bok.ahima.org/doc?oid=107773#.WjxlEORy5jo.

HealthIT. 2020. Section 3 Health Information Exchange. https://www.healthit.gov/playbook/health-information-exchange/.

MerlinOne. 2019. What is Metadata Tagging? https://merlinone.com/what-is-metadata-tagging/.

Ortega, D. 2017. The difference between Data Quality and Data Integrity. https://www.blazent.com/difference-data-quality-data-integrity/

Sharp, M. 2020. Secondary Data Sources. Chapter 7 in *Health Information Management Technology: An Applied Approach*, 6th ed. Edited by N. B. Sayles and L. L. Gordon. Chicago: AHIMA.

Wang, M. D., R. Khanna, and N. Najafi. 2017. Characterizing the Source of Text in Electronic Health Record Progress Notes. https://jamanetwork.com/journals/jamainternalmedicine/article-abstract/2629493.

Zhou, L., S. V. Blackley, L. Kowalski, R. Doan, W. W. Acker, A. B. Landman, E. Kontrient, D. Mack, M. Meteer, D. W. Bates, and F. R. Goss. 2018. Analysis of Errors in Dictated Clinical Documents Assisted by Speech Recognition Software and Professional Transcriptionists. https://jamanetwork.com/journals/jamanetworkopen/fullarticle/2687052.

Chapter 3

Introduction to Databases and Data Analytics

Learning Objectives

- Assist in the development of a database.
- Compare and contrast the different types of data analytics and their roles in the analysis and improvement of healthcare delivery and services.
- Develop and manage the data dictionary.
- Develop queries to retrieve data contained in the database.
- Read and understand an entity-relationship diagram.
- Identify the primary key contained in an entity.
- Differentiate between a data repository and a data warehouse.
- Expound on the ways that data mining can be useful.
- Complete simple normalization of data.
- Differentiate between the various types of data.

Key Terms

Aggregate data 37
Boolean search
Clinical data repository (CDR)
Certified Health Data Analyst (CHDA)
Clinical document architecture (CDA)
Computer-aided software engineering (CASE)
Conceptual data model
Continuity of Care Document (CCD)
Continuity of Care Record (CCR)
Data analytics

Data control language (DCL)
Data definition language (DDL)
Data dictionary
Data content standards
Data field
Data flow diagram (DFD)
Data manipulation
Data manipulation language (DML)
Data mart
Data mining
Data modeling
Data repository
Data scrubbing

Data set
Data standards
Data stewardship
Data warehouse
Database
Database administrator (DBA)
Database management system (DBMS)
Database table
Descriptive analytics
Entity-relationship diagram (ERD)
File
Foreign key
Health informatics

Hierarchical database model	Network database model	Record
Java	Normalization	Standards development
Key field	Object-oriented database	organization (SDO)
Logical data model	model	Structured query language
Mask	Online analytical processing	(SQL)
Metadata	(OLAP)	Systematized Nomenclature
Multidimensional database	Predictive analytics	of Medicine Clinical Terms
model	Prescriptive analytics	(SNOMED CT)
National Information	Physical data model	Use case
Standards Organization	Primary key	Vocabulary standards
(NISO)	Query	Wildcard search
Natural language queries	Query by example (QBE)	

Introduction to Databases and Data Analytics

The world is run by data. No decisions can be made without it. In order to make a well-informed decision, quality data is essential. HIM professionals are, by the very nature of their education and background, always involved in some aspect of the characteristics of data quality as mentioned in Chapter 2.

Data analytics is the science of examining raw data with the purpose of drawing conclusions about that information. It includes data mining, machine learning, development of models, and statistical measurements. Analytics can be descriptive, diagnostic, predictive, or prescriptive. **Descriptive analytics** use a group of statistical techniques to describe data such as means, frequency distributions, and is used to describe the characteristics of a specific group or population. In this age of the coronavirus disease pandemic of 2019 (COVID-19), descriptive analytics would identify the segments of the population most at risk for contracting the disease. **Diagnostic analytics** helps a healthcare organization determine why something happened. Diagnostic analytics tools such as dashboards and data mining are introduced later in this chapter. For example, if the patient volume has gone down, you can investigate types of patients, age of patient, physician admissions, and other attributes to identify the reason for the decline such as losing a physician practice on your medical staff that admitted a lot of patients. **Predictive analytics** is a process to identify patterns that can be used to predict the odds of a particular outcome based upon observed, historical data – think of the daily weather forecast. Predictive analytics can forecast the hospitalization rate and ventilator demand to help healthcare organizations prepare for the increase in admissions. **Prescriptive analytics** uses information generated from descriptive and predictive analytics and modelling to determine a strategy for the best outcome and/or to suggest a course of action to solve a problem. Once the COVID-19 pandemic slows or ends, prescriptive analytics will be used to improve the preparation and mitigation efforts that government and healthcare organizations must do to lessen the impact of the next pandemic (Brinkman 2019).

Many people think that health informatics and health data analytics are the same thing. There is a fine but definite difference between the two. Health data analytics involves database management and statistical techniques to manipulate acquired data to show trends and patterns in medical diagnoses, patient services, and impacts on the health of a community. Analytics, as the name implies, uses collected data to examine, investigate, and evaluate the status of whatever subject is at hand.

Health informatics however, uses information systems and technology to better and more efficiently deliver healthcare services, manage health organizations and personnel, and perform strategic planning. Health informatics uses the data generated by health data analytic techniques to make decisions that impact the processes, technology, and people who must collaborate to make better decisions for the benefit of the target population. **Health informatics** is the application of information generated by health data analytics techniques (Clack, et al 2017).

To perform any type of data analysis, **aggregate data** must be gathered. In healthcare, aggregate data is data extracted from individual health records and combined to form information about groups or patients that can be compared and analysed. This aggregate data is then fed into a database so that statistical analysis can be performed. Examples of aggregate data are number of Medicare patients, average length of stay for July, postoperative infection rate, and average age of patients. A **database** is defined as an organized collection of locally related data, text, references, or pictures in a standardized format, typically stored in a computer system for multiple applications. Healthcare organizations collect and store a tremendous amount of administrative, financial, and clinical data. A database can assist the healthcare organization in many ways, including the following:

- Facilitate data sharing
- Streamline workflow
- Assist in clinical decision making
- Provide information for managerial decision making
- Provide data for data analysis

Databases allow data to be stored in one place and accessed by many different systems and end-users. This consolidation reduces the redundancy of data and improves data consistency because data are entered into the database once, and any screen, report, or system can access that data element. One-time data entry improves the consistency of data, which improves data quality and, ultimately, patient care. Additionally, the use of a database allows for the standardization of data forms, names of data elements, and documentation, which makes moving from transitioning between various screens and various information systems (ISs) easier for the users.

A database requires a **database administrator (DBA)** to manage it. The DBA is the individual responsible for the technical aspects of databases. The DBA is responsible for designing the database as well as managing the database after implementation (Amatayakul 2016, 414). **Data stewardship** is the formalization of accountability and a continuum of stewardship responsibilities across the data life cycle and across the enterprise. Data stewardship is carried out by a network of designated employees who are responsible for managing, collecting, viewing, storing, sharing, disclosing, and otherwise making use of personal health information. **Health data stewardship** is the management and responsibilities of an activity according to its established goals and objectives, regulatory and accreditation conditions, and other organizational obligations to guarantee that health information is used appropriately (Johns 2020, 93). A data steward is responsible for all the policies and procedures that govern the use of information within a healthcare organization, provide operational management of the information systems using healthcare organization data, ensure processes for data integrity, and protect the privacy and security of healthcare organization and health information (Hebbar 2017). HIM professionals can easily transition into data stewardship positions because they have always been intimately involved in the collection, quality evaluation, maintenance and storage, and security of patient data. They understand not only the what, where, when, and how, but also the why of health information (Downing 2016).The **certified health data analyst (CHDA)** credential identifies practitioners who have the knowledge to acquire, manage, analyze, interpret, and transform data into accurate, consistent, and timely information while balancing the healthcare organization's strategic vision with day-to-day details. CHDA-credentialed professionals exhibit broad organizational knowledge and the ability to communicate with individuals and groups at multiple levels, both internal and external (AHIMA 2020).

A major reason why healthcare professionals need quality data and information is to evaluate and improve performance or personnel and institutions. The "Triple Aim" concept was developed by the Institute for Healthcare Improvement (IHI) (2020) to achieve this goal. The three aspects of Triple Aim are:

- Improve the patient experience of care
- Improve the health of the population
- Reduce the per capita cost of healthcare

Aggregate data and databases help clinicians and administrators use this information to change practice guidelines, streamline activities, and improve the financial stability of the organization. Figure 3.1 below shows how the use of various data activities helps to achieve the concept of Triple Aim in healthcare.

Figure 3.1. Data and triple aim goals

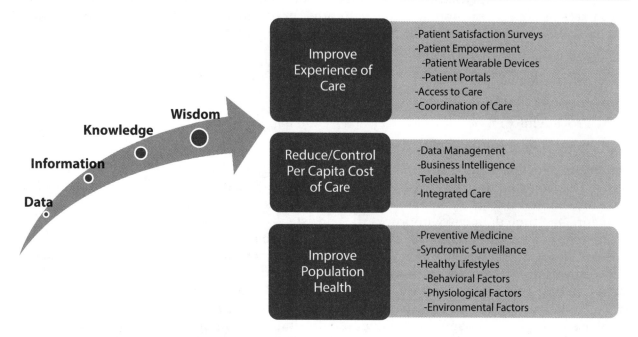

Source: Campbell, 2018.

Requirements for Establishing a Database

The healthcare organization must develop a database that meets its needs. These needs are identified by researching the needs of the users and the external stakeholders, such as the Joint Commission, state licensing agencies, and the Centers for Medicare and Medicaid Services. The data elements stored in the database must meet the requirements of data sets. A **data set** is a list of recommended data elements with uniform definitions that are relevant for a particular use. For example, the Uniform Hospital Discharge Data Set (UHDDS) is used by acute-care hospitals to capture and report the minimal data required for all inpatient discharges. The UHDDS includes patient name, discharge disposition, date of admission, diagnosis and procedure codes, and much more. As this is only the minimum amount of data to be collected, the healthcare organization can add other data elements to meet the needs of the organization, such as accreditation, research, state licensure, and other needs. The data elements may be administrative, such as patient name and health record number; financial, such as the charge for the hospital room or the laboratory test performed; or clinical, such as history of present illness or follow-up plan.

Once all the necessary individual data elements are determined, a common **data definition** should be developed for each data element. As discussed in chapter 2, this definition would be utilized to collect data consistently throughout the healthcare organization. For example, time of discharge could be the time that the discharge order is written, the time the discharge is entered into the IS, or the time the patient walks out of the hospital.

In addition, it may be necessary to make sure the data used in databases is complete, comprehensive, and accurate, but not to the point of redundancy. To do this, it may be necessary to perform data scrubbing. According to Campbell (2018), "**data scrubbing** or cleansing involves the detection, removal, and correction of incorrect, incomplete, or poorly formatted data in health information technology systems. It deals with the detection and elimination of duplicate or redundant information, mistakes during data entry, invalid values, or non-populated values within each information system." A good example of this are the duplicate entries within a master patient index (MPI). One can think of the MPI as technically the initial dataset leading into the EHR, these duplicates within an MPI could lead to incorrect counts as to volume and may influence workload calculations and productivity standards. Another example would be the correction of structural errors. A data set may include fields stating "N/A" or "Not Applicable". These can be read as two separate entities but they mean the same thing. Data scrubbing or cleansing would identify this error and correct it so that either of those entries in a data field would have the same meaning.

Database Management System

A database cannot function without a **database management system (DBMS)** to manipulate and control the data stored within the database to meet the needs of the user. It controls the ability to create, read, update, and delete data stored in the database. There are six DBMS functions, listed as follows:

- Moving where data is stored in database
- Managing concurrent data access by multiple users, including provisions to prevent simultaneous updates from conflicting with one another
- Managing transactions so that each transaction's database changes are an all-or-nothing unit of work. In other words, if the transaction succeeds, all database changes made by it are recorded in the database
- Support for a query language, which is a system of commands that a database user employs to retrieve data from the database
- Provisions for backing up the database and recovering from failures
- Security mechanisms to prevent unauthorized data access and modification (Oppel 2004)

The parts of the DBMS include data definition language, data manipulation language, data control language, and data dictionary.

The **data definition language (DDL)** is used to create the tables within a relational database (defined later in this chapter). It translates how data are stored in the computer from the physical view (physical structure of the database) to the logical view (one that is understandable by the user). It is "used to define data structures and modify data. For example, DDL commands can be used to add, remove, or modify tables within a database" (HIMSS 2017, 64).

The **data manipulation language (DML)** is used to retrieve, edit data in a relational database. The DML accesses, makes changes to, and retrieves data from the database. These capabilities can easily be performed in a database without the user being an experienced computer programmer. It is a "family of computer languages, including commands permitting users to manipulate data in a database" (HIMSS 2017, 70). To retrieve data, a query is generated. As discussed earlier, the term query is used to describe selecting records that meet specific criteria. Queries may also perform calculations on the data, such as calculating the average length of stay. Queries can also screen data for inclusion or exclusion. Four user methods to access data contained in the database are natural language queries, query by example, structured query language, and data dictionary. The **data control language (DCL)** controls access to data within a database.

Natural Language Queries

Natural language queries use common words to tell the database which data are needed. For example, the user may enter a query by typing "list all of the patients whose principal procedure is 0F140D3." This command would generate a list of patients who had the principal procedure. Another example may be, "how many patients were discharged on October 1, 20XX?" To process the query, the system searches key words in the question to fulfill the request. Some ISs may allow the use of voice recognition, thus eliminating the need to type in the request.

Query by Example

Query by example (QBE) is a query method whereby the user only has to point and click to choose tables and fields contained in the database. The IS then allows the user to choose whether the entries that meet those criteria should be included or excluded from the query. For example, the user may choose the patient table and discharge date as the field. The user can then tell the IS to include patients discharged January 1, 20XX through January 31, 20XX. Only the patients with a discharge date within that range would be included in the results of the query. **Boolean search** capabilities such as "and," "or," and "not" may be used in the QBE database to narrow down the data to specifically what the user needs. For example, the query could retrieve patients who had a principal diagnosis of cholecystitis "and" a principal procedure of laparoscopic cholecystectomy. Truncation, such as the **wildcard search**, may be used to look for variations in the word (Oracle n.d.). For example, the user could search for patients whose admission date is greater than, or before, a specific date. The wildcard would be used to indicate that the query should identify data that meet the partial information provided. For example, a query of 0F140D% would retrieve all codes that start with the specified characters such as 0F140D3, 0F140D4, 0F140D5, 0F140D6, and so on. Other query tools include the greater than (>) and less than (<) options to retrieve data that meets the criteria 0F140D. Different characters may be used as wildcards in different databases.

Structured Query Language

A common data retrieval tool is **structured query language (SQL),** the standard language for the relational database. SQL defines data elements, manipulates data, and controls access. The data definition components of SQL allow the user to create tables, delete tables, and show how something is viewed. **Data manipulation** allows the user to add and delete rows in a table and to sort, find, and compare. Another function of the data manipulation component is to update data. SQL is the programming language that manages a user's access and what the user can do. Examples of SQL commands typed by the programmer are CREATE TABLE, SELECT, WHERE, COUNT, and UPDATE (Oppel 2004).

An SQL query that assumes a table with the name Patients and the columns ID, FirstName, LastName, and DateAdded can be used as follows:

- To retrieve all the records and all the columns

  Select * from Patients
- To retrieve all the records and only the FirstName column

  Select FirstName From Patients
- To retrieve all the records and all the columns ordered by LastName Descending

  Select * From Patients Order By LastName desc
- To retrieve all the records and all the columns that were added before 1/1/2014

  Select * From Patients Where DateAdded < '1/1/2014'
- To select only the records where the FirstName is equal to Mark

  Select * From Patients Where FirstName = 'Mark'

Data Dictionary

The **data dictionary** is a descriptive list of the names, definitions, and attributes of data elements to be collected in an IS or database whose purpose is to standardize definitions and ensure consistent use. It also helps to control the quality of data. The data dictionary improves data consistency because it ensures that fields have the same meaning and format throughout the organization. It helps create consistent data field names, data field definitions, field length, and element values (AHIMA 2017, 7). Examples of how the data dictionary supports data consistency are provided in Table 3.1.

Table 3.1. Examples of how data dictionary assists in data consistency

Data Element	Example
Field name	The unique identifier given to a specific patient encounter is called encounter number in all ISs, not account number and not billing number.
Field definition	Discharge time is the time the order was written, not the time the discharge is entered into the system or the time that the patient leaves the nursing unit.
Field length	The field length of the account number is 10 digits in all ISs, not 8 in some and 12 in others.
Element values	The insurance type for Medicare is M in all ISs, not MCR.

The data dictionary assists in improving

- Data quality
- Data integrity
- Documentation
- Data analysis
- Data reuse (AHIMA 2016)

The data contained in the data dictionary is known as metadata. **Metadata** is descriptive data that characterize other data to create a clearer understanding of their meaning and to achieve greater reliability and quality of information. Some of the metadata contained in the data dictionary includes, but is not limited to, the following:

- Names of data elements
- Definition
- Source of data
- Length of field
- Allowable range as appropriate
- Valid values
- Access restrictions
- Length of field (Amatayakul 2017, 315)

Metadata is often referred to as "data about data," but this definition oversimplifies the concept. A better definition is "structured information used to increase the effective use of data" (Johns 2020, 83). It includes the electronic time stamp of when data was created, accessed, or manipulated. See Figure 3.2 for an example of metadata in a data dictionary for a relational database.

Figure 3.2. Metadata for a relational database

emlployee_id	first_name	last_name	nin	department_id
44	Simon	Martinez	HH 45 09 73 D	1
45	Thomas	Goldstein	SA 75 35 42 B	2
46	Eugene	Cornelsen	NE 22 63 82	2
47	Andrew	Petculescu	XY 29 87 61 A	1
48	Ruth	Stadick	MA 12 89 36 A	15
49	Barry	Scardelis	AT 20 73 18	2
50	Sidney	Hunter	HW 12 94 21 C	6
51	Jeffrey	Evans	LX 13 26 39 B	6
52	Doris	Berndt	YA 49 88 11 A	3
53	Diane	Eaton	BE 08 74 68 A	1
54	Bonnie	Hall	WW 53 77 68 A	15
55	Taylor	Li	ZE 55 22 80 B	1

Data

Metadata

Column	Data Type	Description
emlployee_id	int	Primary key of a table
first_name	nvarchar(50)	Employee first name
last_name	nvarchar(50)	Employee last name
nin	nvarchar(15)	National Identification Number
position	nvarchar(50)	Current postion title, e.g. Secretary
department_id	int	Employee depamtnet. Ref: Departmetns
gender	char(1)	M = Male, F = Female, Null = unknown
employment_start_date	date	Start date of employment in organization.
employment_end_date	date	Employment end date. Null if employee sti

Source: Dataedo, 2018.

The **National Information Standards Organization (NISO)** advises that metadata should be used to sustain interoperability. Interoperability is the ability of different information technology systems and software applications to communicate; to exchange data accurately, effectively, and consistently; and to use the information that has been exchanged. Metadata makes it easier to find, acquire, use, and effectively manage the data within the healthcare organization's information systems. Metadata identifies when an entry was created and who created it, from where it was accessed, and all changes made to the file or document. During an information breach investigation, a single employee's electronic activity or the activity that occurred at a single workstation or terminal can be audited. This recommendation is also advocated by the Office of the National Coordinator (ONC) for Health Information Technology in that metadata supports data integrity for health information exchange (HIE) (Dolezel 2015).

Metadata can prove the integrity of a healthcare organization's records by identifying the creation, changes, access, and security of the information to ensure its quality and trustworthiness. As previously mentioned in chapter two, there are three types of metadata:

- Descriptive metadata addresses specific data elements acquired and used by the information system. The data dictionary established for all the datasets within the information system is an example of descriptive metadata.

- Structural metadata is the process of acquiring, storing, manipulating, and displaying data. Data models, such as entity-relationship diagrams (ERD) and dataflow diagrams (DFD) are diagrammatical or graphic tools used to help program the system and to identify areas of inefficiency.

- Administrative metadata is programmed in the information system in order to generate data about the usage of the information system, such as audit trail and activity reports. The audit trail identifies tasks such as who accessed the information system or when and where someone performed a certain data function. Administrative metadata also includes decision support functions wherein the information system assists in helping to assemble, manipulate, and prioritize data and make recommendations about specific courses of action that can be taken to address an identified issue (Amatayakul 2016, 438). For example, audit trails can identify when a data entry error was made and who made it. Analyzing this type of data entry error activity may show how often it occurs and which employee(s) is(are) responsible. This information could be used in training employees.

There are several data items that are important within the realm of metadata. These items are important because it shows when the data was created and by whom. It alleviates any questions regarding who recorded the information or if any data had been altered, which would call into question the integrity and security of the data. These items are the user name, identification number, patient name, health record number, the name or IP address of the computer where and when the data was accessed, the date and time information was manipulated, printed, or downloaded, and what documents or reports were accessed or manipulated (Biedermann and Dolezel 2017, 445).

The data dictionary may also control if a mask is used and, if so, what form it takes. Table 3.2 shows an abbreviated sample of a data dictionary. The data dictionary defines any masks to be used. A **mask** is a format in which data are displayed. This display is different from how the data are stored in the database. For example, if a patient's home telephone number is entered as 5555555555, numbers could appear as (555) 555-5555. Another example of where a mask could be used is social security number. The social security number of 123456789 could be entered and it appears in the system as 123-45-6789.

Table 3.2. Abbreviated data dictionary

Field Name	Last Name	First Name	Health Record Number	Date of Birth	Gender
Data type	Text	Text	Text	Alphanumeric	Alphanumeric
Format	A–Z	A–Z	0–9	MM-DD-YYYY	M, F, U
Field size	25	25	10	8	1
Range			0000000001– 0009999999		
Required	Yes	Yes	Yes	Yes	Yes

Vocabulary Standards

Vocabulary standards, a list or collection of clinical words or phrases with their meanings, address the problem of multiple ways to define, classify, and represent language. "Language generally refers to a system of communication using an arbitrary set of vocal sounds, written symbols, signs, or gestures in conventional ways with conventional meanings" (Amatayakul 2017, 289). Medicine has its own language. There are many terms used in medicine that can have multiple synonyms. For example, the terms "medical" and "therapeutic," "curative" and "drug," and "medication" and "pharmaceutical" can be used relatively interchangeably. The use of synonyms can make it difficult to identify patients with a specific disease or condition. Several terms fall into the concept of vocabulary standards, including language, vocabulary, terminology, and nomenclature:

- Language is a system of communication used by a group of people.
- Vocabulary is all the terms that can be used for communication within the area of specialization.
- Terminology means the words used for a specific purpose.
- Nomenclature is a system used to assign names. (Amatayakul 2017, 289–290)

Vocabularies require terms to be evaluated for inclusion. Each term included in the vocabulary should have a unique meaning; however, it should be noted that synonyms are linked within the vocabulary, such as the examples listed above. Terminologies, in general, are a set of terms representing the system of concepts of a particular subject field. A clinical terminology provides the proper context and usage of clinical words as names or symbols. Terminologies, along with classification systems, are necessary to support the EHR, personal health record (PHR), and population health reporting as well as quality reporting (Palkie 2020, 146). PHRs are discussed in more detail in chapter 9. Vocabularies and terminologies can have overlapping terms due to synonyms and eponyms. This is one of the challenging aspects of medicine and the application of EHR and diagnostic software to interpret unstructured (and sometimes structured) text from a physician or other healthcare provider.

Systematized Nomenclature of Medicine

As stated previously, nomenclature refers to systems that use established rules that assign the names used in a particular field. The use of a nomenclature allows for comparison and aggregation of data (Amatayakul 2017, 294). The most widely recognized nomenclature in healthcare is the Systematized Nomenclature of Medicine (SNOMED). It was developed in 1975 by the College of American Pathologists, but maintenance was transitioned to the International Health Terminology Standards Development Organization in 2007. The current version, **Systematized Nomenclature of Medicine Clinical Terms (SNOMED CT),** is the most comprehensive, multilingual clinical healthcare terminology in the world. SNOMED CT contributes to the improvement of patient care by underpinning the development of EHRs that record clinical information in ways that enable meaning-based retrieval.

SNOMED CT is used for the EHR, research, and clinical decisions. The information that SNOMED CT captures includes items such as diagnoses, procedures, signs, symptoms, and cause of injury. SNOMED CT has a concepts table that consists of more than 352,000 concepts, 450,000 medical descriptions, and one million concept interrelations, each of which has a unique meaning and format definition such as 98 degrees versus 98°. It also contains description tables with more than a million language descriptions or synonyms (this allows for flexibility in expressing clinical concepts). A relationships table contains over 1.3 million semantic relationships (ONC 2017f). These relationships are important to data retrieval (Amatayakul 2017, 294). See figure 3.3 for a short example of how clinical information is coded in SNOMED CT.

Figure 3.3. SNOMED CT working behind the scenes in an EHR

In the following excerpt from an EHR, a few of the applicable SNOMED CT codes are noted in parentheses to illustrate what SNOMED CT is doing behind the scenes. It is automatically identifying standard terms and tagging them for future references.

Office visit for a 64-year-old established female patient being seen for review and follow-up of non–insulin-dependent diabetes, obesity, hypertension, and chronic right-sided congestive heart failure. Complains of shortness of breath and admits to dietary noncompliance. Patient's heart failure is assessed (blood pressure measures, level of activity assessed, clinical signs and symptoms of volume overload assessed, respiratory status assessed, and weight recorded). She is counseled concerning diet and current medications adjusted.

- -81531005 | Type II diabetes mellitus in obese (disorder)|
- -59621000 | Essential hypertension (disorder)|
- -66989003 | Chronic right-sided congestive heart failure (disorder)|
- -26700087 | Dyspnea (finding)
- -129832003 | Noncompliance with dietary regimen (finding)|
- -46973005 | Blood pressure taking (procedure)|
- -398636004 | Physical activity assessment (procedure)|
- -422834003 | Respiratory assessment (procedure)|
- -424753004 | Dietary management education, guidance, and counseling (procedures)|
- -182838006 | Change of medication (procedure)|

Source: Giannangelo 2015.

CHECK YOUR UNDERSTANDING 3.1

1. The best choice for field type to assign the health record number is _____.

   a. Alphanumeric
   b. Numeric
   c. Autonumbering
   d. Alphabetic

2. The term used to describe breaking data elements into the level of detail needed to retrieve the data is

   a. Normalization
   b. Data definitions
   c. Primary key
   d. Database management system

3. Information collected on a single patient is found in a _____.

   a. File
   b. Record
   c. Row
   d. Field

4. The term used when queries are limited by words such as "and" is:

   a. Boolean search
   b. Natural language queries
   c. SQL
   d. Data dictionary

5. Identify the component that defines the length of a field.

   a. Data manipulation language
   b. Data definition language
   c. Data dictionary
   d. Data control language

6. The user entered the social security number as 123456789 and it was displayed as 123-45-6789. This is an example of a _____.

   a. Query
   b. DBMS
   c. Mask
   d. Wildcard

7. Which of the following is not an example of any of the three aspects of "Triple Aim"?

   a. ABC Hospital increased its profit margin by 7%
   b. XYZ Hospital was able to decrease the radiology wait time by 20% by improving training of scheduling staff
   c. ABC Hospital decreased its nosocomial infection rates by installing hand sanitizers at elevators and stairways
   d. XYZ Hospital showed a 5% decrease in Type II diabetic patients after coordinating menu plans with local grocery stores

(Continued)

CHECK YOUR UNDERSTANDING 3.1 (*Continued*)

8. In order to better prepare for hurricane season, Sunshine Hospital uses a variety of statistical models to help them figure out how to streamline the admissions process for emergency patients, determine what type of backup generators would meet their needs during a blackout, and determine which additional clinical staff will be needed during future disasters. This type of analytics is referred to as

   a. Simplistic
   b. Descriptive
   c. Predictive
   d. Prescriptive

9. Edward is responsible for evaluating the content of the new COVID-19 database. The number of cases in the database do not match up with the initial numbers from the Infection Control Department. He is reviewing all entries to determine if there are any duplicate or repeat entries, if all data fields are entered correctly, and to identify any missing data points. The process he is performing is called:

   a. Data mining
   b. Data scrubbing
   c. Data modeling
   d. Data stewardship

10. Amanda is an HIIM professional with 10 years' experience in a variety of healthcare settings. When she discusses her role in a healthcare organization she talks about managing personnel and processes that protect patient information, meets all federal, state, and accrediting rules and regulations, for acquiring, storing, and releasing information to authorized requestors. These activities are also known as:

    a. Data mining
    b. Data scrubbing
    c. Data modeling
    d. Data stewardship

11. Part of Jackson's job as the privacy officer is to examine who, when, and where patient data was put into the EHR. Where would Jackson find this information?

    a. Metadata
    b. Data repository
    c. Data mining
    d. Data warehouse

Data Modeling

Data modeling is the process of determining the users' information needs and identifying relationships among the data. The model should be based on the organization's strategic plan and should identify the data elements to be collected and the relationship between them. It contains all of the entities appropriate for the healthcare organization and shows the technical database structure to be used in the database. There are three levels of data models—conceptual data model, physical data model, and logical data model.

The **conceptual data model** is not tied to a particular database model, but rather defines the requirements for the database to be developed. This conceptual data model is the basis for the logical and physical data models.

The **physical data model** shows how the data are physically stored within the database. The users are not involved with this level of the database because of its technical complexity.

The **logical data model** is a "complete representation of data requirements and the structural business rules that govern data quality in support of project's requirements" (HHS n.d., 1). In other words, it ensures that the data are available and in a useful format for the intended purpose. For example, the nursing department would look at the data differently than the HIM department and the HIM department would look at it differently than the marketing department.

The data-modeling tools used in the logical data model vary by the type of database involved, but may include the entity-relationship diagram. Data modeling generally includes the entity-relationship diagram or the semantic object model. The **entity-relationship diagram** (ERD) is a common type of data modeling that focuses on relationships between entities. An entity is a person, location, thing, or concept that is to be tracked in the database. In healthcare, entities would include such items as patient, physician, and laboratory test. Each entity has attributes, which are facts or data about the entity. Some examples of attributes of the entity patient include:

- Health record number (primary key)
- Last name
- First name
- Middle initial
- Street address
- City
- State
- Zip code
- Home phone
- Cell phone
- Work phone
- Date of birth
- Social security number

Each entity would have a unique identifier. A patient's unique identifier could be the health record number. In an entity-relationship diagram, entities are linked together to show relationships between the two. There are several types of relationships, such as one-to-one, one-to-many, and many-to-many. An example of a one-to-one relationship is a lab test and its result. The following are examples of the one-to-many relationships:

- A patient may have many physicians.
- A patient may have many laboratory tests.
- A physician may have many patients.

In a many-to-many relationship a patient can have many lab tests and a lab test can be performed on many patients. Additional examples of these relationships are shown in figures 3.4 and 3.5.

Figure 3.4. One-to-one relationship: Patient has one attending physician

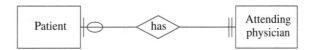

Figure 3.5. Many-to-many relationship: Patients can have many consulting physicians and consulting physicians can have many patients

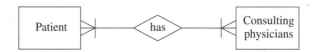

Data-Modeling Tools

A number of tools can be used to create the data model. **Computer-aided software engineering (CASE)** is designed to create many of the diagrams and other tools used in the data model. CASE can develop tools such as the entity-relationship diagrams described as well as **data flow diagrams (DFDs)**. A DFD is a diagram that shows how data moves (input, storage, output) within the system. The DFD is a way to show management and other nontechnical users the system design. It is also a way to introduce the overall design of the system without getting bogged down in the details. These details can be shown on other diagrams. Unfortunately, developing and updating a DFD are time-consuming, and the DFD may be difficult to design if the user does not have the necessary level of detail or if the data flow is constantly changing.

Another tool for data modeling is the use case. The **use case** is a technique that is used to develop scenarios based on how users will use the data and functionality to assist in developing ISs that support the information requirements. These ISs include the databases that support them. For example, a use case might be created to show how the user would retrieve information or generate a report. Specifically, it might show how to create a list of healthcare claims requiring coding. This use case identifies the data elements needed, the flow of information, and more.

Common Database Models

The database model is a description of the structure used to organize data in a healthcare-related database such as an electronic health record. This is different from data modeling, which is the process of determining what data is needed. There are a number of database models available, including relational, hierarchical, network, object-oriented, and multidimensional (Morley and Parker 2017, 505–506).

Relational Database Model

The most common database model used is the relational database model. In the relational database, data are stored in tables. It is named for the relationships that are created when there are data elements, such as health record number, in common between the tables. The **database table** contains all data related to a particular subject or concept, such as a patient, and is made up of the records and fields. In the table, the data are stored in rows and columns much like a spreadsheet. The data in a database is stored in a file. A **file** is a collection of digital data stored in the database. In healthcare, a file contains information on patient care, patient accounts, employee files, or another subject. Within the file are multiple records.

Within the relational database model, each row in the database table is called a record. A **record** is all the data that has been collected on an individual patient, employee, patient account, or a specific transaction. This data is stored in a data field. A **data field** is a predefined area within a healthcare database in which the same type of information is usually recorded. Examples of data fields collected in healthcare include patient last name, health record number, gender, diagnosis, procedure, and date of birth. The computer screen should provide a definition of the field, instructions on how to enter data into the field such as format, and valid characters.

The data collected in each field can take a number of formats based on the type of data. Types of fields include the following:

- Alphabetic fields accept only alphabetic characters. Data elements of this field type include patient name and city.

- Numeric fields accept only numbers that can be calculated. This would include charges, but would not include zip codes and the health record number, as these numbers cannot be calculated (added, subtracted, and so on).
- Alphanumeric fields accept alphabetic characters, numbers, or a combination of the two. Examples of alphanumeric fields include street address, zip codes, and phone numbers.
- Time and date fields contain only a date or time or a timestamp.
- Autonumbering fields create a unique number that will never be assigned again. This could be the health record number or a unique number assigned to a patient visit.

Before the data elements go into a database, the fields should be normalized. **Normalization** is breaking the data elements into the level of detail desired by the healthcare organization. For example, last name and first name should be in separate fields, as should city, state, and zip code. This allows the user to search or otherwise manipulate any of the data elements. Conversely, if the city and state were stored in the same field, the user would not be able to run reports or query the database based on state; because the name of the city varies widely in length, the computer does not know where the city ends and where the state begins. For example, the name of the city of Opp, Alabama is much shorter than San Luis Obispo, California. The latter also has three words in the name, so the computer cannot be made to look for a space or a number of characters. By breaking the city and state into different fields, searches by city or state can be done with ease. See table 3.3 for examples of normalized and unnormalized data.

Database administrators and others are able to display information about the data onscreen when a user has a request for particular data. The information is requested through a **query**, which is a search for data that meet specific criteria the user requests within subsets of the database. The queries sort and filter the data to display all records that meet the criteria for user review. For example, the user could query all patients discharged by Dr. Smith in 20XX. The patients could then be sorted by diagnosis, procedure, date of discharge, or other data element that exists in the database. If the results of the query are too voluminous, the criteria for the search can be narrowed to provide further filtering for a more desirable result. For example, the patients who received an appendectomy could be limited to Medicare patients or Dr. Smith's patients.

Table 3.3. Examples of normalized and unnormalized data

Normalized Data	Unnormalized Data
Last name	Last name, first name
First name	Middle initial
Middle initial	Address
Address	City, state, zip
City	
State	
Zip	

Key Field

A **key field** is a field in a table that holds a unique identifier to ensure that each data entry in the database table is different. This unique identifier is generally called the **primary key**. In the electronic health record (EHR) and other clinical ISs, this unique identifier is typically the health record number. Within the database, the tables organize the information from all records into rows and columns or cubes and use the primary key to locate the information. With the use of the primary key such as the health record number (in the patient table), then all of the patient's health information can be linked together.

When a primary key from one table (such as patient table) is found in another table (such as encounter table), the latter is called a **foreign key**. For example, the patient table would have a primary key of health record number but the physician table primary key may also be in the table so that the patient's attending physician can be identified. Once the attending physician is identified, then all of the physician's information, such as specialty, address, and phone number, can also be retrieved. Other examples of primary keys found in healthcare are a billing number or a physician identification number.

When a certain data field is designated as a primary key, this means that a search for certain criteria values of this field will speed up the process. Furthermore, in a relational model two tables can be matched by using the search criteria, so searching can be done across tables. The relational database has a number of advantages. First, it is flexible because the file is not tied to a specific application. The relational database allows the database administrator to control access to certain tables in order to provide security for the data contained in that database. Also, because data are entered only once, data consistency and quality are improved. This one-time data entry improves not only the quality of the data but also the efficiency of the healthcare organization. Finally, because data are stored in a single location, the user will have the most current data available. See table 3.4 for an example of the table in the relational database.

Table 3.4. Example of table in a relational database

Medical Record Number	Last Name	First Name	DOB	Admitting Date	Discharge Date
123456	Smith	Harry	10/10/1963	04/17/2018	04/21/2018
234567	Jones	Patricia	11/08/1956	05/14/2018	05/27/2018
345678	Adams	Georgia	01/31/1930	04/23/2018	04/25/2018
134534	Warren	Mallory	03/12/2008	05/01/2018	05/04/2018

Source: ©AHIMA.

Hierarchical Database Model

The **hierarchical database model**, like the name implies, structures the data in a hierarchy very similar to that used for an organizational chart. To use the analogy of a tree, the trunk of the tree would be the starting point or the initial query by the user, and as the search narrows or goes forward, each branch of the tree becomes smaller, progressing outward toward the leaves of the tree, which represent the end point of the search. Each piece of data in the database is called a node. Pointers indicate where in this tree structure the data are stored. A parent-child relationship is created by the relationships developed by the pointer. The relationship can be described as one-to-many. This means that a parent can have many nodes but a child can have only one parent (Harrington 2016, 604).

As mentioned before, in the hierarchical data model, access to data starts at the top of the hierarchy and moves downward. For example, in figure 3.6, the hierarchy moves from patient, to laboratory test, and then to name of test. In that example, the node patient is parent to three child nodes. These three nodes are laboratory test, attending physician, and radiology examination. The node laboratory test has four child nodes. Then at the next level, laboratory test becomes a parent to four children: name of test, date of test, time of test, and test results.

The hierarchical database model is not always user-friendly because it may require developers of the IS to predetermine the queries that will be needed rather than write a query ad hoc (as needed). Another disadvantage of this model is that the user must understand both the physical and logical data models (Abdelhak and Hanken 2016, 299).

Figure 3.6. Example of a hierarchical data model

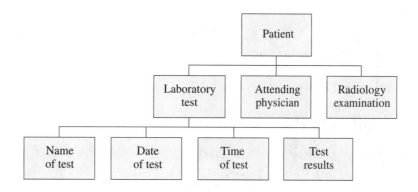

Source: ©AHIMA.

Network Database Model

The **network database model**, illustrated in figure 3.7, uses pointers to connect data. The nodes are called owners and members rather than parent and child nodes, as in the hierarchical database model. A member node in the network database model can have more than one owner, unlike in the hierarchical database model (Abdelhak and Hanken 2016, 299).

Figure 3.7. Example of a network database model

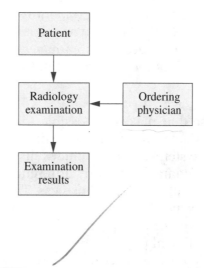

Source: ©AHIMA.

Object-Oriented Database Model

The **object-oriented database model** handles text, images, audio, video, and other objects. These images and other nontext items are stored as objects. An object is the basic component in an object-oriented database that includes both data and their relationships within a single structure. Each data element is called a variable. The object-oriented database uses programming tools such as **Java**, a programming language that was designed to be used on the Internet and that runs some of the functions of Internet applications. When the users access the webpage, a window appears asking the user to install the Java applet, which are programs that reside on HTML web pages.

Two concepts related to the object-oriented model are encapsulation and inheritance. Encapsulation is defining the characteristics of an object. For example, a laboratory test would have a name, test result, time, and date. In the object-orientated database, an object can inherit properties from another object when the characteristics are similar. This characteristic is called inheritance. An example of this is physician and resident physician. Both have the data elements of name, address, specialty, phone number, and others in common as they are both physicians (Abdelhak and Hanken 2016, 300).

Multidimensional Database Model

A **multidimensional database model** is used in data warehouses. The data are collected from multiple sources, such as other databases, and then summarized. This enables data analysis using a wide range of data. The multidimensional database is designed to quickly access this summarized data (Morley and Parker 2017, 506).

Data Repository and Data Warehouse

Data in healthcare organizations are collected in many different systems, both clinical and administrative. The data from these ISs are frequently centralized into a single database. Two options for this single database are the data repository and data warehouse.

Data Repository

A **data repository** is an open-structure database (not dedicated to the software of any particular vendor or data supplier) in which data from multiple ISs are stored so that an integrated, multidisciplinary (includes a variety of healthcare providers) view of the data can be achieved in a single source. The data repository is updated by the various ISs in real time, thus providing users with access to the most current information available. This real-time access to data is called online or real-time transaction processing.

The data repository may store clinical, administrative, and financial information data. Other data repositories store one specific type of data. For example, a data repository for a laboratory or pharmacy IS stores only clinical information. This centralized data repository is called a **clinical data repository (CDR)**. For example, a query could identify all of the patients who took a specific medication and had to be admitted to the hospital as a result of an adverse effect. CDRs that use object-oriented databases may include video, audio, images, and other types of data. The primary key and secondary keys are used to link the data between the various data repositories.

Data Warehouse

A **data warehouse** is a database that makes it possible to access data from multiple databases and combine the results into a single query and reporting interface. Like the data repository, it stores data from many different systems, and it includes historical and current information. Data warehouses hold an abundance of data from many different source systems and are designed for specific types of analyses, such as patient care or business. The source systems will vary depending on how the data warehouse will be used. For example, a data warehouse may be designed to look for trends in patient care. This type of data warehouse will require information from all of the clinical ISs, the financial IS, the clinical provider order entry, and other ISs. These systems would be chosen for inclusion in the data warehouse because they provide data on the care provided to the patient, the costs of that care, the tests ordered, and the alerts identified. It does not include systems like the chart locator and chart deficiency systems used in the HIM department because these systems have no bearing on identifying trends in patient care.

Additional uses of a data warehouse in healthcare include identifying best practices in patient care, such as which medication is the most effective; identifying data that can provide the competitive advantage, such as which services or physicians generate the most revenue; and improving efficiency. A data warehouse can also be used in quality management to look for trends in problem areas, such as nosocomial infections; identifying patterns in coding practices such as comparing hospital medical necessity denials to national rates; looking for particular diagnoses, procedures, services, or physicians that may have a compliance problem; and investigating other HIM-related issues.

The data warehouse is updated daily rather than in real time like the EHR or the data repository. There should be a predetermined policy about the frequency of the updates and how long data should be retained.

Data Mart

A **data mart** is a subset of the data warehouse designed for a single purpose or specialized use. The data mart performs the same type of analysis as a data warehouse; however, the scope of the data is narrower. The healthcare organization may choose to develop the data warehouse before the data mart, or the data mart can be developed first, or both can be developed at the same time. This order of development depends on the needs of the organization. Examples of how a data mart may be used include patient satisfaction and medical research. Patient satisfaction would not require the patient-specific information that would be stored in the data warehouse, but it would include the types of services, the nursing unit, and other basic information in addition to the patient survey or other patient satisfaction information collected. The data mart can be used in research because it can be used to provide deidentified information and the limited information required to conduct the research and thus can protect the confidentiality of the patient by providing only the minimum information necessary.

Data Mining

Data mining is the process of extracting and analyzing large volumes of data from a database for the purpose of identifying hidden and sometimes subtle relationships that would be unnoticed without the analysis. Data mining may also be called database exploration or information discovery. Data mining is important because it turns data into meaningful information. Data mining requires sophisticated software, tools, and techniques, such as anomaly detection, association rule learning, cluster analysis, classification analysis, and regression analysis:

- Anomaly detection: In anomaly detection, the goal is to identify data that does not follow expectations. This can be used to identify fraud and or other issues that need investigation.

- Association rule learning: This type of data mining identifies interesting relationships between two concepts in the database. For example, it may identify that patients who are treated with drug A have a better outcome than patients who are treated with drug B.

- Cluster analysis: Cluster analysis is identifying concepts that have traits in common. For example, monitoring the treatment practices of physicians for a specific diagnosis or procedure.

- Classification analysis: Classification analysis is a method of identifying important information about the data in the database by grouping data much like grouping diagnoses and procedures. This grouped data can then be used in the cluster analysis described earlier.

- Regression analysis: This method identifies the dependency between two (or more) variables, one being the outcome or dependent variable, the other being the influencing or independent variable. A regression analysis could determine how much influence hypertension or diabetes has on the outcome of a COVD-19 patient's survival.

Once the data pattern, dependency, or trait has been identified, the healthcare organization must decide how to use the information.

Figure 3.8 shows the results of data mining from the large national database from the Healthcare Cost and Utilization Project. (HCUP). This graph not only shows Florida pediatric Emergency Department visits by payer/insurance type, but it also covers a 12-year period that includes the transition from ICD-9-CM to ICD-10-CM.

Figure 3.8. Example of results from data mining

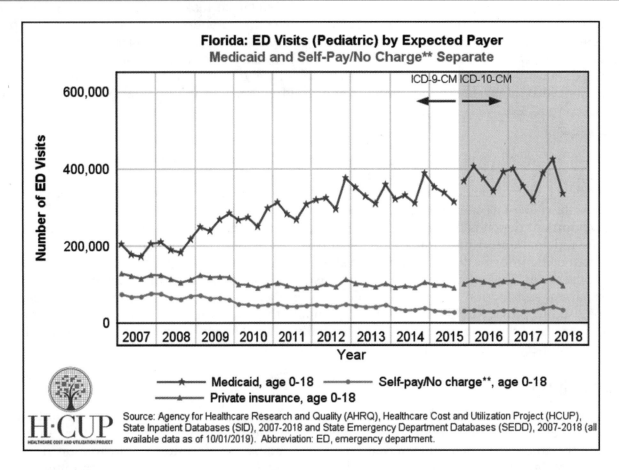

Source: HCUP, 2019.

Online Analytical Processing

Online analytical processing (OLAP) is a data access architecture that allows the user to retrieve specific information from a large volume of data. The use of OLAP turns the data warehouse into a decision support tool because it can analyze large amounts of data quickly. It does this in one of three ways: drilling down into the data, rolling up, or "slicing and dicing." Drilling down is going deeper and deeper into the data. For example, drilling down could entail looking at the cancer rate from across the country, then at the cancer rate Georgia, then in Macon, and then within the zip code 31052. Rolling up refers to the aggregation of data, which is just the opposite of drilling down. "Slicing and dicing" is looking at the data from multiple viewpoints. For example, a healthcare organization could look at their reimbursement by payer type (Medicare, Medicaid) and then look at it by service (medical, surgical, obstetric) (Hall 2015, 477). OLAP enables the healthcare organization to use operational data that it already has in order to make strategic decisions.

Common Uses and Examples in Healthcare and Health Information Management

Healthcare organizations collect an abundance of data and retain these data for years. Unless the data are turned into information, they have no real value to the healthcare organization. HIM professionals work together with database administrators, other information technology staff, and the end users to ensure that the data stored within the data warehouse will meet the needs of the users. The HIM professional is often a liaison between the information technology staff and the end user. The HIM professional can be involved in data mining by defining the data to be collected and stored in the data warehouse. The HIM professional can build data quality into the databases contained in the data warehouse. This can be done by building a data dictionary, populating drop-down boxes, building edits, and by building other data quality measures into the system. Examples of how data mining can be used in healthcare, including HIM, include identifying

- Best practices in patient care
- Medication adverse effects
- Potential fraud and abuse violations
- Patterns of mortality and morbidity
- Patterns of denials

Having this type of information enables the healthcare organization to use new information to improve services, patient care, and other functions. As more data are entered, the healthcare organization can continue to run analyses to determine if other patterns appear.

CHECK YOUR UNDERSTANDING 3.2

1. In a database model the concept of patient is an example of a(n) _____.

   a. Entity
   b. Relationship
   c. Data flow diagram
   d. CASE software

2. Identify an appropriate tool to illustrate how data moves through the IS.

   a. Data dictionary
   b. Entity-relationship diagram
   c. Data flow diagram
   d. Data standard

3. An attribute is _____.

   a. An assumption about an entity
   b. A fact about an entity
   c. Defined by the data dictionary
   d. A type of data model

4. The database model that uses a table as the basis for the design is _____.

   a. Relational
   b. Network
   c. Hierarchical
   d. Object-oriented

5. Identify the tool that shows how users will use the IS.

   a. Data flow diagram
   b. Use case
   c. Data model
   d. OLAP

Real-World Case 3.1

Janice has been given the responsibility of creating and managing the data dictionary for the laboratory IS that is being implemented. There are a number of existing ISs that have their own data dictionaries. The data from the laboratory IS will be part of a clinical data repository. She decided that she needs to start from scratch to make the data dictionary the best it can be. She is reviewing the data dictionaries from the other ISs used at the healthcare organization but she does not always use the same terminology and format that are used in the other ISs.

Real-World Case 3.2

Lewis-Beck Medical Center is a 650-bed acute care hospital in north Florida. In response to the COVID-19 pandemic, it is developing a database of all inpatients and outpatients who have come to the healthcare organization for treatment. Much like cancer registries, the COVID-19 registry will attempt to track patients for the rest of their lives. It collects data about their hospital admission: length of stay, level of care (general medical or ICU), medications, radiology and lab resources, testing status, attending physicians/hospitalists, discharge status, etc. In addition, if patients were treated on an outpatient basis, either through the Emergency Department or through the COVID-19 clinic, encounter data (like the inpatient data) is collected. Not only will this database be used to develop after action plans and to evaluate hospital functioning, but also to collect data on any residual or sequela diagnoses that patients may develop due to their exposure to COVID-19.

REVIEW QUESTIONS

1. The role of the database management system is to _____.

   a. Control and manipulate the database
   b. Collect data
   c. Report data
   d. Delete data when the need for it is over

2. An advantage to a database is that it _____.

   a. Controls the data stored in it
   b. Reduces redundancy
   c. Stores data using flat files
   d. Establishes data sets

3. The date of birth is an example of a _____.

   a. File
   b. Record
   c. Data field
   d. Key field

4. Select the key field for the physician entity.

   a. Last name
   b. Address
   c. Unique identifier
   d. Date of birth

5. Identity the tool that can be used to retrieve a list of all of Dr. Smith's patients.

   a. Data definition
   b. Data dictionary

REVIEW QUESTIONS (*Continued*)

    c. Metadata
    d. Query

6. Data about data is known as _____.

    a. Metadata
    b. Data definition
    c. Query
    d. Mask

7. The data model that addresses the data requirements is the _____.

    a. Logical data model
    b. Conceptual data model
    c. Relational database
    d. Physical data model

8. The hierarchical database relationships are called _____.

    a. Structured
    b. Parent and child
    c. Table
    d. Owners and members

9. Java is used in the _____ database.

    a. Relational
    b. Object-oriented
    c. Multidimensional
    d. Hierarchical

10. Data repositories are _____.

    a. A proprietary database
    b. Used solely for clinical data
    c. A database used solely for video and audio
    d. An open-structure database

Abbreviations/Acronyms Matching

American National Standards Institute

1. ANSI   A. a programming language designed for databases

2. SNOMED *44*   B. method to request information from a database where the uses points/clicks to choose tables and fields

3. DFD *48*   C. a US-based standards organization

4. CHDA *37*   D. an organization that establishes criteria for data so that it is consistent across countries, vendors, etc.

5. SDO   E. subset of clinical data in a data repository

6. CCR *199*   F. a data modelling technique that shows the relationship between entities

(*Continued*)

REVIEW QUESTIONS (*Continued*)

7. QBE 40   G. a data modelling technique that shows how and where data proceeds through a process

8. CDR 62   H. the most comprehensive medical vocabulary in the world

9. ERD 47   I. credential that identifies skills and knowledge or data analytics

10. SQL   J. a data set that follows the patient to the next healthcare provider so that care can continue

References

Abdelhak, M., and M. A. Hanken. 2016. *Health Information: Management of a Strategic Resource*. St. Louis, MO: Saunders Elsevier.

Amatayakul, M. K. 2017. *Health IT and EHRs: Principles and Practice*, 6th ed. Chicago: AHIMA.

Amatayakul, M. K. 2020. Health Information Systems Strategic Planning. Chapter 13 in *Health Information Management: Concepts, Principles, and Practice*, 6th ed. Edited by P. Oachs and A. Watters. Chicago: AHIMA.

American Health Information Management Association. 2020. Certified Health Data Analyst (CHDA). http://www.ahima.org/certification/chda

Biedermann, S. and D. Dolezel. 2017. *Introduction to Healthcare Informatics*, 2nd ed. Chicago: AHIMA.

Brinkmann, B. 2019. Comparing Descriptive, Predictive, Prescriptive, and Diagnostic Analytics. https://www.logianalytics.com/predictive-analytics/comparing-descriptive-predictive-prescriptive-and-diagnostic-analytics/

Campbell, A. et al. "Beyond the Basics for Health Informatics Professionals". *Journal of AHIMA* 89, no. 8 (September 2018): 58–63.

Clack, Lesley; Houser, Shannon H.; Kadlec, Lesley; Mikaelian, Raymound; Tabisula, Braden; Zeglen, Margie. "Data Analytics and Informatics are Two Separate Disciplines (And Why This Matters to HIM)" Journal of AHIMA 88, no. 10 (October 2017): 20–24.

Dataedo. 2018. What is Metadata (with examples). Accessed 5/31/2020. https://dataedo.com/kb/data-glossary/what-is-metadata

Department of Health and Human Services (HHS). n.d. Practices Guide: Logical Data Modeling. Accessed February 5, 2018. https://www2.cdc.gov/cdcup/library/hhs_eplc/26%20-%20Logical%20Data%20Model/EPLC_Logical_Data_Model_Practices_Guide.pdf.

Dolezel, D. Metadata Offers Roadmap to Structured Data. http://bok.ahima.org/doc?oid=107555#.WnPfH6inFRY.

Downing, K. 2016. Importance of Data Stewards in Information Governance. http://bok.ahima.org/doc?oid=301584#.WnPf7ainFRY.

Hall, J. A. 2018. *Accounting Information Systems*. 10th ed. Boston, MA: Cengage Learning.

Harrington, J. 2016. *Relational Database Design and Implementation*. 4th ed. Cambridge, MA: Elsevier.

Healthcare Cost and Utilization Project. 2019. HCUP Fast Stats - State Trends in Emergency Department Visits by Payer. Accessed 5/31/2020. https://www.hcup-us.ahrq.gov/faststats/State PayerEDServlet?state1=AZ&type1=PY00B&combo1=s&state2=FL&type2=CN01P&combo2=s&expansionInfoState=hide&dataTablesState=hide&definitionsState=hide&exportState=hide

Health Information Management Systems Society. 2017. *HIMSS Dictionary of Health Information Technology Terms, Acronyms, and Organizations*, 4th ed. Boca Raton, FL: CRC Press.

Health Level 7 (HL7). 2017. About HL7. https://www.hl7.org/about/index.cfm?ref=nav.

Hebbar, P. 2017. Who Is A Data Steward And What Are His Roles And Responsibilities? Accessed 9/7/2020. https://analyticsindiamag.com/data-steward-roles-responsibilities/.

International Standards Organization (ISO). 2018. About ISO. https://www.iso.org/about-us.html.

Johns, M. 2020. Data Governance and Stewardship. Chapter 3 in *Health Information Management: Concepts, Principles, and Practice*, 5th ed. Edited by P. Oachs and A. Watters. Chicago: AHIMA Press.

Morley, D., and C. S. Parker. 2017. *Understanding Computers: Today and Tomorrow, Comprehensive*, 16th ed. Boston, MA: Cengage Learning.

Office of the National Coordinator for Health Information Technology (ONC). 2017a. Health IT Curriculum Resources for Educators EHR Functional Model Standards, Component 9 Networking and Health Information Exchange, Unit 3 National and International Standards Developing Organizations. https://www.healthit.gov/topic/health-it-resources/health-it-curriculum-resources-educators.

Office of the National Coordinator for Health Information Technology (ONC). 2017b. National and International Standards Developing Organizations. https://www.healthit.gov/providers-professionals/health-it-curriculum-resources-educators.

Office of the National Coordinator for Health Information Technology (ONC). 2017c. Standards to Promote Health Information Exchange. https://www.healthit.gov/providers-professionals/health-it-curriculum-resources-educators.

Office of the National Coordinator for Health Information Technology (ONC). 2017d. Standards for Developing Organizations. https://www.healthit.gov/providers-professionals/health-it-curriculum-resources-educators.

Office of the National Coordinator for Health Information Technology (ONC). 2017e. Health Data Interchange Standards. https://www.healthit.gov/providers-professionals/health-it-curriculum-resources-educators.

Oppel, A. 2004. *Databases DeMYSTiFieD: A Self-Teaching Guide*. Emeryville, CA: McGraw-Hill Osborne.

Oracle. n.d. Performing Query-by-Example and Query Count. Accessed February 5, 2018. https://docs.oracle.com/cd/A60725_05/html/comnls/us/fnd/10gch314.htm.

Orlova, Anna; Rhodes, Harry B.; Warner, Diana. "Standardizing Data and HIM Practices for Interoperability" Journal of AHIMA 87, no. 11 (November 2016): 54–58 [web expanded version].

Palkie, B. 2020. Clinical Classifications, Vocabularies, Terminologies, and Standards. Chapter 5 in *Health Information Management: Concepts, Principles, and Practice*, 5th ed. Edited by P. Oachs and A. Watters. Chicago: AHIMA.

Panoply. 2020. Data Mart vs. Data Warehouse. Accessed 5/31/2020. https://panoply.io/data-warehouse-guide/data-mart-vs-data-warehouse/

System Selection

Learning Objectives

- Identify the steps in the system selection process.
- Develop the request for proposal.
- Explain how the decision matrix will assist in the most appropriate selection for the healthcare entity.
- Collect data to be used in the systems analysis process.

Key Terms

Acceptance testing
Alpha site
Best of breed
Best of fit
Beta site
Bidders' conference
Buy-in
Change management
Chief analytics officer
Chief information officer (CIO)
Chief medical information officer
Closed-ended questions
Cloud computing
Critical path
Delivery date
Escrow
External scanning
Feasibility study
Flowchart
Force majeure

Functional requirements
Gantt chart
Go-live
Information systems project steering committee
Information system strategic planning
Intangible benefits
Integrated information systems
Interface
Internal scanning
Legacy system
Observation
Open-ended questions
Payment milestones
PERT chart
Project
Project definition
Project management
Project manager
Project team

Prototyping
Request for information (RFI)
Request for proposal (RFP)
Scope creep
Site visits
SMART methodology
Software license
Source code
Status reports
Structured interview
Sunset
Systems analysis
System development life cycle (SDLC)
System selection
Tangible benefits
Termination
Testing
Unstructured interview
User task force
Warranties and guarantees
Weighted decision matrix

Today most healthcare organizations have existing information systems (IS). The concepts outlined in this chapter can be used for replacing existing or an IS implementing new ISs. Existing ISs are often referred to as legacy systems. Legacy systems are a type of information system that uses older technology but may still perform optimally. Replacement of legacy systems are done for many reasons such as the legacy system no longer meets the needs of the healthcare organization or the vendor has sunset the information system. Sunset is the term used when a vendor is no longer going to maintain an IS after a specified date. The date typically provides the healthcare organizations with time to select and implement a new IS before the legacy system is no longer supported.

System selection is determining which IS will be purchased. The system selection process begins with the idea that the healthcare organization should consider obtaining a particular IS, such as the master patient index. The process continues until the contract has been signed. The complexity of the system selection process varies widely, from selecting a standard off-the-shelf software product like a word processor to the very complex implementation of an electronic health record (EHR) system. The length of time required thus varies from a few minutes to a year or more. The number of people involved will also vary based on who is impacted by the IS and the complexity of the IS to be selected.

System selection is part of the **system development life cycle (SDLC)**, a model used to represent the ongoing process of developing (or purchasing) ISs. The SDLC is a structured process that can be useful by identifying users' needs and alternatives, selecting the IS, system implementation, and other steps in managing IS. SDLC requires the involvement of people throughout the healthcare organization, including those who use the information system. The use of people throughout the healthcare organization who are impacted by the healthcare organization ensures that the needs of all the users and the healthcare organization are met. There are a number of different models for the SDLC. The one used in this chapter (shown in figure 4.1) has six steps: Project planning, system analysis, information system design, information system implementation, evaluation of implementation, and information system maintenance. The focus of this chapter will be the first three stages: project planning, system analysis, and information system design.

Figure 4.1. System development life cycle (SDLC) diagram

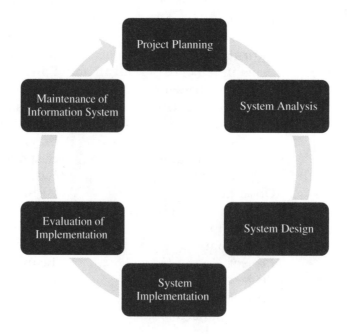

Source: ©AHIMA.

Project Planning

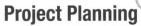

During the planning and analysis phase of the SDLC the project is defined, a formal structure for project management is created, and the needs of the healthcare organization are identified. The phase begins with initiation, which is when the decision is made to obtain the IS. This decision may come about because of an IS strategic plan, the obsolescence of an existing IS, or some other reason.

One thing to keep in mind during the planning process is that any IS selected should support the healthcare organization's business objectives. An example of a business objective for a healthcare organization might be to provide high-quality care. The specific IS to be implemented should be identified and prioritized during the IS **planning** process, as more ISs are usually identified than the healthcare organization's resources can handle. **Information system strategic planning** is the development of a strategy related to the information including needs of an organization and defining the ISs that best meet those needs. The information strategic plan should support the business plan for the healthcare organization. For example, if a healthcare organization business objective is to meet a goal of improved quality of care, then the healthcare organization should look for an IS that would support this goal, such as the EHR or clinical provider order entry (CPOE). The EHR would improve the quality of care because of the immediate access to patient information, as well as the use of alerts and other features. The CPOE would improve care because the orders would be immediately available to the ancillary department, and the healthcare provider would be able to take advantage of reminders and alerts regarding contraindications, the need for laboratory tests to monitor blood levels, and so on. Part of the IS strategic planning process is performing a needs assessment. The needs assessment evaluates the need for the various ISs under consideration. The needs assessment should include a comparison of costs to benefits received.

Steps included in the planning and analysis phase are as follows:

1. Planning
2. Organizing the project
3. Defining scope of project
4. Systems analysis

Planning

Planning is the most critical step in the system selection process. A major IS selection requires a lot of collaborative work by many people across a healthcare organization. A lack of planning can cause problems with the information system, which can ultimately cause the IS to fail or delay the implementation date, thus costing the healthcare organization money and wasting resources. An example of poor planning is ordering hardware without evaluating the space. Hardware installation can be delayed when there is not enough electrical wiring, inadequate space, or some other problem with the physical plant. The most common reasons for failure are:

- Lack of clear objectives
- Poor planning or management of the project
- Unrealistic expectations
- Trying to do too much at once
- Lack of training and support
- Failure to obtain early employee buy-in
- Poor data quality in IS database
- Not planning for the changes or going beyond the scope of the project
- Inadequate hardware and/or network
- Poor selection of software (Fay Business Systems Group 2016)

Another reason for failure is the lack of end-user involvement. Employees who are involved in the system selection and implementation are more likely to embrace the IS than those who are not as they have had a say in the process.

If a healthcare organization spends more time and energy from the beginning of the IS selection project, it will be better positioned to succeed. Adequate planning is demonstrated, in part, when the healthcare organization has the necessary staff, money, and other resources, as well as an understanding of what is needed and identification of desired outcomes from the outset of the project. Planning for an IS is a complex process and involves the following:

- Conducting a feasibility study
- Setting the budget
- Setting the goals and objectives
- Identifying the project manager and team
- Obtaining buy-in from management and users

Conducting a Feasibility Study

A **feasibility study** is conducted by the healthcare organization to determine if a proposed IS is an appropriate option to meet the objectives of the healthcare organization. For example, the healthcare organization could investigate the feasibility of implementing an EHR to support an objective to improve the quality of care. The study examines the costs, the benefits, and any expected problems and then determines whether or not to proceed with the proposed IS. The benefits should be both tangible and intangible. **Tangible benefits** are easy to quantify in dollars and include eliminating duplicate tests, no longer having to purchase health record file folders, and not microfilming paper records. **Intangible benefits** cannot be quantified monetarily. An example of an intangible benefit would be improved quality of care. If the benefits outweigh the costs, then the project should be considered.

This phase would also address factors other than financial. These would include whether or not a healthcare organization is ready for the change, if the necessary infrastructure is in place, if the necessary resources are available (such as staff), and if the desired information system is legal. A change in an information system has a significant impact on the healthcare organization but the people within the organization. The healthcare organization must be prepared for this change. The implementation of the information system may require upgrades to networks. There may be changes in laws required. For example, there was a time when state laws required signatures to be in ink which would prohibit digital signatures. For more on digital signatures, refer to chapter 9.

Setting the Budget

Developing the budget for a system selection project is important as cost is a key determining factor in deciding whether or not to implement an IS. The budget should be comprehensive and as accurate as possible because it is used in the decision-making process. The budget should include system selection and implementation expenses (one-time expenses) as well as the cost of maintaining the IS for a specified period of time (on-going expenses), such as two to five years. The budget should include the software licensing fee, staff required to maintain it, additional hardware, cost of software, upgrading infrastructure, hardware, training, renovations to the physical plant, maintenance of the IS, project management, consultant expenses, and travel expenses for site visits. The ongoing maintenance cost includes the annual software licensing fee, cloud storage, hardware leasing, plus other expenses.

Goals and Objectives

Goals and objectives for the IS must be established as part of the planning process. The goals and objectives identify what the healthcare organization wants to accomplish with the implementation of the proposed information system and how these goals will be achieved. These IS goals should be based on the healthcare organization's business goals. As with any goals, they should be realistic and attainable.

One strategy for writing goals is the **SMART methodology**, which stands for

- **S**pecific,
- **M**easurable,
- **A**ttainable,
- **R**elevant, and
- **T**ime-based

A specific goal tells you the what, who, where, when, which, and why. A measurable goal provides something that you can use to compare the actual outcome to the goal to determine if it has been met. An attainable goal is one that you have the skills and resources to accomplish. A relevant goal is one that, while challenging, can be accomplished given the time and other factors. A time-based goal is one that provides a deadline to meet (Johns 2020, 90).

Examples of SMART goals include the following:

- To provide new employee orientation to 100 percent of new hospital employees within 1 month of their hire date
- To reduce the number of hospital staff by five by the end of next March
- To reduce the amount of discharge not final billed (DNFB) report to $500,000 within six months
- To reduce the number of duplicate tests by 25 percent by the end of the fiscal year

Goals will be determined by the type of IS and the needs of the healthcare organization. Once established, goals should be used to identify which information best meets the desired outcomes.

Once the IS is implemented, it should be evaluated regularly thereafter as to whether it met and will continue to meet or exceed the stated goals and objectives. For example, the support and evaluation will identify whether the duplicate tests were reduced by 25 percent or whether staffing was reduced by five.

Identifying the Project Manager and Project Team

The project manager and project teams are an important part of project management. **Project management** is a formal set of principles and procedures that help control the activities associated with implementing a usually large undertaking to achieve a specific goal, such as an IS project. Project leadership including the project manager and the project team members should be identified before the project begins. A project team is a collection of individuals representing various disciplines, such as billing, clinician, administration, or information technology assigned to work on a project. Their role is important because they are responsible for ensuring that the system implementation plan is carried out according to the project manager's specifications. The project team members' skills will vary according to the needs of the project. For example, implementation of an EHR will require information technology staff, health information management (HIM), physicians, nursing staff, and other clinical users of the IS. A project team is composed of people who are assigned to work on the project either part time or full time. The project team will be discussed in detail later in this chapter.

The **project manager** is in charge of leading the project and therefore must have an understanding of the IS being implemented. The project manager must have strong skills in a multitude of areas, such as project management, leadership, organizational skills, and conflict management. The project manager is responsible for ensuring that the project plan stays within the designated timeline, issues are resolved, desired outcomes are met, and customer satisfaction is achieved.

Many project managers have the project management professional (PMP) certification. This PMP demonstrates knowledge of project management topics. These topics cover project management content from initiation of the project until completion (Project Management Institute 2015).

Obtaining Buy-in from Management and Users

It is critical that the healthcare organization's upper management support the project from the very beginning of the process. If management shows support for the IS, the employees will follow suit and support it. However, if management displays discontent or lack of support, the employees will most likely resist the change. Support can be shown by attending meetings; talking about the IS's benefits to the healthcare organization, its employees, and customers; and generally demonstrating that the IS is valued. Communication is critical at this stage. Staff and everyone to be affected by the IS should receive ongoing updates on the decisions, changes, and expectations. The more staff members are informed about the EHR or other projects, the less likely they will be to resist because they will know what to expect. If staff who will use the information system are asked for their feedback, they will feel valued and will be more likely to support the IS.

Change management is the formal process of introducing change, getting it adopted, and diffusing it throughout the healthcare organization. Although some people welcome change, most have a natural aversion to it. A great deal of change management involves reducing these fears and preparing them for what is to come. For example, if people are afraid, they will lose their jobs with the implementation of new technology, these issues must be addressed. Administration must be open and honest about layoffs, changes in job roles, and other related changes.

Administration should be seen as a strong supporter of the IS. If administration does not publicly support the IS, then the employees may follow the administrator's lead and not see its value. It is important to the success of the IS that both administration and employees buy into the IS.

Employees should be kept current on the implementation process: they want to know what the IS will do for them, when training will occur, and the overall progress of the implementation, including any issues. This can be done in a number of ways, such as employee newsletters, announcements at meetings, and so forth. Employees should be involved in the process whenever possible. Several ways of doing this are discussed later in the chapter. Employees should have realistic expectations about what the IS can and cannot do so that they will not be disappointed when the IS is implemented. Thus, user preparation will make them more comfortable with the IS when it is implemented.

All processes related to the IS must be reviewed and modified to accommodate the new IS. This means changes to policies and procedures, possibly changes in organizational structure, and any other changes needed to support the new IS.

Organization of the Project

Once the decision is made to implement an IS, the project's formal organizational structure must be put in place. A **project** is a plan and course of action that will address a specific objective, made up of a series of activities and tasks with defined start and stop dates. The plan has targeted objectives and deliverables to be accomplished. The project will need specific resources assigned to it in order to be completed; a project frequently has a separate budget that sets limits on spending. Another resource assigned to a project is staff. As discussed previously, a project team is assigned to the project. Temporary employees may be hired to either assist in the implementation or assume the tasks of staff members who have been reassigned to the project. An example of a project is the implementation of the EHR. Members of the EHR project would involve many different types of professionals including physicians, nurses, other healthcare providers, HIM professionals, computer programmers, network technicians, and many more.

The level of organization for the project depends on the level of complexity of the IS being implemented. If it is a small department IS, it may only require two or three people to implement. Major ISs that impact the entire healthcare organization can take hundreds of people to select and implement the IS. In large projects, frequently subcommittees are responsible for small areas of the project. The subcommittees meet and work on their segments of the project. The chair of the subcommittee then reports back to the full project committee. Table 4.1 shows examples of what is and what is not a project.

Table 4.1. Examples of what is and what is not a project

Not a Project	Project
Monthly reports	Implementation of IS
Routine software update	Creating a security plan
Backing up data	Creating a business continuity plan

Source: ©AHIMA.

Project Team

Most, if not all, IS projects require a project team of individuals to successfully implement the IS. The number of individuals needed and the composition of this team vary from project to project, depending on the needs of the implementation. For example, if the healthcare organization is implementing an encoder for use only in the HIM department, the project team should include the appropriate people in HIM and the IS. The project team would not need to include physicians, nurses, risk managers, or laboratory staff.

If the healthcare organization is implementing a CPOE, the project team would need representatives from the physician staff as well as from the HIM, nursing, laboratory, pharmacy, and other departments who are impacted to ensure that the IS is properly planned and developed. The project team works with the project manager to implement and manage the project. This project team will meet periodically, based on project needs, to discuss progress of the project and any issues that arise.

An HIM professional should frequently sit on the project committee because the IS may impact the HIM department directly or indirectly, and having an HIM professional involved in the process will help ensure that the department's needs are addressed. Additionally, the HIM professional serves as a consultant and source of information for compliance, privacy, security, legal, and other concerns. For example, the HIM professional can assist with retention, privacy, security, data quality, and documentation issues, among many other considerations of the IS, which may ultimately affect the HIM department.

The major participants in the project management team are the IS project steering committee, project team, the user task force, the vendor, the project manager, and possibly one or more consultants.

The **information systems project steering committee** is responsible for every IS acquisition project in the healthcare organization. Each project team will report back to the steering committee. The steering committee's role is to ensure that the strategic IS is being efficiently and effectively implemented and that the project stays on target. This committee is frequently led by the **chief information officer (CIO)**. The CIO is generally at the executive level and is responsible for all information resource management functions at the healthcare organization. The IS department, HIM, and other information management–related departments frequently report to the CIO. The CIO must have strong management skills. Although the CIO is not always a technical role, the individual must understand enough about information technology to ensure the proper management of the information systems. Other team members may be administrators, managers, project managers, and other leaders in the healthcare organization.

Two other roles that may be involved in the IS project steering committee are the chief medical information officer (CMIO) and the chief analytics officer (CAO). Both the CMIO and CAO are upper level managers in the healthcare organization. The CMIO acts as a liaison between physicians and the information technology staff. The CMIO is also responsible for the information systems used by physicians. The chief analytics officer utilizes information to make business decisions.

The **user task force** is a group of users, who will ultimately be using the IS, who test the IS and perform other project-related tasks for which the committee receives feedback. These users are generally on loan from various departments to assist in the project. Some members of the user task force may be deployed as needed for **testing** (performing an examination or evaluation) and other tasks, whereas others are pulled out of their departments for the duration of the project. This reassignment may last a year or more, depending on the project.

The vendor representative is the expert on the IS and so will be an extremely valuable team member. This individual will be the liaison between the healthcare organization and the leadership at the vendor's company. The vendor representative knows the product and can be a valuable resource with regard to how best to implement and use the IS. Additionally, the vendor representative can give the project team information on what has (and has not) worked for other healthcare organizations. This information can help the healthcare organization recognize and use best practices and help it avoid costly mistakes. If not scheduled to be on-site during a meeting, the vendor representative may need to attend via telephone conference in order to provide expertise.

If the healthcare organization decides to hire a consultant, the consultant will be a valuable member of the project team as well. The consultant should not have ties to a particular vendor's product, but rather be objective to help the healthcare organization obtain the product that best meets its needs. The consultant should have experience in system selection and implementation.

The project manager is responsible for coordinating the individual project, monitoring the budget, managing the resources, conducting negotiations, and keeping the project on schedule. These roles require the project manager to have technical, analytical, and people skills. The project manager should be skilled in conflict resolution, communication, and project management. Leadership skills are also important because the project manager must be able to develop a consensus and manage meetings for the project team. The project manager would have to handle any problems that arise during the implementation.

Defining Scope of Project

The healthcare organization must define what the accomplished project is. The **project definition** is determined during the project planning process to tell the healthcare organization exactly what it is trying to do with the IS being implemented and the expected outcomes. The healthcare organization must identify:

- The purpose of the IS (such as patient care documentation)
- How the system links to the healthcare organization's business strategy (such as provide quality of care)
- The goals for and scope of the project (The scope for the EHR might be to document inpatient care. There would be multiple goals for an inpatient EHR. An example is that documentation will be available immediately after care.)

The scope of the project determines exactly what work is—and is not—to be included in the project based on resources available. Identifying the project's definition is important to prevent scope creep. **Scope creep** happens when items not included in the original scope are added after the project has begun. For example, a project starts out to implement an EHR in a medical clinic and then the decision is made to add the EHR to the outpatient surgery area. The needs of these two areas are different, so more time and resources would be required. These additions to the project will increase the time needed for the project, the money allocated and the resources (training resources, staff, and so forth) required to accomplish it. Scope creep occurs because of:

- Failure to make the project deliverables clear
- Failure to establish clear project requirements

- Changes to deliverables midproject
- Stakeholders who are not "all in"
- Failure to communicate adequately (Teamgantt 2020)

To help keep the project on target and avoid scope create the project team should:

- Know the desired end resolve from the very beginning of the project
- Create comprehensive project plan that is followed as closely as possible
- Be able to say no when asked to tack on additional requirements.
- Communicate impact on timeline
- Have formal process for changing the scope of the project (Teamgantt 2020)

Project Plan

Once the healthcare organization knows what it plans to do, the project team can begin dividing the project into specific activities or tasks. The project team may start out with a basic skeleton of a project plan and continue to add substance to it as they go along. This project plan should describe each task to be completed, how it will be completed, who is responsible for its completion, when a task should begin, and when the task should be finished. The basic components of the plan are as follows:

- Feasibility study: This study defines the objectives and need for the project and justifies the plan.
- Resources: This component identifies the resources needed to meet the objectives of the plan. Resources include money, time, staff, and space.
- Design: In the design stage, the project team identifies the specific details required to implement the plan. For every task identified, the plan must provide the start and end dates and a person responsible. If the project requires programming, the team must establish the standards that will be used in writing the program.
- Hardware and software procurement: This stage ensures that the healthcare organization has all of the hardware and software needed and that any missing components arrive in a timely manner. For example, hardware delivery may take six weeks, so ordering needs to be done early in the process so that the project is not delayed because the hardware is not available.
- Transition: The transition phase prepares the healthcare organization for the conversion from the legacy system to the new IS. The transition stage includes not only the actual conversion of data (discussed later in the chapter) but also preparing staff for the change (discussed later in the chapter).
- Implementation: The implementation stage includes the steps to be taken to prepare for the implementation and the actual conversion to the new IS. For specifics on implementation, refer to chapter 5.
- Evaluation and maintenance: The support and evaluation stage begins immediately after implementation is complete. The project team must evaluate itself to prepare for the next project. It should also include an evaluation process to determine if the objectives of the project were met and how the process could have been improved. For specifics on evaluation and maintenance, refer to chapter 5.

Project Management Tools

A number of tools can be used to control the project. These tools include Gantt charts, project evaluation and review technique (PERT) charts, project plans, trouble tickets, and status reports.

The project plan provides details for how to accomplish a project and guides the project team on activities, timing, costs, and the sequencing of activities. The project plan could include project tools such as the Gantt chart and the PERT chart.

The **Gantt chart** is a project management tool that records specific tasks, their start and end dates, the person responsible for the tasks, and any connections between tasks. The Gantt chart (see figure 4.2) can easily show which tasks are behind schedule, which are on target, and which are ahead of schedule. A **PERT chart** (see figure 4.3) is a management tool that evaluates the tasks, the dependencies on other activities, the activity sequence, and the time required to complete the task. Because the PERT chart shows interdependencies between tasks, it will help determine

Figure 4.2. Sample Gantt chart

	Task	Assigned To	Start	End	Dur
	Information System Implementation	Abigail Jones	8/25/21	10/14/22	298
1	Identify project manager		8/25/21	9/9/21	12
1.1	Identify project manager	Abigail Jones	8/25/21	9/7/21	10
1.2	Identify project team	Abigail Jones	9/8/21	9/9/21	2
2	System Analysis		9/10/21	12/2/21	60
2.1	Conduct systems analysis	Gail Johnson	9/10/21	12/2/21	60
3	Request for Proposal/Selection		12/3/21	4/21/22	100
3.1	Create RFP	Gail Johnson	12/3/21	2/3/22	45
3.2	Distribute RFP to vendors	Gail Johnson	2/4/22	2/4/22	1
3.3	Receive RFP submissions	Gail Johnson	2/5/22	2/7/22	1
3.4	Review RFP	Project Team	2/8/22	2/25/22	14
3.5	Site visits	Project Team	2/26/22	3/17/22	14
3.6	Check references	Steve Taylor	3/18/22	4/6/22	14
3.7	Make decision on information system	Project Team	4/7/22	4/15/22	7
3.8	Negotiate contract	Chief Information Officer	4/16/22	4/20/22	3
3.9	Sign contract	Chief Information Officer	4/21/22	4/21/22	
4	Hardware/Software		4/22/22	4/26/22	3
5	Order hardware	Bob Adams	4/21/22	4/22/22	2
6	Site preparation	Sam Moore	4/16/22	4/21/22	4
7	Install hardware	Brandon Burke	4/23/22	5/3/22	7
8	Install software	Daphne White	5/4/22	5/16/22	9
9	Configure settings	Daphne White	5/21/22	5/25/22	3
10	Implementation Process		5/26/22	10/14/22	102
10.1	Create routine reports	Jared Dodd	5/26/22	7/6/22	30
10.2	Develop/revise screens	John Burgur	6/11/22	7/22/22	30
10.3	Develop training plan	Elise Harrison	6/11/22	7/22/22	30
10.4	Identify data conversion needs	Robert Williams	6/11/22	6/15/22	3
10.5	Write interfaces	Robert Williams	6/16/22	7/14/22	21
10.6	Create user manual, training materials, and policies and procedures	Elise Harrison	7/23/22	9/23/22	45
10.7	Conduct testing	Fred Simpson	7/24/22	9/3/22	30
10.8	Correct errors identified in testing	Robert Williams	9/4/22	10/14/22	30
10.9	Train the trainers	Elise Harrison	8/7/22	8/26/22	15
10.9.1	Conduct training	Elise Harrison	8/7/22	8/26/22	15
11	Go-live	Project Team	8/27/22	8/29/22	1
12	Acceptance testing	Project Team	8/30/22	10/10/22	30
13	Evaluation of implementation	Project Team	9/1/22	9/14/22	10

The timeline columns for 2021 show weekly increments: 8/22, 8/29, 9/5, 9/12, 9/19, 9/26, 10/3, 10/10, 10/17, 10/24, 10/31, 11/7, 11/14, 11/21, 11/2[8].

Figure 4.3. Sample PERT chart

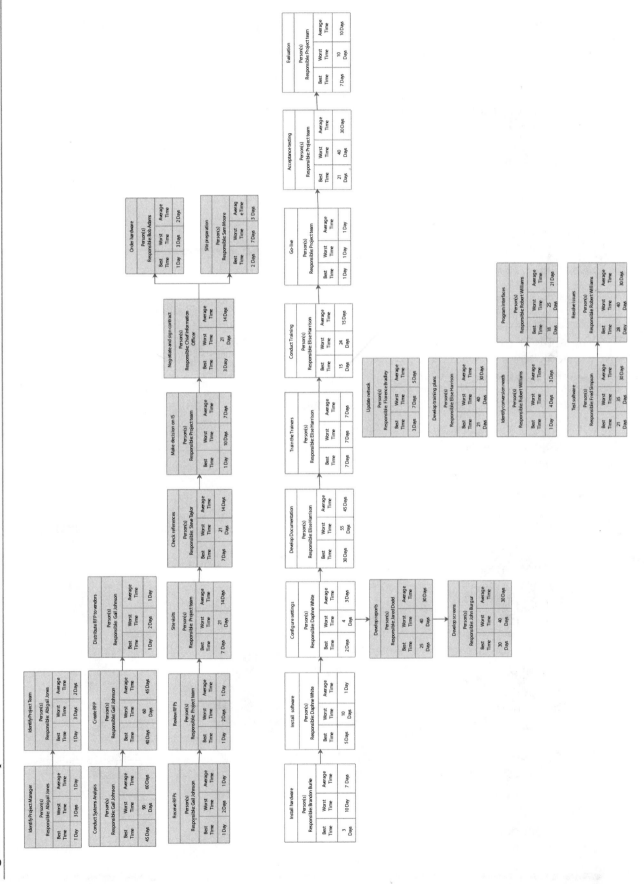

whether the implementation date is slipping because of delinquent tasks. This slippage is shown by review of the **critical path**, which shows the longest amount of time to complete the project. If key tasks along the critical path are delayed, the critical path itself lengthens, thus lengthening the duration of the project.

Status reports are periodic updates on the current state of the project, what has been accomplished, and what issues have been encountered. Solutions for the issues should be identified in the report. Status reports are typically directed to the information project steering committee to keep that group informed on the project's progress. The status report is generally written by the project manager, but could be written by a designee.

Additionally, software applications can be used to help manage a project. Project management software can create the Gantt and PERT charts as well as other types of tools for the project team to review. It can also track how much of each task is complete (0 to 100 percent), who has been given the responsibility for each task, the beginning and ending dates, the sequencing of tasks, and more.

CHECK YOUR UNDERSTANDING 4.1

1. Identify a project.

   a. Completing a monthly report
   b. Implementing the EHR
   c. Making minor changes to a policy and procedure
   d. Utilizing the MPI to update information

2. Researching the possibility of implementing a new information system is known as _____.

   a. Project definition
   b. Project plan
   c. Feasibility study
   d. Status report

3. The PERT chart shows if there is slippage in the implementation date. This slippage is shown by _____.

   a. Dependencies
   b. Gantt chart
   c. Project plan
   d. Critical path

4. A tool used for project management is _____.

   a. Transition plan
   b. Design plan
   c. Gantt chart
   d. Feasibility study

5. The original plan was to create an EHR that will be used for the emergency department, but now the EHR must be used for all outpatient services. This is an example of _____.

   a. Scope creep
   b. Project plan
   c. Project definition
   d. Project tool

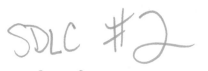

Systems Analysis

Systems analysis is an important process of collecting, organizing, and evaluating data on the healthcare organization and the information that it needs. Systems analysis should be performed early in the project as it helps the project team determine the data, storage, reporting, and functionality needs of the healthcare organization. In systems analysis, the healthcare organization determines what users need from the proposed IS. This stage reviews the current processes of the healthcare organization, the proposed processes, and the desired **functional requirements**. Functional requirements describe the functionality that an IS should be able to perform.

To identify the needs of the healthcare organization, the project team would look at the existing ISs and the needs of the users and identify and evaluate alternatives. During systems analysis, users are asked questions such as:

- What do you like about the current information system?
- What problems do you have with the current information system?
- What changes do you foresee that will impact this information system?
- What information do you need from the information system?
- What functions would you like to see in the new information system?

Answering these questions helps the project team understand the current IS and how it meets or does not meet the needs of the users. An IS will be used by the healthcare organization for many years and therefore must be adequate both at the time of go-live and in the foreseeable future. **Go-live** is the official time and date that the healthcare organization begins using the new IS.

To identify the needs of the healthcare organization for the foreseeable future, the project team needs to understand the environment in which the information system will operate. No one can see into the future with certainty, but internal and external environmental scanning can identify some issues that must be addressed. **Internal scanning** entails identifying changes within the healthcare organization that will impact the IS, such as if new services or new clinics will be implemented. **External scanning** is identifying changes outside of the healthcare organization that will impact the healthcare organization. The healthcare organization may be aware of pending legislation, trends, or other issues that may impact the IS under consideration. Understanding the environment helps ensure that the IS will work today and for the expected future. Examples of what might be found during internal and external scanning is in Table 4.2.

Table 4.2. Example of internal and external scanning findings

Example of Internal Scanning Findings	Example of External Scanning Findings
New services to be opened (e.g. new cardiovascular surgery services)	Potential legislation (federal, state, and/or local)
Current services to be closed (due to low numbers and/or profit)	Changes in community (e.g. aging population, new major employer, declining population)
Changes in medical staff (e.g. new physician group)	New competitor

Source: ©AHIMA.

Questionnaires, interviews, observations, flowcharts, and other data collection tools may be used to obtain the data needed to answer these questions. The planning team should collect data from all levels and types of users. The needs of the clerical users will be very different from the needs of management users. Many managers believe they know the needs of their staff, but many of them know what the policy states, not what is actually happening. The information gathered should include all aspects of the information system such as data elements, reports, privacy, security, and overall functionality.

Questionnaires allow for a large number of users to provide input about the needs of the IS as the results are easy to collect and analyze. This is especially true if closed-ended questions are used so that the responses can be tabulated quickly and easily. Closed-ended questions can be answered with yes or no, Likert scales, and other limited choice responses. Likert-scales are great for obtaining the users' beliefs regarding a statement. An example of a Likert scale begins with a statement such as: "On a scale of 1 to 5, with 1 being 'strongly agree' and 5 being 'strongly disagree,' rate the following statement." An example of a belief could be, "The new EHR will improve the efficiency of the healthcare organization." An example of a typical closed-ended question could be, "Do you generate reports as a part of your job?" Obviously, the response to this question is limited to yes or no. Computerized tools make the aggregation and analysis of the responses quicker. The downside of questionnaires is that the correct questions may not be asked, so there may be gaps in the data collected and the information needed. The use of open-ended questions may help fill some of these gaps, but they slow down the aggregation of data and data analysis. Open-ended questions are designed to get more information from the participants as they can expand on their response; however, the project team must collect, read, and analyze each statement individually. An example of an open-ended question is "How does the current information system help you in your job?"

Interviews are powerful tools for obtaining information. There are three types of interviews: structured, unstructured, and semistructured. In the structured interview, everyone is asked the same questions. This improves analysis of the findings but does not encourage the interviewee to talk openly about pertinent issues, thus taking the risk that important data will be overlooked. In the unstructured interview, the interviewer does not have a list of questions but rather gets the interviewees talking about their jobs, their data needs, and other issues related to the IS. The semistructured interview is a combination of the structured and unstructured formats. There are questions that interviewees are asked, but they are also encouraged to discuss in detail their jobs, data needs, and other issues related to their IS needs. The unstructured and semistructured formats make it harder to identify trends and to analyze data, but major issues that could have been overlooked otherwise may be identified.

Typically, two members of the project team are needed to conduct interviews because one person interacts with the interviewee and the other person takes notes. Because of the increased staffing needed to interview, the amount of time required to collect and analyze the data, and the need to meet with users individually, interviews are very time-consuming, which makes them costly. This means that the planning team may interview fewer individuals than would be involved with questionnaires.

Observation is watching an action being performed. It is useful in determining what employees are actually doing. This is important because supervisors or others frequently tell the interviewers what they think is happening but in reality, something very different is occurring. The use of observation is a way to validate what the interviewee has been told. If using observations, each observation session should be short because the observer can be disruptive to the work environment. Also, observation sessions should be scheduled throughout the day because different tasks may be performed at different times.

Flowcharts may be used to illustrate the flow of information within the healthcare organization (see figure 4.4). The flowchart uses standardized symbols to demonstrate the steps performed. Problems and inconsistencies may be identified through the development and analysis of the flowchart. The process on the flowchart would depend on the type of IS being developed but could represent the flow of the health record in the HIM department, the flow of a physician query, or the steps in denial management. The flowchart would identify critical points in the process as well as problem areas. This information can be used to improve new processes implemented along with the new IS.

Figure 4.4. Sample flowchart

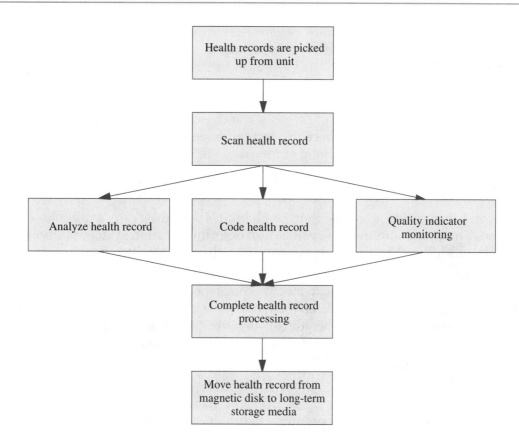

Many healthcare organizations use a combination of questionnaires, interviews, observations, and other data collection tools to obtain the best information. The use of multiple tools also allows the project team to involve more users and at the same time obtain detailed, validated information. The large number of participants helps to foster buy-in from the users. Buy-in refers to the acceptance of the information system and recognizing its value to the user and to the healthcare organization. Users who buy in to the information system are more supportive and less likely to resist the changes that the information system brings to their jobs.

It is a mistake to ignore or give only minimal attention to systems analysis during the system implementation process. Systems analysis is critical because it forces the healthcare organization to evaluate itself and to look at how it does business. This understanding will help select the IS that will best meet the needs of the healthcare organization.

System Design

After the project itself has been decided on and the formal structure has been created, a number of decisions have to be made. The design of the information system should reflect IS objectives, output specifications, input specifications, database design, and expected costs. The requirements identified in systems analysis are used to create specifications for the IS. The specifications will be used for programming the IS if developed in-house or for evaluating vendor systems. The design should specify what data are collected, from where the data will originate, and in what format the data should be stored as well as the size of the database and amount of activity expected. Once the specifications are developed, they should be presented to administration for approval. The design phase includes determining who will build and maintain the system, choosing between integrated and interfaced ISs, and making the decision on which IS will be selected.

Determining Who Will Build and Maintain the Information System

One of the critical decisions to be made during the planning process is whether a healthcare organization should build the information system itself, purchase it from a vendor, or use vendor services such as cloud computing. **Cloud computing** is the delivery of computational services (e.g., analytics, storage, and application sharing) by a vendor over the Internet. In cloud computing the information system operates on a computer that is owned and maintained by a vendor. This IS is at the vendor's location, not the healthcare organization, so the IS and its data must be accessed remotely. To do this, a user logs into and accesses the IS exactly as if the data center were located in-house. The data center is the area where the computers and other hardware that run the various IS operations are kept. Advantages to cloud computing are as follows:

- Flexibility: Cloud computing can handle variances in patient workload. It can provide multiple methods of security to protect the patient information and where data is stored.

- Efficiency: Information systems that use cloud computing are available from virtually anywhere. The cloud computing organization does information system maintenance such as data backups and the healthcare organizations only pay for what they use.

- Strategic value: Since healthcare organizations do not have to manage the information system, they have more time to address other concerns. Since the cloud computing organizations focus on the information systems, they can keep them current which can give the healthcare organization the competitive edge over other healthcare organizations (IBM nda). For example, they can advertise that they have the "latest and greatest" information systems to help attract patients.

- Scalability: Scalability enables the expansion or reduction of information technology resources as it is needed by the healthcare organization (Vonnegut 2017).

- Lowering costs: The healthcare organization will save money in several ways. It will not have to purchase computers, pay for computer maintenance, or hire employees with specialized skills.

The cloud computing method is favored by healthcare organizations that do not have staff with the necessary skills to develop and maintain an IS. A disadvantage of cloud computing is that the user may not have as much control over the IS. For example, the scheduling of maintenance and upgrades is up to the host. Another disadvantage is that the healthcare organization is that cloud computing is "renting" the IS. It is not investing in its own structure and therefore would have to make a large investment should it ever decide to bring the information system in-house.

When the decision is made to utilize cloud computing, the healthcare organization must sign a contract with the cloud computing organization. This contract should cover a number of topics including: services provided, ability to the cloud computing organization to utilize the data, confidentiality, and terminal of contract (Eddu saver 2019).

The second option would be for the healthcare organization to build the IS. If a healthcare organization decides to build an IS, it would be designed to meet the specific needs of that healthcare organization. Creating a **prototype** is a way to quickly design and develop an IS. With prototyping, programmers quickly develop an IS, show it to the users, obtain feedback, make revisions to the program, and continue this cycle until the IS is developed. Although this is an option for system design, most IS designs are much more formal and detailed. The IS would have the look and feel that is desired as well as the desired functionality. There are, however, disadvantages:

- It could take longer to develop as the healthcare organization is building it from scratch.

- The planning must be more detailed than if purchasing an IS to facilitate development of the information system.

- If the healthcare organization loses the staff that developed the information system, it may be difficult to upgrade the information system to meet the needs of the healthcare organization over time or to troubleshoot any issues that arise.

- There could be high development costs due to the amount of work required.

The final option, which most healthcare organizations choose, would be to purchase a predeveloped software system from a vendor. The vendor has invested millions of dollars in research and development and has a support system to assist the healthcare organization in the implementation of the IS being purchased. As with other options, there are advantages and disadvantages. An information system purchased from a vendor may not be exactly what the healthcare organization wants, but it would be faster to implement, and the healthcare organization would benefit from extensive research and development conducted by the vendor.

When working with a vendor, the healthcare organization may have the opportunity to be an **alpha site**. An **alpha site** is the first healthcare organization to implement the information. The healthcare organization generally receives a discount in exchange for participation in the development of the IS. Because the IS is still being developed, the healthcare organization may face problems with the implementation that would not be encountered with a more mature version of the same IS. It also takes more time than a typical implementation. The healthcare organization may also be asked to be a **beta site**. Beta sites are the next healthcare organizations who subsequently implement the IS. Many of the problems have been resolved with the alpha site, but these beta sites are likely to encounter numerous problems as well.

Choosing Between Integrated and Interfaced Information Systems

If the decision is made to purchase an IS from a vendor, the next decision is whether the product should be integrated or interfaced.

Integrated Information Systems

Integrated information systems are separate applications that are designed to work together. Data are entered into one IS and then are accessible to the other ISs. Many healthcare IS vendors use this model to interface systems used by healthcare organizations. This type of IS is much easier to manage than an interfaced IS because of the lack of interfaces. Integrated ISs collect, store, and retrieve information from the same database. The ISs have a similar screen design, which makes moving from one IS to another easier for the user. The decision to purchase software from a single vendor is frequently called **best of fit**.

Interfaced Information Systems

In an interfaced IS, the products are not designed to work together, but rather are linked through an interface. An **interface** takes data from one information system and plugs that data into another IS. In other words, an interface acts as a bridge between two ISs or databases to translate data into each IS's respective language. An interface has to know what data to retrieve, where the data are located in the first database, whether any data manipulation has to be performed (and, if so, what that manipulation is), and where the data will be entered into the second database. If the interface is not working, the ISs will not be able to share information until the problems with the interface are resolved.

Although an interfaced IS takes more effort to manage, many healthcare organizations choose this method because users can choose the various products that they want instead of choosing a single vendor's product that, for example, may have a wonderful encoder but an inadequate laboratory IS. Choosing the ISs based on functionality rather than by vendor is called choosing the **best of breed**. With best of breed, the healthcare organization chooses the best information system for their needs regardless of the vendor. In other words, they may choose the Registration-Admission-Discharge-Transfer (R-ADT) from vendor A, the clinical provider order entry information system from vendor B and the EHR from vendor C. For more on these information systems, refer to chapters 7, 8, and 9 respectively.

System Selection

The healthcare organization must identify what they demand from an IS, such as specific functions and compatibility with existing ISs. This information is used to determine which IS best meets the needs of the healthcare organization. There are a number of steps in the system selection process:

1. Request for information and proposal

2. Evaluation of the proposed IS

3. Selection of an IS

4. Contract negotiation

Some of the steps in the SDLC are sequential, but others can be performed concurrently. For example, the development of the request for proposal can be begun during the earlier systems analysis process, but it would not be finalized until after the process has been completed. It is imperative to remember that throughout the project, the plan itself is a working document and will continuously change and evolve.

Request for Information and Request for Proposal

The **request for information (RFI)** is a formal document requesting information on IS. The RFI asks the IS vendor for basic information about the product and how the IS would meet the requirements outlined in the RFI. The RFI can be used to select minor IS, or the information gathered in the RFI can be used to determine who will receive the more rigorous **request for proposal (RFP)**, a type of business correspondence asking for very specific product and contract information that is often sent to a narrow list of vendors that have been preselected after a review of requests for information during the design phase of the SDLC.

The RFP is a much more detailed document than the RFI and is critical to the selection process. The purpose of the RFP is to give the vendor all the information needed to propose an IS that meets the needs of the healthcare organization. The RFP describes what IS is needed, the healthcare organization, and the desired functions. Common components of the RFP are:

- Letter of introduction
- Information for potential vendors
  - Information about bidders' conference
  - Description of healthcare organization
  - Patient (or other) volume statistics—historical and future or projected growth
- Description of the system
  - Technical requirements
  - Functional requirements
  - Interface requirements
- Required format of response
- Instructions for RFP
- Request for sample documentation
- Request for sample contract
- Request for vendor profile
- System testing requirements
- Request for sample resumes of implementation staff
- System selection criteria
- Training requirements
- References

Letter of Introduction

The letter of introduction is a cover letter that is sent to the vendor along with the RFP. The letter introduces the vendor to the RFP and identifies who the vendor should contact at the healthcare organization. It may also provide some information that did not make it into the RFP. The letter also specifies the date, time, location, and other information of the bidders' conference.

The **bidders' conference** is a meeting for vendors to come to the healthcare organization to ask questions about the RFP, the healthcare organization, and other important points. This meeting enables all of the potential vendors to hear the same information and to get all of their questions answered so that they can completely respond to the RFP.

Information for Potential Vendors

The description of the healthcare organization section provides the vendor with enough information about the healthcare organization to enable the vendor to properly respond to the RFP. This information includes the size of healthcare organization, number of employees, number of employees who would use the system, and number of locations that would use the IS. This section also should describe the healthcare organization's existing ISs so that the vendor can respond concerning how it can work with the existing information system.

It should also include patient (or other) volume statistics that would be related to the IS (see table 4.3). The statistics may include number of discharges, number of surgeries, number of emergency department visits, and the number of outpatient visits—whatever is needed for the proposed IS.

Table 4.3. Sample of requested volume

Healthcare Organization Volume Statistics	Number
Average number of discharges per day	45
Average number of emergency department visits per day	60
Average number of outpatient surgeries per day	25
Average number of outpatient visits per day	125
Average number of pages—inpatient discharge	100
Number of synchronous users	75
Number of locations software is to be used	12

Source: ©AHIMA.

Description of the Proposed Information System

In the proposed system section, the vendor describes the IS that it is proposing to meet the needs of the healthcare organization. The vendor should describe the infrastructure required, licensing, the capabilities of the IS, the benefits that would be realized, and all pertinent information.

As stated earlier, the functional requirements identify the desired functions of the IS, which makes this a significant part of the proposal. This document is developed during the systems analysis process and outlines all of the functions expected of the proposed information system. The functions should include all aspects of the information, including but not limited to, individual data elements, data entry methods, reporting, management of the system, functionality, and technical issues. Technical issues can include topics such as the type of database used and the ability to work with a certain operating system or interface with existing products.

Each functional requirement is listed. The vendor indicates whether the function is available, is available with customization, will be available in the future, or is not available. The healthcare organization will take this same list of functional requirements and use it to evaluate the proposal. There are at least two ways to classify each functional requirement. The first way is to designate each functional requirement as mandatory or desirable. Some proposals use three categories: mandatory, desirable, and luxury. Another option is to develop a numeric rating system in which each function is scored based on its importance. For example, each function is rated on a scale of 1 to 5 (1 = unimportant, 5 = highly important). The functional requirements qualifying the availability of each function are part of the RFP, but the evaluation rating is not. The functional requirements are used in the system evaluation to determine if a vendor has all of the functionality and to determine if the missing functionality is important. For example, if there is a functional requirement to combine duplicate health record numbers, and it is missing from one of the products under review, the rating would help the reviewer determine whether this is a serious gap. For an example of functional requirements refer to Table 4.4.

Table 4.4. Example of functional requirements

Function	Mandatory	Desirable	Luxury
Add new patients	X		
Edit existing patient demographics	X		
Add new patient visit	X		
Discharge patient	X		
Transfer patient internally	X		
Utilize retinal scan for security			X
Data analysis functions		X	

Source: ©AHIMA.

Other RFP Requirements

The required format of response tells the vendor what the healthcare organization requires regarding the proposal. For instance, the healthcare organization might require a specified number of paper copies and an electronic copy of the RFP in a specified format; it may limit the number of pages or the design of the document; it may even provide an electronic template for the vendor to complete. The instructions for proposal may include rules regarding whom the vendor can talk to at the healthcare organization, the deadline for submission, and a statement that the vendor must assume responsibilities for the expenses to complete the proposal as well as the expenses for any on-site demonstrations, along with expenses for proposal preparation.

The request for sample documentation and for a sample contract is simply a request for a copy of the documents. The vendor profile is a description of the vendor and is designed to ensure that the company is financially sound. This is important because the vendor needs to be around for many years to provide technical support and any updates needed. The RFP asks for information on the number of installations of similar ISs the vendor has performed, financial viability of vendor, and the number of years the product has been available.

IS testing requirements would outline the expectations the healthcare organization has regarding testing. The proposal would provide the types of testing to be performed and the role of the vendor in that testing.

Many healthcare organizations request sample résumés from the vendor's staff, which provide details of the experience and qualifications of the staff who could be assigned as consultants to that particular project. These sample résumés are used to ensure the vendor has experienced staff members who can support the healthcare organization throughout an implementation. It is not a guarantee that any of the individuals represented would be assigned to the project, but rather a representation of the experience that the vendor's employees have.

The RFP should specify the system selection criteria. These criteria would include major evaluation methods, such as findings from the demonstration, findings from site visits (visiting a healthcare organization that has already implemented the system), review of the RFP, costs, expected benefits, and reliability of vendor's products. It would not include rankings of importance and other details that the project team will utilize to make the final decisions.

Finally, the RFP should request the training recommendations for the IS, including the number of people trained by the vendor, cost of training, the estimated time it should take to train each user, types of training required, and other recommendations regarding the training process.

Evaluation of Proposed Information Systems

The evaluation process used to select an IS should be established during the planning process. The process should have multiple components, including:

- Onsite and online demonstrations
- Site visits
- Review of RFP
- Reference checks

Onsite Demonstrations

In an onsite demonstration, the vendor brings its product to the healthcare organization, either as a demonstration version or a full version of the product. Project team members and other users gather to view the IS and to ask questions of the sales team. The idea is to have as many users and members of the project team as possible watch the demonstration to see what the IS can and cannot do. All attendees should bring to the demonstration situations they encounter in their daily tasks and ask how the IS would handle it. Examples of situations are admitting Medicare patients, ordering medication, and merging duplicate health records – whatever is appropriate for the specific IS.

The on-site demonstration allows for multiple user involvement and is an important opportunity to learn about the information. This may be the only chance for some team members or other users to see the IS before implementation; not everyone can go to site visits to see the IS in a live environment.

Site Visits

Site visits are a great way to view the products in a live environment. A site visit usually consists of a small group of team members visiting a healthcare organization, preferably one that is similar in size and characteristics, that has the product implemented to observe the IS in use. During the visit, the project team asks the healthcare organization's staff questions about the IS. Often the salesperson for the product will attend the site visit to answer questions and ensure that the project team obtains the information needed to make a decision. Seeing the IS operating in a real environment is quite different from a demonstration environment and thus gives the project team a much more realistic view of the IS and how it works.

Reviewing RFP Responses

The vendor spends a lot of time responding to an RFP, so the RFP should only be sent to the vendors who are seriously being considered. Responding to the RFP is time consuming and therefore very expensive for the vendor. The number of RFPs submitted is typically limited to three to five vendors. The vendor's proposal should be received by a designated person, generally the project manager. The project manager then coordinates the review of the proposals. The healthcare organization also spends hours reviewing the RFP responses because for major IS purchases, the responses could fill a three- or four-inch binder. A spreadsheet is frequently developed to assist in the analysis of the RFPs, and this enables the decision makers to compare key information between products side by side making which facilitates decision making.

Some of the information that could be included in the spreadsheet includes cost, compatibility with existing information systems, the level to which the system meets functional requirements, and the reaction to site visits.

A sample comparison is shown in table 4.5.

Table 4.5. Sample of comparisons among vendors responding to RFP

System Capabilities	System A	System B	System C
Works with existing hospital IS	Yes	Yes	Yes
One-time costs	$654,000	$498,500	$576,000
Ongoing costs (3 years)	$65,000	$89,000	$79,000
Hardware needed	File server	File server	File server
Works with existing database	Yes	Yes	Yes
Number of years vendor in existence	31	12	6
Number of installations	123	26	2
RFP shows financial viability	Yes	Yes	Yes

Source: ©AHIMA.

Reference Checks

The healthcare organization should contact several other healthcare organizations where the product is currently in use. These reference checks are a great way to learn if other healthcare organizations are satisfied with the product without the expense and time it takes to go to on-site visits. The vendor will provide a list of references, and the evaluating healthcare organization should try to obtain a complete list of client sites from the vendor or independently identify client organizations that are not on the reference list. Best practices recommend that the evaluating project team contact healthcare organizations from the vendor's reference list, as well as healthcare organizations that are clients of the vendor but are not included on the reference list, including any site visit personnel. The reference list may contain only customers who are satisfied with the product and leave off the unsatisfied ones. Healthcare organization not on the list may be identified through the corporate offices, networking, or cold calls. Notes from these reference checks should be collected and used as part of the decision-making process. See Table 4.6 for examples of questions that might be asked during a reference check.

Table 4.6. Examples of questions for reference checks

What issues with the information system have you encountered?
What issues with the vendor have you encountered?
What words of wisdom do you have for someone considering this information system?
If you had it to do over again, would you select this information system?

Source: ©AHIMA.

CHECK YOUR UNDERSTANDING 4.2

1. The information system must meet documentation standards. This needs to be listed as part of the _____.

   a. Functional requirements
   b. Gantt chart
   c. Project definition
   d. PERT chart

2. Identify the tool that gathers data from many people on their information system needs.

   a. Observation
   b. Questionnaires
   c. Interviews
   d. Flowchart

3. The healthcare organization is trying to determine who they will send a RFP to. Identify the tool that can assist in this decision.

   a. RFI
   b. External scan
   c. Flowchart
   d. Vendor profile

4. The SDLC phase that identifies the functions that are needed in an IS is _____.

   a. Planning and analysis
   b. Design
   c. Implementation
   d. Maintenance and evaluation

5. Justify the decision to be an alpha site.

   a. All of the problems have been worked out of the IS at this point.
   b. Although the IS is new, many of the issues have been resolved by the beta sites.
   c. It will enable us to meet federal and state laws.
   d. It allows the healthcare organization to play a significant role in the design of the IS.

SDLC #4

Selection of an Information System

It is the responsibility of the project team to review the responses to the RFP and other evaluation tools to determine which IS will best meet the needs of the healthcare organization. To prevent disagreements over which system to choose, there should be a quantifiable means of evaluating the ISs. One way is to assign points to the RFP review, site visits, observations, and other evaluation methods. If a point system is used during the evaluation process, then the system with the highest number of points should theoretically be the best IS and therefore the one that is chosen. However, this is not always the case, because a vendor may have the overall highest score but have low scores in some important functions; the selection team should not only consider the total points but each individual task as well.

A useful method of ascertaining the best EHR product and vendor is a **weighted decision matrix**, a method used to help select an IS based on what features are the most important to the healthcare organization. For example, compliance with privacy and security requirements is more important and deserves a higher weight than the ability to change the color of the screen. Points are typically awarded and the system with the highest number of points is the frontrunner for selection. The project team is responsible for determining the criteria to rate the EHR systems chosen. It is best to limit the number of EHRs in the weighted decision matrix; otherwise, it would become unwieldy. Three comparisons are usually sufficient. The objectives of the EHR system RFPs are an excellent beginning for choosing the criteria used in the decision matrix. Additional measurable and demonstrable criteria can be formulated by the project team with input from stakeholders.

The project team should perform the following steps to create the weighted decision matrix:

1. Determine objective, measurable, and quantifiable criteria against which the EHR system can be evaluated. Most of these criteria should come from the objectives of the RFP.

2. Assign weight for each criteria. The higher the weight, the more important the criteria.

3. Rate how each EHR meets each criterion on a rating system such as 1 = lowest to 5 = highest.

4. Multiply each EHR rating by the criteria weight. The answer is the score for that criterion and EHR.

5. Total the numeric products for the EHR system for all the criteria.

6. The EHR system with the highest complete score is the one that best meets the healthcare organization's criteria better than the other EHR systems evaluated from their RFPs.

As shown in table 4.7, EHR System Vendor #2 has scored the highest and therefore best meets the criteria established by the project team for selecting an EHR for the healthcare organization and therefore should be considered unless there is a reason not to.

Contract Negotiation

Once the decision of which IS to purchase has been made, the contract negotiation process begins. Some healthcare organizations start negotiations with more than one vendor. Based on the initial meetings, the healthcare organization chooses one vendor to continue with negotiations. Typically, a contract team, not the project team, negotiates the contract. The negotiating team should include at least the CIO and an attorney; however, with a minor implementation, the HIM director may work with a member of administration. A minor IS might be a encoder/group information system that is used only by the HIM department, is quickly and easily implemented, and has a simple contract. A major implementation would involve multiple areas of the healthcare organization, a significant period of time to implement, and a complex contract. The goal of the contract negotiations is a

Table 4.7. EHR system vendors decision matrix example

Criteria	Criteria Weight (1 = low, 5 = high)	EHR System Vendor #1 Rating based on (1 = low, 5 = high) Criteria Weight X Rating	EHR System Vendor #2 Rating based on (1 = low, 5 = high) Criteria Weight X Rating	EHR System Vendor #3 Rating based on (1 = low, 5 = high) Criteria Weight X Rating
Criteria #1: System price	4	Rating: 3 Score: 3*4 = 12 out of possible 20	Rating: 5 Score: 5*4 = 20 out of possible 20	Rating: 1 Score: 1*4 = 4 out of possible 20
Criteria #2: EHR certification	5	Rating: 4 Score: 4*5 = 20 out of possible 25	Rating: 4 Score: 4*5 = 20 out of possible 25	Rating: 4 Score: 4*5 = 20 out of possible 25
Criteria #3: Vendor stability	3	Rating: 5 Score: 5*3 = 15 out of possible 15	Rating: 4 Score: 4*3 = 12 out of possible 15	Rating: 4 Score: 4*3 = 12 out of possible 15
Total EHR weighted rate	—	47 out of a possible 60	52 out of a possible 60	36 out of a possible 60

Source: ©AHIMA.

win-win situation. The healthcare organization wants a good product at a reasonable cost that is implemented in a reasonable time period. The healthcare organization should not try to secure the product under such strict requirements that the relationship with the vendor is negatively impacted from the beginning. With many of these installations, the healthcare organization will be working with the vendor for 10 years or longer; therefore, it is in the healthcare organization's best interest to create a good working relationship. The healthcare organization should not accept the sample contract provided by the vendor because this contract is written in favor of the vendor. The negotiation team is responsible for working with the vendor to develop a contract that works for both parties.

Some of the clauses covered by the contract include:

- Software license
- Delivery dates
- Warranties and guarantees
- Responsibilities of each party
- The state whose laws govern the contract
- Cost
- Payment milestone
- Force majeure
- Escrow
- Termination (of contract)
- Version of software to be installed
- Penalties
- Acceptance testing

- Maintenance and updates
- Training
- Documentation

A **software license** describes what the healthcare organization can do with the software. It controls the locations that can use it, who can use it, and how it can be used. It may also include how many users can access the IS and if the IS is used solely by one department or the entire healthcare organization. The healthcare organization is prevented from using the IS in a way outside the license.

Delivery dates are the dates that the software and hardware will be delivered to the healthcare organization. The inclusion of these dates in the contract is important because nothing can be done until the software is available and installed at the healthcare organization. Warranties and guarantees are affirmations the vendor makes for which they are held accountable. Samples of warranties are:

- Vendor has the legal right to sell software.
- If it is found that the vendor does not have the right to sell the software, then the vendor is legally responsible.
- IS will be available 99.9 percent of the time.
- IS will perform query within 3 seconds.
- Technical support will respond within 30 minutes.

It is important to detail the responsibilities of each party in the contract (see table 4.8). This helps ensure that no problems will arise later over who is responsible for what. This information will be used in the negotiation of the price. The more participatory a vendor is during implementation, the more the vendor should be paid.

Table 4.8. Sample allocation of responsibility list

Task	Responsible Party
Train the trainer(s)	Vendor
Train end users	Healthcare organization
Develop interfaces	Healthcare organization and vendor
Design screens	Healthcare organization
Testing	Healthcare organization and vendor

Source: ©AHIMA.

Contract law varies by state; therefore, the contract must specify which state's laws cover the terms of the contract. The vendor generally asks for the laws of its state and the healthcare organization asks for its state, so negotiation is required.

The cost of the IS is one of the last clauses negotiated. The amount of money paid to the vendor will be based on the responsibilities of the vendor, the number of users specified in the contract, and other clauses. The healthcare organization should require a fixed price so it knows exactly what the cost of the IS will be. Healthcare organizations should never pay the entire negotiated amount or a large percentage of the cost up front; rather, the contract should then establish **payment milestones** (see table 4.9). A payment milestone is an action that triggers payment to the vendor.

This payment is a specified percentage of the total cost of the IS. This must be negotiated and spelled out in the contract. Typical milestones include delivery of software, go-live, and acceptance testing. A significant percentage of the payment should be held until acceptance testing is complete. Failure to do so could result in the vendor moving to the next installation and not responding in a timely manner to any outstanding issues. If there is a significant amount of money involved, the vendor is more likely to be responsive to the needs of the healthcare organization.

Table 4.9. Sample milestones for payment

Milestone	Percentage of Vendor's Payment
Signing of contract	20 percent
Delivery of software	10 percent
Commencement of testing	10 percent
Go-live	30 percent
Completion of acceptance testing	30 percent

Source: ©AHIMA.

Force majeure is a legal term that refers to "an event or effect that cannot be reasonably anticipated or controlled" (Merriam-Webster 2020). This contract clause is designed so that the parties of the contract cannot be held accountable to a deadline if there was an "act of God" that prevented compliance. For example, if an IS is being implemented and the world is experiencing a pandemic during the process or a tornado hits the hospital two days before the implementation date delaying implementation, the vendor would not be held accountable for any penalties as specified in the contract.

Healthcare organizations have the need to protect themselves in the event the vendor goes bankrupt. One way to do this is to place a clause in the contract that requires the vendor to place the source code in escrow. **Source code** is the programming code that was used to develop the information system. **Escrow** is a situation in which a third party holds a copy of the software in case the vendor goes bankrupt. This means that if the vendor goes out of business, the healthcare organization can obtain access to the source code behind the software so that they can maintain the IS themselves or hire someone else to do so. The vendor prefers this method as well because it does not want its trade secrets to be widely available.

Termination of the contract becomes important if the product or vendor does not meet the needs of the healthcare organization. This clause allows the vendor or healthcare organization to void the contract with appropriate notice. There should also be a period of time, such as five years, in which the contract is in force unless cancelled earlier by either party. This clause may require a 30- or 60-day notice to the other party in the event of a cancellation.

The version of software that will be delivered to the healthcare organization should be specified in the contract. The vendor will know when the next version is scheduled for release. Depending on the time frame of implementation, the healthcare organization may receive the current version or the new version. The contract may also state that the healthcare organization will install the current version but will receive the upgrade to the new IS as part of the contract or at a reduced cost.

The contract should specify penalties for both the vendor and the healthcare organization for failure to meet the dates specified in the contract. Penalties vary widely and can be monetary or in the form of free training, free software modules, or other forms. The penalties should be serious enough to keep the parties on target, but not so punitive they would seriously risk the financial stability of either party. For example, one healthcare organization had negotiated such a tight time frame with major penalties that the IS department essentially did not do anything other than implement the new IS and keep the current ISs operational for an entire year. If departments needed assistance with the IS, they were told to hire someone to do it for them. Placing this amount of pressure on the vendor or the project team is not the purpose behind the penalties in the contract. The purpose is to keep everyone on task and on target.

Acceptance testing is a type of testing that occurs after the go-live date. It tests the IS to confirm that it is working as expected as per the contract, RFP response, and any other documentation. It is a critical part of the IS implementation because it establishes whether the terms of the contract have been met regarding performance and functionality. For more information on testing see chapter 5. The contract must spell out what outcomes are acceptable. These outcomes will be used to determine when the acceptance testing is complete and the vendor can receive payment. ISs are constantly changing. Maintenance must be an ongoing responsibility for both the vendor and the healthcare organization. The contract should spell out the responsibilities of both parties. The contract should also specify if upgrades to the IS are included in the contract and the costs for those upgrades. Exactly what is included in maintenance is spelled out in the service-level agreement as maintenance occurs after implementation (Mirman 2019). The upgrades are necessary as they assist the healthcare organization in remaining compliant with accreditation, regulations, and other mandates. The information system updates also repair any issues found in the IS and keeps the information system operational. Because a healthcare organization frequently has multiple vendors with maintenance agreements with each, the concept of cotermination is being included in contracts. This allows the healthcare organization to renew agreements at the same time regardless of the effective dates of the service (IBM ndb).

Training responsibilities of the vendor, including issues such as the number of people to be trained, where they will be trained, the cost of the training, and the length of the training, should be specified in the contract. The training should include whether the training will be e-learning, remote or face to face. The contract should also spell out the ongoing training needed after implementation and the associated expenses.

The contract should include the type of documentation provided by the vendor to the healthcare organization. This documentation generally includes technical manuals for technical support as well as user manuals.

CHECK YOUR UNDERSTANDING 4.3

1. Identify an appropriate tool for analyzing the RFPs that have been submitted.

   a. Trouble ticket
   b. Spreadsheet
   c. Gantt chart
   d. Weighted decision matrix

2. The vendor went out of business two years after the healthcare organization implemented the information system. The decision is made to continue with the existing information system for now but they will need to take over making updates to the information system. Identify the section of the contract that addresses this.

   a. Warranty
   b. Force majeure
   c. Escrow
   d. Payment milestone

CHECK YOUR UNDERSTANDING 4.3 (*Continued*)

3. The desired outcome for contract negotiation is a contract that _____.

   a. Completely benefits the healthcare organization
   b. Contract that benefits the vendor
   c. Is a win-win for both parties
   d. Is based on the laws of the vendor's state

4. The healthcare organization decided to develop their own information system using an iterative process. The strategy chosen is _____.

   a. Escrow
   b. Warranty
   c. Prototype
   d. Force majeure

5. The contract states that we can only utilize the information system at our main hospital. The portion of the contract that limits use to location is known as _____.

   a. Escrow
   b. Warranty
   c. Guarantee
   d. Software license

Real-World Case 4.1

XYZ Hospital just learned that their current EHR is being sunsetted and will no longer be supported by the IS vendor starting in two years. In the hospital's rush to select an IS, it decided to take some short cuts. These short cuts included:

- Creating a committee of only three people to select the system
- Not going on a site visit
- Not performing systems analysis
- Deferring planning until after the contract is signed

These shortcuts were recommended by the chief executive officer of XYZ Hospital. The logic behind his recommendation to defer planning was that there will be some time after the contract is signed but before the software is available, so the planning can fill in this time period. The contact with a vendor was signed yesterday so the planning is ready to commence.

Real-World Case 4.2

ABC Health Clinic has been conducting system analysis for a new clinical provider order entry system (CPOE) for several months now. They have made a firm commitment to the project and now they have some significant decisions to make before they can move to selecting the new information system. They need to determine who will build the information system and whether the information system should be integrated or interfaced.

The clinic has a practice management system and plan to implement an electronic health record after the CPOE is implemented. Because of this, they have a small information technology staff. Most of these staff members stay busy helping with the day to day issues such security, backups, personal computer problems, and so forth, but one of the staff members has experience with implementing information systems.

REVIEW QUESTIONS

1. Identify the step that would help the healthcare organization learn of changes within the healthcare organization that might impact the needs of an information system.

   a. Internal scanning
   b. Request for proposal
   c. Request for information
   d. External scanning

2. One of the goals of the IS under consideration is to improve patient care. This is an example of a(n) _____.

   a. Project definition
   b. SMART goal
   c. Intangible benefit
   d. Tangible benefit

3. Justify the need to have a HIM professional on the EHR information system project team.

   a. It is mandated by Joint Commission
   b. It is mandated by CMS
   c. The HIM professional documents daily in the EHR
   d. The HIM professional can address issues related to HIM

4. The hospital has gone into a partnership with an IS vendor. The hospital will be the first healthcare organization after the alpha sites to utilize the EHR under development. The hospital is known as a(n) _____.

   a. Alpha site 2
   b. Beta site
   c. Project plan
   d. Critical path

5. Before the project began, the healthcare organization decided to implement an EHR that will be used at all three of the hospitals owed by the organization. This is an example of a(n) _____.

   a. Acceptance test
   b. Project definition
   c. Scope creep
   d. Feasibility study

6. The vendor's right to sell a product is an example of a(n) _____.

   a. Warranty and guarantee
   b. Force majeure
   c. Acceptance test
   d. Source code

7. The healthcare organization has decided to purchase all of the ISs from one vendor. This strategy is known as _____.

   a. Best of the best
   b. Best of breed
   c. Best of fit
   d. Best of choice

REVIEW QUESTIONS (*Continued*)

8. The strategy that links two information systems from different vendors is known as

    a. External scanning
    b. Best of breed
    c. Integrated
    d. Interfaced

9. Identify the type of evaluation of an information system that sees the actual information in action.

    a. On-site demonstration
    b. Site visit
    c. Reference checks
    d. Reviewing RFP responses

10. The information strategic plan should support

    a. The users
    b. Internal scanning
    c. The business strategic plan
    d. External scanning

References

American Health Information Management Association. 2017. *Pocket Glossary of Health Information Management and Technology*, 5th ed. Chicago: AHIMA.

Eddu saver. 2019. Key Components to Creating a Great Cloud Provisioning Contract. https://www.eddusaver.com/key-components-to-creating-a-great-cloud-provisioning-contract/.

Fay Business Systems. 2016. The Top 10 Reasons Why Software Implementations Fail. https://fayebsg.com/2016/10/the-top-10-reasons-why-software-implementations-fail/.

IBM. nda. Benefits of Cloud Computing. https://www.ibm.com/cloud/learn/benefits-of-cloud-computing.

IBN. ndb. Contract Cotermination. https://www.ibm.com/support/knowledgecenter/SSYQ89_10.1.1/com.ibm.help.ecm_userguide.doc/C_ContractCotermination.html.

Johns, M. 2020. Governing Data and Information Assets. Chapter 3 in *Health Information Management: Concepts, Principles, and Practice*, 6th ed. Edited by P. Oachs and A. L. Watters. Chicago: AHIMA.

Merriam-Webster. 2020. Force majeure. Merriam-Webster Dictionary Online. https://www.merriam-webster.com/dictionary/force%20majeure.

Mirman, E. 2019. The Ultimate Guide to service-Level Agreements (SLAs). https://blog.hubspot.com/blog/tabid/6307/bid/34212/how-to-create-a-service-level-agreement-sla-for-better-sales-marketing-alignment.aspx

Project Management Institute. 2015. Project Management Professional (PNP) Examination Content Outline. https://www.pmi.org/-/media/pmi/documents/public/pdf/certifications/project-management-professional-exam-outline.pdf?v=6c1b35af-231d-481f-9522-efe6c46e2636.

Teamgantt. 2020. What is Scope Creep, and How can You Avoid It? https://www.teamgantt.com/guide-to-project-management/taming-scope-creep.

Vonnegut, S. 2017. Scalability in the Cloud: How Organizations Win with the Cloud. https://www.stratoscale.com/blog/cloud/scalability-cloud-organizations-win-cloud/.

System Implementation

Learning Objectives

- Identify the steps in system implementation.
- Make recommendations for the testing and implementation of the information system.
- Develop training materials and conduct training classes for users.
- Recommend conversion needed for data being transferred from existing system.

Key Terms

Computer-assisted instruction (CAI)	Reengineering	Train the trainer
	Setting configuration	Trouble ticket
Data conversion	Site preparation	User interface design
Graphical user interface (GUI)	System evaluation	User preparation
Information system (IS)	System implementation	
Information technology (IT)	Test environment	

In chapter 4, the system development life cycle (SDLC) was introduced and the first three stages were discussed. In this chapter, the last three stages, system implementation, evaluation of implementation, and maintenance of information system, will be covered.

System Implementation

System implementation is the process of preparing and launching the information system (IS) that has been selected for use. System implementation of complex information systems such as the EHR is a laborious process. There are many tasks involved. Some of these steps can be completed concurrently, whereas others must have one or more of the steps preceding them completed before proceeding. For example, software cannot be installed if the hardware has not been installed first. It is the responsibility of the project manager and the project team to keep the project on track (financially, timing, and so forth) using Gantt and PERT charts (as discussed in chapter 4) and other project management skills.

These steps are controlled by decisions made in the first three steps described in chapter 4. These steps are also shown in Figure 5.1.

Figure 5.1. Steps in implementation

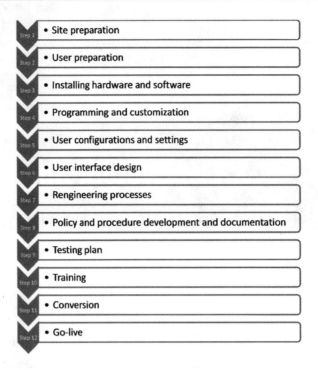

Source: ©AHIMA.

Site Preparation

Site preparation requires making any needed changes to the physical location where the computer, workstations, printers, or other hardware will be installed. The needs of site preparation vary widely, from construction of a new building, to renovation of an old one, to use of existing structures and upgrades to the infrastructure. Modifications needed may require the installation of special air conditioning or floors designed to run cables under it, added security measures, or more electrical outlets, to name a few. However, site preparation may be as simple as moving existing hardware around to make room for the new. The nursing units, the health information management (HIM) department, and other locations may need to be renovated to add space for computer terminals, barcode printers, network printers, and other hardware. The data center, where computers will run the IS, must be completed first because the nursing units and other departments will not use the IS until go-live. In addition to the physical plant, the healthcare organization network may need to be updated to accommodate the extra traffic resulting from the new information system.

Failure to properly prepare the site and infrastructure will result in delays in the installation of hardware and software, which will in turn delay the entire implementation plan of the information system. For example, a healthcare organization might attempt to plug in the hardware and not have an available electrical outlet to use, thus delaying the project.

User Preparation

User preparation involves providing the users with enough information about the IS being implemented so that they are prepared both psychologically and through training to use the new information system. This stage is a part of the change management process discussed in chapter 4 and continues throughout the project. It is important for IS users to be notified and updated throughout the system selection and implementation process. The users need to know that the IS is being implemented and should have an accurate understanding of what to expect from the expected IS and what is expected of them. Many people fear change when new ISs are installed;

therefore, these fears must be addressed. For example, they may have a fear of change because it takes them out of their comfort zone. They may fear that their position will be replaced with the information system and more. Management must be open and honest with the users regarding expectations, downsizing, changes in job descriptions, and other concerns. The information provided to the users must be accurate; otherwise, users will lose trust in the manager's word. Sometimes a new information system is promoted so intensely that users expect more than the IS can provide. These unrealistic expectations lead to disappointment and, in turn, a lack of support from the users. There should be as many users involved in the IS selection and implementation as possible to obtain their support. Their involvement can be through the systems analysis function, being part of the implementation team, assisting in testing, and other ways. Even those users not involved in the selection and implementation need to have realistic expectations. Their expectations can be managed through training, articles in the healthcare organization newsletter, updates at department meetings, and other formal and informal means of communication. If the IS does not live up to the user's expectations, they may not use the IS to its fullest or take the time to use it properly; thus impacting the overall success of the implementation.

Installing Hardware and Software

Because it may take several weeks to receive hardware (computers, monitors, servers, and so on), staff needs to plan accordingly and place the order early. The most critical piece of hardware is the file server or other computer storage component that will house the application software. System implementation may be delayed if the file server or other hardware is not available according to the project plan since the process cannot proceed without the file server.

Once the hardware arrives, it will need to be set up and installed in the data center. Computers will also need to be installed in the nursing units, training rooms, and other locations according to the project plan. The printers, network, scanners, and other hardware will also need to be installed.

The software will then need to be loaded onto the file server, mainframe, or other computer in the data center. Some applications require software to be used on an individual user's computer. If this is the case, the software will have to be installed on all authorized computers prior to implementation, especially for development and testing. Any failures in the site preparation will be identified in this stage.

The application software will be provided to the healthcare organization by the computer vendor based on the date specified in the contract. The version of the software provided will also be controlled by the contract. If the vendor is late in sending the software for installation, the implementation of the IS will be delayed.

Programming and Customization

Programming may or may not be required, depending on the type of IS, complexity of the IS, and whether the healthcare organization is purchasing an IS or programming one themselves. If the IS interfaces with other ISs to share information, such as patient demographics or other information, the interfaces will have to be programmed. See chapter 4 for more information on interfaces. If the healthcare organization is converting data from another IS, computer programming will have to be done to perform **data conversion**. Data conversion is the process whereby data are copied from the existing IS, manipulated into the format required by the new IS, and entered into the new IS. This is done through an interface.

The data conversion may be performed by a computer programmer or a Certified Health Data Analyst (CHDA). The CHDA is an AHIMA certification that specializes in "knowledge to acquire, manage, analyze, interpret, and transform data into accurate, consistent, and timely information, while balancing the "big picture" strategic vision with day-to-day details" (AHIMA 2020).

This data conversion mapping from one format to another is critical to data quality as well as sharing of data. For example, if a health record number is stored in the current information system as a 10-digit number (0000123456) and the new IS requires a 12-digit number, then two more leading zeroes would need to be added to the number (000000123456). This conversion will be done immediately before the new information system is implemented. The programming of the interfaces has to be written and tested so that it is ready to convert the data.

The healthcare organization may want to have the vendor customize some functions to better meet its needs. Although customization may better prepare the IS to meet the needs of the healthcare organization, there are reasons why the healthcare organization should not customize the software beyond what is already built into the IS:

- It will be expensive to have the vendor customize the software. There may be annual costs to maintain the customization in addition to the upfront costs.
- The vendor may not be able to address issues with the information system.
- The vendor may no longer provided updates
- There may be additional security risks (PCD Group 2018).
- The information system may become unstable which may result in data integrity and documentation issues.

User Configurations and Settings

Most computer software purchased by healthcare organization generally provides some flexibility in the implementation of the IS. This flexibility is allowed through setting configuration. **Setting configuration** is the entry of the desired behaviors of the IS into tables or setting fields. For example, if the IS will keep track of the patient type, the hospital determines if patients will be classified as inpatient, outpatient, emergency department, testing, outpatient surgery, or other patient types. The healthcare organization may even be able to determine that "I" means inpatient.

The project team sets up the specifications by filling in tables and other fields with the desired setup. They will also be able to update tables that provide their reimbursement rates, tax identification number, national provider identifier, or other appropriate values. Other settings may include time frame before bills drop, data and format of claims submitted to fiscal intermediary, and what fields are required. The settings will ensure that the IS works according to the needs of the healthcare organization.

It can take minutes or months to get all the specifications and tables updated, depending on the complexity of the specifications and the IS. An example of a table that must be uploaded is the user table. In this table, each user's information must be entered into the IS, including their username, initial password, location, type of access, and permissions as to what they can perform within the IS. For example, Mary Smith may have access to the laboratory results, but she can only view these results—not delete or modify them. Determining who has access to what information and what they can do with it is a time-consuming task. More on access controls is available in chapter 12.

User Interface Design

The IS may allow the healthcare organization to make changes to the computer screen so that it works the best for the healthcare organization. **User interface design** means developing screens of an IS to meet the needs of the user and to promote job efficiency. To accomplish this goal, team members involved in this process must be aware of the needs of the users and the work they perform. Reasons why the healthcare organization may want to change the computer screen include the following:

- No single screen contains the data needed to make data entry or viewing efficient.
- The vendor's screens do not have data elements in a logical order for the workflow of the users.

- The existing screens are too cluttered for the users' preference.
- Changing the screen will improve the process workflow.

There are rules to follow when designing screens used in information systems. The fields should be in a logical sequence to facilitate data entry. The logical flow of data helps the users locate information. For example, if reviewing a screen containing basic patient demographic information, the address, city, and state would be located together in that order rather than address at the top and city beneath other data elements. The flow of data entry should be appropriate for the language. For example in the United States, it would be from left to right and top to bottom. Other countries may read right to left or other flows. Screens, like paper forms, should have a title and a control number to manage the screen. The title of the screen should be descriptive of the data contained on the screen such as "Lab Results." Screens should be simple to use and have a standardized terminology across screens to facilitate data entry, training, and data quality. For example, the health record number should be called the same name on all screens—not medical record number on one and health record number or patient identifier on another. Screens should also have the same look and feel so that the user can easily move from screen to screen. A standardized look and feel for a screen include the same colors, location of key data elements such as patient name, and same location and terminology for key buttons such as "Next Screen." Instructions can be posted on the screen where necessary to assist users. Color, or reverse video can be used to draw the user's attention to important data such as allergies. In reverse video, the font is the normal color of the background and the background is the normal color of the font. These special features should be used sparingly so that the user's attention is drawn to the information displayed. The color of the screen and text should be comfortable for users to view for long periods of time. For example, red and bright neon colors are typically used only sparingly as it can put a strain on the user's eyes. An example of good screen design is seen in figure 5.1 and an example of poor screen design is seen in figure 5.2. In figure 5.1, the data elements are listed in a logical order, there is a descriptive title for the screen, it has a screen number, and the buttons are clear in their function and are in a logical location. In figure 5.2, the data fields are not in a logical order nor are the buttons, and the screen does not have a title.

Figure 5.1. Example of good screen design

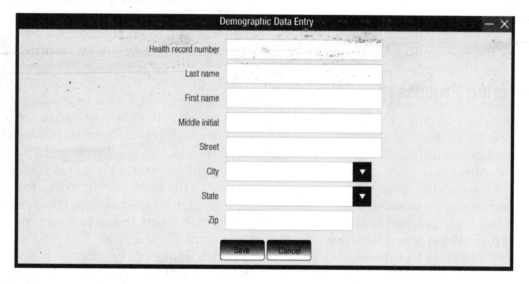

Source: ©AHIMA.

The screen design may include designing computer views for various types of users. This flexibility would allow nurses to see new orders, care plans, or other information first; the cardiologist and neurologist would have first access to cardiac and neurologic tests, respectively.

Figure 5.2. Example of poor screen design

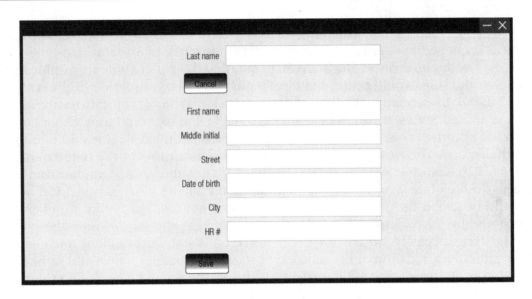

Source: ©AHIMA.

A **graphical user interface (GUI)** is a term used to describe the interaction of users and the computer whereby the user clicks on icons, menus, and other tools to assist in the use of the IS. Frequently, these icons are shown on a toolbar. Icons provide shortcuts to functionality within the information system, along with buttons and menus, allowing the user to command the software to perform specific tasks.

The HIM professional must work with the information technology professionals to ensure the screens in the IS are designed to support quality data entry. Information technology (IT) is the field that includes hardware, software, and databases. Information systems (IS) is a broader term that includes information technology as well as the staff and processes needed to operate and manage them (Florida Institute of Technology 2020). One of the ways this can be done is through required fields. A required field does not allow the user to proceed until it is completed. Not all fields should be required because not all fields apply to all patients. For example, obstetrical data fields would not be required for male patients. If a field is identified as required inappropriately, the users would become frustrated and may resort to entering erroneous data to be able to proceed. For more on data quality, refer to chapter 2.

Reengineering Processes

Reengineering is evaluating the way the healthcare organization does business in order to improve efficiency. Reengineering is a task that is frequently overlooked in the efforts to implement the IS. Every task and preconceived notion must be challenged. The question "why" should be asked over and over. Everything is subject to evaluation and change, without exemption. This is challenging to employees who are comfortable with the status quo. Some of the tasks performed by the employees have been performed for years. The reason behind the task may be outdated, but the task continues because the employee is afraid to stop. The implementation of a new IS is a perfect time to critique the tasks performed to try and improve efficiency, costs, and effectiveness.

The employees may feel threatened and intimidated because of the changes impacting their jobs, but reengineering is a necessary part of the IS process. The healthcare organization cannot implement an IS and expect the work processes to remain the same. The healthcare organization will need to change procedures, update the policy and procedure manual, change workflow, eliminate unnecessary tasks, and add new tasks. Failure to do so can decrease efficiency rather than maximize the benefits the IS affords. The IS changes the way a healthcare organization conducts business and impacts the manual processes and workflow as well as their overall interaction with the computer. The policies and procedures tested during the testing phase should contain the revised processes.

Policy and Procedure Development and Documentation

After the reengineering is completed, the policy and procedure manual must be updated to reflect the new way of doing business. Policies and procedures should blend together the manual processes and decision-making processes. Management and maintenance of the information system itself must also be clearly outlined. These policies frequently cover backups, downtime policies for routine maintenance, upgrades, testing of upgrades, and disaster planning.

The policies and procedures need to address how the IS will be used by the various users throughout the healthcare organization such as coding professionals, admission clerks, and other staff. In addition, the healthcare organization must create training manuals and user guides for reference. These materials will be available to the users as resources on how to use the information system, how to incorporate it into their jobs, and how to identify how their jobs have changed.

CHECK YOUR UNDERSTANDING 5.1

1. Controlling how an IS behaves is impacted by _____.

   a. Interfaces
   b. Policies and procedures
   c. Reengineering
   d. Setting configurations

2. Critique this statement: Data elements on a computer screen should be read from right to left and top to bottom.

   a. This is a true statement.
   b. This is a false statement as it should be read from right to left and bottom to top.
   c. This is a false statement as it should be read from left to right and top to bottom.
   d. This is a false statement as it should be read from left to right and bottom to top.

3. Making room for new computers is part of the _____ process.

   a. Site preparation
   b. System selection
   c. Flow charting
   d. Reengineering

4. The current information system's health record number field allows 8 characters. The same field in the information system being implemented allows 12 characters. This is handled through _____.

   a. Data conversion
   b. Site preparation
   c. Policies and procedures
   d. Setting configuration

5. Identify the process that helps maximize the functionality of the new information system.

   a. GUI
   b. Policies and procedures
   c. Conversion
   d. Reengineering

Testing Plan

All components of the IS will need testing before the go-live. Testing helps the implementation team identify any problems with the information system so that they can be corrected. This is a cyclical process, so the team will test the IS, identify problems, fix problems, and test the information system again. The test cycle will continue until all problems have been resolved. Testing requires careful and detailed planning to ensure that complete and accurate testing is carried out in a timely manner.

Types of Testing

Many types of testing must be performed in preparation for an IS implementation. The types of testing include the following:

- Interface testing: Ensures that the interfaces function properly. The healthcare organization must test to confirm that data from the source system are transferred into the new IS in the correct field and in the right format. Data to be transferred vary by IS, but commonly include the patient's name, health record number, date of birth, and other demographic information. Other types of data that may be transferred include laboratory tests, radiology results, and any other data that are collected.

- Integration testing: Ensures that all hardware, including computers, printers, and scanners, work together as they should. Examples of testing to be performed include the ability to scan documents, print a report, or scan a barcode. Some computers may have limitations placed on their abilities for privacy, security, or other reasons. For example, the healthcare organization may choose not to print laboratory results on the nursing units to protect confidentiality, thus forcing users to look up the most current results available.

- Application testing: Ensures that every function of the new IS works as it should. Application testing also ensures that the IS meets the functional requirements and other required specifications in the request for proposal (RFP) or contract. Application testing should also ensure that every conceivable situation that the computer will be used to address can be handled. The project team must also test the reports to ensure that the data and statistics contained therein are correct.

- Documentation testing: During the implementation process, a number of documents, including user guides, policies and procedures, and training materials, are created. These documents should be followed during the testing process to ensure that the instructions in the documents are accurate. In testing the documentation, the tester follows and tests the IS documentation that will be provided to the users. Errors in the documentation will be identified and corrected so that the user will have the proper instructions.

- Conversion testing: Ensures that the project team is able to transfer data from the old IS to the new IS. Conversion testing will confirm that the data conversion is performed correctly. Testing usually begins with a small amount of real data that have been copied. After the initial test has been run, the project team would fix any problems, rerun the test, and then continue to add larger and larger amounts of data. This testing will continue until the project team is certain that the problems have been resolved prior to the actual data conversion.

- Training testing: The project team should train a group to see how well the training materials, agenda, format of training, time allotted for training, and other attributes work. Changes are made to the training process as needed before real training begins.

- Volume testing: Most of the testing performed on the application is done with a handful of people sitting at an IS trying to identify problems. The IS may work fine with a small group of people, but most ISs are used by large groups of people simultaneously. To test the IS in as real an environment as possible, volume testing should be performed. Volume testing gets as many people to use the IS at one time as possible. Volume testing confirms that the IS and the network can handle the large volume of users and data. The user task force as well as other users throughout the healthcare organization can be brought in for volume testing. The project team will need to recruit as many users as possible to use the IS at the same time.

- Parallel testing: Running parallel tests is used for both testing and facilitating the transition of data and business processes. Unlike most other testing, parallel testing occurs when the new IS is operational. This is not a required test, but can be a valuable one. In parallel testing, the healthcare organization runs the old and the new ISs simultaneously and compares the reports and data from the two information systems to validate both performance and synchronization. For example, the healthcare organization could compare the number of admissions for a specific date, the number of tests ordered, or the number of times that a test was ordered. Because of the extra resources needed to operate both ISs, this test is frequently omitted. The benefit to parallel testing is that if the new IS does not work as expected and the healthcare organization has to shut it down, then the existing IS is current, thus not impacting the operations of the healthcare organization.

- Acceptance testing: Like parallel testing, acceptance testing occurs after go-live. It is a time to verify that the IS is working as expected in a live environment. It gives the healthcare organization time to confirm that the new IS meets response time, functional requirements, and other standards guaranteed in the contract. (Amatayakul 2017, 267).

Test Plan

The testing plan is a document that covers areas such as what is to be tested, who will be involved in the testing, dates of testing, documentation of testing results, and types of testing. The testing must continue until all problems have been fixed. The testing must include the documentation created for use with the IS as well such as training materials, policies and procedures and more.

The testing plan should create a realistic **test environment**, which is an exact duplicate of the IS in use, excluding the live data. In this test environment, changes can be made to the IS and then tested to see what happens. For example, the settings in the test system environment should be the ones that the healthcare organization will utilize during operation. The testing plan will identify a "laundry list" of functions that must be tested before the IS is implemented. One way to test the functions is scenario or use-case testing, during which users bring real-life situations to be addressed by the IS. These scenarios should be documented in the plan. The use of scenarios allows the user to think through how a situation will be handled by actually using the IS. Scenario testing thoroughly tests the information system because it addresses entries into the IS, tasks, and output.

Testing Documentation

Many healthcare organizations use what is frequently called a trouble ticket to report problems encountered during the testing phase. The **trouble ticket** is a form that is used to give specific information on problems encountered. The information provided may include the screen where the problem occurred, function being performed, error message received, data entered, report with incorrect data, or other problems encountered. The information provided must be as detailed as possible so that the problem can be replicated by the project team. The trouble ticket is logged into some type of tracking system when received, assigned a tracking number, and assigned to the appropriate project team member to solve. Once the problem has been resolved, the resolution is recorded, and the IS testing begins again. The project team cannot just test the part that was broken because the change that was made to fix the problem may have broken something else.

Training

Training is crucial to the success of the implementation process. There needs to be a well-designed training plan that addresses the timing and methods used to train the users. The plan must be properly executed or negative repercussions can occur. Users may feel like they are reverting back to being a novice employee after being an expert in their position. Job security may be another concern. Individuals who are most concerned with the new ISs are often those who have little experience with computers. Communicating with employees and keeping them informed of changes, impact, and expectations of their position will help prepare them for training.

The learning curve is different with each employee. Learning ability is impacted by age, maturity level, and experience. People have different preferred learning styles—auditory, visual, and so forth. Because of these factors, instructors should use a variety of methods that will accommodate all learning styles.

Instructors and trainers should have a basic understanding of adult learning principles and practice them in the development and implementation of training. Some key adult learning principles are:

- Adults like being responsible for their own decisions: They resent not having control, so the instructor should let the learners have a say in the program. This can take the form of helping to set the agenda, deciding which of two or three activities to do, strategies to use, and so on.

- Adults are experienced: Adult learners come to the training session with a lot of experience and knowledge upon which they can draw. Not all adults have the same knowledge and experience. The instructor and students can learn from each other. The varied backgrounds and knowledge can make for an interesting discussion and an improved learning experience.

- Adults need to know why: Instructors should get into a habit of telling the adults why they need to do something or why they need to learn what they are being taught. They need to know why something is important just as much as they need to know how to do it.

- Adults need to see relevance: Adults do not want to waste their time. They want to learn what they need to know for the immediate future. The instructor will need to tie the class material to what the individuals in the course will be doing. In other words, do not teach nurses how to do something with the IS that only the HIM department will be doing in the future. The nurses need to know what they will be doing. If adult learners do not see relevance to themselves, they will not be motivated to learn.

- The adult needs to be ready to learn: Training sessions may be mandatory and the learners may show up physically to the session, but they cannot be forced to learn. The instructor must engage the learner and encourage the desire to learn.

- The learner has to be motivated to learn: Some healthcare organizations have motivated learners by making them take a competency test at the end of the training session. This test makes the learner use skills they learned in class. Learners are motivated because the healthcare organization sometimes ties employment to successfully completing this test. These tests are generally very easy, but occasionally some people cannot pass them. These users are usually given a second or third chance before they are terminated. The threat of termination is not the best motivation because motivation to learn should come from within; however, the healthcare organization must know that the users are competent to use the ISs.

A separate training environment or sandbox is frequently created so that users can "play" with the information during and after training. This would allow for fake patients to be added to a database for users to practice using the information system without harming actual patient data.

Planning for Training

There should be someone on the project team who is responsible for planning the complete training process. This trainer has a wide range of responsibilities including developing objectives, developing the training plan, and implementing the training.

The trainer would attend project team meetings in order to keep up with the status of the project. The trainer needs to know when training will be needed, the type of training needed, and also be a superuser (or expert) on the new IS. With this knowledge, the trainer will be prepared to develop the training program necessary to teach others to use the IS. The trainer is responsible for sharing and providing the necessary knowledge needed to prepare other trainers to teach as well.

The trainer will also work with the training staff from the vendor. The vendor's staff knows the product well and will be able to offer the project team suggestions on different teaching methods directly related to the IS. The vendor should provide the trainers with resources that can be customized for the healthcare organization.

The trainer will be working with both administration and end-users during the training planning and training implementation stages. These interactions make the trainer an excellent liaison between the two groups. The trainer will be able to communicate expectations of administration to users as well as communicate the fears and concerns of the users back to administration.

Contents of the Plan

The project team should create a training schedule that allows everyone who needs training to participate. The schedule should include sessions for all work shifts, including day, evening, night, and weekend shifts. The training plan should contain learning objectives that show both trainer and trainees what will be accomplished throughout the training sessions. The training plan should also outline the agenda, which describes the functions of the IS that will be covered, how they will be covered, and how much time will be spent on each topic. Teaching tools such as presentations, hands-on training, demonstrations, and computer-assisted instruction (CAI) are to be used during training.

The training plan should also address the content that will be covered, such as rollout schedule, policies and procedures, confidentiality, and security. When planning content, trainers need to determine each trainee's level of computer literacy before deciding what training is needed. Based on how many students will attend each session, the number of trainers and training sessions can be determined. The planners will also have to determine the necessary resources, such as a training room, computers, Internet access, training database, data projector, and handouts.

Not all users need the same training, so the training will be designed in modules based on the areas of content. Two examples are by department (such as nursing) or by function (such as order entry). In other words, the planner needs to decide whether the session will teach all nurses together or will teach people how to look up test results and have everyone who needs to know how to do this included in the same session. The division of the training into modules will impact the number of teachers, the schedule, and the training materials.

Selecting the Training Location

Not every trainer is fortunate enough to have a dedicated training space. Trainers may be forced to reserve computer classrooms throughout the healthcare organization. A room would not be necessary if online training is utilized.

Scheduling the Training

Scheduling can be a very complicated task because trainers have to conduct different training classes required by patient care providers, administrative office staff, and other groups of users. Follow-up sessions after go-live should be offered as well to answer any questions that the users have once they start using the IS.

Many healthcare organizations are open 24 hours a day, 7 days a week, and thus, employees work a variety of shifts. Because of this, training must be offered on all shifts, including weekends, to accommodate all employees needing training. The following issues should be considered:

- Breaking modules down into separate classes helps to avoid confusion. If there is more than one class required, the team must make sure that they are offered in a logical format. For example, employees would need to know how to retrieve a patient file before they can learn how to place an order for a patient.

- This is further complicated by the fact that the trainers need to schedule the classes as close as possible to go-live while starting training early enough to get everyone trained in time. Completing training too early is also problematic because the users can forget what they learned before the IS is implemented, thus making the transition difficult for the user and the healthcare organization.

- Length of a session matters. Short sessions tend to work better because users are less likely to become overwhelmed. Also, if they are unaccustomed to sitting down, they may become frustrated by inactivity.
- The training sessions should not be scheduled during holidays because many people take time off, which causes scheduling problems with getting everyone trained.
- Physicians should be scheduled for one-on-one training sessions to accommodate their schedules. It could be early in the morning, at lunch, late in afternoon, in the evening, or on weekends in order to avoid interfering with physicians' office schedules.

Resources Needed

Each user should be provided a handout at the training session. Training materials are excellent resources to remind users how to do some task that may have been forgotten. Several days, weeks, or even months may pass between the initial training session and the implementation of the IS. During that time, users are likely to forget much of the material learned. To help them retain the knowledge acquired in training, the healthcare organization may also want to make the IS available (in test mode) to users for practice throughout this interim period.

Content suggestions for the development of educational materials provided to the students are as follows:

- The objectives should be clearly outlined.
- The agenda for the course should be sent to the scheduled attendees ahead of time. The agenda is subject to change, but acts as a guide to help keep trainers on track.
- Providing information about the IS prior to training offers a useful preview.

Train the Trainer

Train the trainer is a method of training certain individuals who, in turn, will be responsible for training others on a task or skill such as how to use the new IS. These people are generally called superusers. Superusers return to the healthcare organization and train other trainers who will in turn help conduct training sessions.

The user identifies the trainer as an expert on the system and its uses and who is likely to be a go-to resource. This visibility will make the trainer a key player in the hours and days following go-live. Users turn to the trainer with questions and fears.

Conducting the Training

Now that all of the work planning the training is finished, it is time to conduct the class. Instructors should be prepared and check the classroom to make sure it is ready for training—software has been installed, all computers are working, and so on. The trainer should make sure the room is physically comfortable. This means that the room is at a comfortable temperature, has appropriate lighting, and the workstations are ergonomically sound.

Evaluating the Training

Trainers must be evaluated on their delivery, impact, and knowledge of the application to make sure objectives of the training are being met. Objectives vary but typically include whether or not the attendees are learning how to use the information system.

A valuable method for obtaining feedback is to have each trainee complete a written evaluation at the end of the session, answering questions about the overall training and the ability of the trainer. These evaluations can help to identify what is and is not working. Findings may identify needed improvements such as in the handouts, poor instructors, or not enough time for hands-on activities. Findings from the trainee evaluations should be shared with the instructors anonymously to identify any needed modifications and to evaluate the overall training plan performance. Evaluation results should be used to improve the quality and method of training where needed. There is always room for improvement.

The overall training program should also be evaluated on a continuing basis to ensure that goals of training are met. A formal plan for evaluation should be developed prior to the start of the training sessions.

Additional and Ongoing Training

After the training phase and before go-live, the healthcare organization eventually will not need the same number of trainers or frequency of class sessions but they will need some since training does not end. Training needs should be reassessed to determine frequency and specific needs. Training may be reorganized in conjunction with the healthcare organization's human resources department new employee orientation program or it may be separate. Training may be required before an employee is issued a user identification and password.

In a perfect world, the IS on which users are trained would remain the same as the one implemented. However, changes to the IS will be made and are necessary for technology advances, resolving glitches, and other issues. Therefore, training does not end with go-live of the IS. When significant changes are made, training may be needed to update and prepare users for the changes. Also, existing employees may need additional training to learn advanced capabilities, reinforce what they have already learned, or acquire new skills if they transfer to other jobs or their job changes over time.

Computer-Assisted Instruction

Computer-assisted instruction (CAI) is a software program designed to use multimedia and interactive technology to teach a topic. Multimedia can use audio, video, simulation, self-quizzes, and other tools to engage the learner. Drill and practice CAI reinforce material that the learner already knows, whereas problem-solving addresses issues that the learner may face in his or her discipline.

The benefit of CAI is that learners are able to work at their own pace and on their own schedule. They are able to receive immediate feedback on whether or not they do something right. CAI also reduces costs, provides standardized training, and is designed to use multiple learning styles.

The downside is the start-up costs and the amount of time required to develop the training. Also, CAI should not be used when the content changes frequently because the CAI software will require updating with every change.

Documenting the Training

Documentation of all training provided is critical. Attendees should sign into each training session to provide proof of attendance for both employee's and employer's benefit. Copies of all training materials and objectives for the training also should be retained. If a competency test is given, documentation of the results also should be maintained. Some healthcare organizations require users to make a minimum grade on a competency test. Failure to make the required grade would result in termination. Employees are typically able to take the competency test more than once to enable them to retain their position.

Conversion

With most new ISs, a healthcare organization is converting from one IS to another. The healthcare organization cannot ignore the historical data but, rather, must bring some (if not all of it) to the new IS. In an IS implementation, conversion is transferring data from one IS to another while simultaneously making any necessary changes in format or content. A conversion is more difficult than it sounds because systems frequently store data very differently or the healthcare organization may be making changes to how it wants data to be collected. For example, the health record number may be 10 digits in one IS and 12 in the other, or Medicare may be entered as M in one information system and MCR in another. During conversion planning, the project team has to determine how much data are being converted and what data fields will need to be converted from one format to another. The amount of data transferred is a decision that must be made by the healthcare organization. The decision will be influenced by the type of IS, laws and regulations, whether or not the old IS will remain operational, and other issues. Sometimes healthcare organizations decide to transfer data from a specified time period only into the new IS. For example, they may decide to convert only the last two years. Other conversions require all data be transferred. The healthcare organization may also choose to enter data for all time periods, but only selected data elements rather than all data collected.

Once the conversion planning is finished, a program needs to be written that will make the necessary changes. A formal testing plan is required to determine how the project team will test the conversion to work out any problems before go-live. Once the IS is ready for use and the healthcare organization is ready for the IS, the data conversion plan must be implemented to move the existing data into the new information system in the appropriate format. If data conversion is successful, the healthcare organization is then ready to start using the new IS. Healthcare organizations frequently capture the information available in the IS at midnight so that they can determine what data are in the old IS and what data are in the new. A specific time period of transition is useful in case the healthcare organization has to go back to the old IS because the new information system did not work properly. See Table 5.1 for additional examples of conversion.

Table 5.1. Examples of conversion of data

Data Element	Data in Existing Information System	Data Needed for New Information System
Health record number	9 digits: 000123456	12 digits: 000000123456
Date	6 digits: XX/XX/XX	8 digits: XX/XX/XXXX
Service	4 services: Medical, surgical, obstetrics, newborn	8 services: Medical, general surgery, cardiology, obstetrics, orthopedics, cardiovascular surgery, paediatrics, endocrinology, gynecology

Source: ©AHIMA.

In these examples, conversion of the health record number and date is straight forward. With the health record number, three leading zeros are added. With the date either a 19 or a 20 is entered before the date. For example, if the year in the existing system is 63, then 19 is added to the front resulting in the year 1963. Converting the services is more challenging. The existing four services include all of the eight services required for the new information and potentially more such as neurology and nephrology. The question becomes how to map the two data. There are different ways that this can be done. For example, surgical patients in the existing information whose attending physician is a gynecologist could be converted from surgical to gynecology. Sometimes it may take a combination of factors. For example, a pediatrician may treat pediatric patients and newborns. In that case, the information system would need to consider additional data to determine the service such as both the attending physician and either the birthdate or diagnosis code for newborn. See Table 5.2 for an example of how the patient type might be mapped.

The outpatient patient type would be mapped based on services provided. As this example only gives two patient types for outpatient services, it would depend solely on whether or not the patient had surgery or not.

Go-Live

As stated in chapter 4, **go-live** is the official time and date that the healthcare organization begins using the new IS. Sometimes go-live may be called deployment especially in cloud computing

Figure 5.2. Examples of patient type mapping

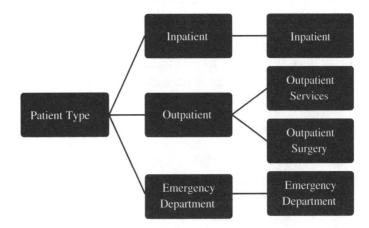

Source: ©AHIMA.

(discussed in chapter 4). The go-live is generally scheduled for a time when the healthcare organization is the least busy. For example, a hospital will generally go-live during the night shift because there is less activity at that time.

Go-Live Models

Go-live strategy generally refers to how an application will be implemented throughout a healthcare organization (such as the rollout to each departmental in a designated sequence). There are three types of go-live strategies: phased, pilot, and big bang. There are two turnover strategies: straight turnover (also known as direct turnover) and parallel processing. These strategies are discussed in the following sections.

Phased Approach

One go-live strategy is the phased approach. In this method, the implementation starts with one module of the IS and then gradually other modules are added. A module is a subset of an IS, such as pharmacy orders in a CPOE system. All units, departments, and other entities utilize the information system, but they only use it one module at a time. For example, a hospital could start using their order entry system by ordering medications only. After the medication ordering is successful, then laboratory will be added, and so on. With an electronic document management system, hospitals frequently start scanning emergency department records, then outpatient surgery, and then other record types until they work their way up to inpatient records. The advantage of this method is that staff is not overwhelmed by trying to do everything at once and the impact on the staff is lessened. The disadvantage is that it takes an extended period of time to finish the start-up process, which disrupts the operations of the healthcare organization.

Pilot Method

The next approach is the pilot method in which only one nursing unit, department, or other entity starts using the new IS at a time. Once consistently successful, the next group is implemented. For example, the 3W nursing unit starts ordering everything using the new IS, but nobody else uses the information system. They continue to utilize the existing information system. The next unit scheduled would be unit 3E and then other units would be rolled out. Again, this method is designed to limit the impact on the healthcare organization.

Big Bang Method

The last method, the big bang method (also called the cutover method), is the riskiest. With this method, the healthcare organization stops using the old IS and starts using the new information system. It is the riskiest because the healthcare organization may not have the old information system as a backup and the new IS is being used all over the hospital.

Straight (Direct) Turnover

With straight turnover, the former information system and processes cease with the implementation of the new IS. There is a risk here if the new IS has to be aborted; however, it is more cost effective and reduces the work load significantly because there is no duplication of efforts.

Parallel Processing

Parallel processing entering data in both the old and new IS for a specified period of time such as two weeks. This allows the users to keep the database current in both information systems. Although parallel processing works well, it is labor intensive and therefore expensive. Because the old IS is in place and current, this approach provides a safety net and has the least amount of risk involved.

Planning for Go-Live

Whichever method is chosen, planning is critical because IS implementation cannot interfere with patient care. Certain steps should be taken no matter which plan is selected.

Initial Support

There should be a member of the project team in every unit or department when the IS goes live. These project team members should be highly visible to one another; for example, they could wear matching shirts. Project team members are needed to answer questions and generally ensure that the IS start-up runs as smoothly as possible. Trainers play an important role not only in the training but also during go-live, which means they are a key part of the implementation presence throughout the healthcare organization.

Ongoing Support

Initially, someone must be available 24 hours a day, 7 days a week to assist users. The length of time that this intensive support is needed will depend on the magnitude of the IS and how well the implementation is going. Generally, this intensive support is needed for only a few days. There should be a help desk that users can call when help is needed. The amount of coverage will eventually be reduced to the regular help desk support. The project team must be prepared to go back to the old IS if the new one does not work.

System Evaluation and Maintenance

After the new IS is implemented and functioning properly, the project team will need to evaluate how well the implementation went. **System evaluation** is how the healthcare organization determines whether or not the IS functions as expected. The project team needs to learn what did and did not work during the implementation process and determine how they can improve the next implementation. For example, the team may not have started system testing early enough, or maybe there were expenses that were not budgeted for. The project team will also want to know if the healthcare organization met the goals that were established for the project and if the project came in on budget. This evaluation allows the project team to learn from mistakes and from the experience.

After a predetermined time period, the project team will need to determine if the healthcare organization has realized all expected benefits and all of the goals that were established during the planning and analysis phase. For example, did the healthcare organization save the money that was expected, did it reduce the turnaround time on obtaining test results and so forth.

In the immediate support and evaluation period, problems may be found that were not revealed during the system testing and will need to be resolved. Changes may be needed to correct the problems and more testing will be done. Even after the information system is working well, periodic updates will ensure that the IS is current. There will also be routine maintenance and upgrades, such as backing up data, increasing storage capacity, and upgrading hardware and software. As discussed earlier, major information systems have what is called a test system or a **test environment**.

It is in the test environment, and not the production environment, that the software changes can be tested without worrying about problems resulting from the changes. This will enable support staff to solve problems before the update is live; once the IS is working appropriately in the test environment, it can be implemented into the live one.

Also in this stage, there will come a time when the IS is no longer meeting the needs of the healthcare organization. The vendor may stop supporting it, the healthcare organization may need more functionality or users than the current information system will accommodate, and other needs may arise. When this obsolescence occurs, the process begins again.

CHECK YOUR UNDERSTANDING 5.2

1. A new update has been received from the vendor. Before installing it for use by the users, it should be uploaded first into the _____.

    a. Production environment
    b. Test environment
    c. Training environment
    d. Live environment

2. Identify the go-live model in which the old information system and the new information system are used at the same time.

    a. Phased
    b. Pilot
    c. Cutover
    d. Parallel

3. Identify an adult learning principle.

    a. Adults need to see relevance.
    b. Adults like to be told what to do.
    c. Adults learn well even if not motivated.
    d. Adults have the same knowledge and experience.

4. The type of testing that ensures that the new information system can handle the amount of data and number of users is known as _____.

    a. Volume testing
    b. Integration testing
    c. Parallel testing
    d. Application testing

5. The stage when the team determines what they could have done better is known as _____.

    a. Training
    b. Testing
    c. Evaluation and maintenance
    d. Systems analysis

Real-World Case 5.1

Home Health of America is about to implement the new EHR. This EHR will be used by all of the nurses, nursing aides, therapists, and other staff members who work with patients in the patient's home. It will also be accessed in the home office for billing and other administrative purposes. The chief executive officer mandated the big bang go-live strategy. He also mandated that the go-live begin on Monday, which is their busiest day. His thoughts were that if the EHR could handle Monday, then it could handle anything. The users ran into several problems on the first day. Some of the functionality did not work, the cellular connections used to connect to the IS did not work at some of the homes, and the documentation was slow, which prevented the nurses and other care providers from seeing the patients in a timely manner. They had planned for some overtime as they knew that documenting in the new EHR would be slower. The overtime ended up being twice what was expected and they still did not see three of the patients. The decision was made to go back to the paper system while the problems were worked out.

Real-World Case 5.2

The physicians at ABC Clinics decided to implement a new EHR. This was their first EHR and they are excited to take this step. The physicians decided that the fastest way to implement the EHR was to have two-three physicians select the information and then have the information technology staff implement it using the standard settings without input from other users. They decided to utilize the straight turnover strategy. The physicians were shocked at the number of problems that they encountered on the first day of go-live. Some of these issues were as follows:

- The users did not know how to use the information system
- Some fields were required when they should not be
- Some functionality did not work
- Users had to go to multiple screens to enter demographic and other basic data

The physicians had no choice but go back to the paper and work to eliminate the issues.

REVIEW QUESTIONS

1. Installing an update to the information is performed in the SDLC stage of _____.
   a. Planning and analysis
   b. Design
   c. Implementation
   d. Evaluation and maintenance

2. If the healthcare organization wants to avoid risk during go-live, they should choose the _____ go-live strategy.
   a. Straight turnover
   b. Big bang
   c. Pilot
   d. Parallel processing

3. The type of testing that addresses the sharing of data from a source system to the new IS is known as _____.
   a. Interface testing
   b. Integration testing

REVIEW QUESTIONS (*Continued*)

   c. Application testing

   d. Conversion testing

4. Identify the adult learning principle.

   a. Adults do not need content to be relevant to their position.

   b. Adults like to be told what to do.

   c. Adults need to know why.

   d. Adults do not have to be prepared to learn.

5. Identify the true statement about conversion of data.

   a. Conversion of data is only needed in rare instances.

   b. Conversion of data requires interfaces to be programmed.

   c. Conversion of data is only needed in integrated systems.

   d. Conversion of data is only needed when multiple ISs are connected together.

6. Critique this statement: CAI should only be used for training if the training is not expected to change.

   a. This is a true statement.

   b. This is a false statement as CAI is not used in training.

   c. This is a false statement as CAI is inexpensive to create.

   d. This is a false statement as CAI is rarely effective in training.

7. Select the policy that should be adopted regarding screen design.

   a. Bright colors should be used for text on computer screens.

   b. Color should be used throughout the screen to draw attention to the different fields.

   c. Fields should be in logical order.

   d. All fields on a screen should use the same field type.

8. Recommend a go-live model that will allow the healthcare organization to implement all features of the new information system in one department.

   a. Phased

   b. Pilot

   c. Cutover

   d. Parallel

9. The type of testing that ensures that the information system can handle a large number of transactions at the same time is known as _____.

   a. Volume testing

   b. Integration testing

   c. Parallel testing

   d. Application testing

10. User preparation includes preparing users _____ to use a new information system.

   a. Through training only

   b. Psychologically only

   c. Both through training and psychologically

   d. Both through training and knowledge

References

Amatayakul, M. K. 2017. *Health IT and EHRS: Principles and Practice.* Chicago: AHIMA.

American Health Information Management Association. 2020. Certifications & Careers. https://www.ahima.org/certification-careers/certifications/chda/.

American Health Information Management Association. 2017. *Pocket Glossary of Health Information Management and Technology*, 5th ed. Chicago: AHIMA.

Florida Institute of Technology. 2020. Information Systems vs. Information Technology. https://www.floridatechonline.com/blog/information-technology/information-systems-vs -information-technology/.

PCD Group. 2018. The Pros and Cons of Custom Software vs. Off-the-Shelf Solutions. http://pcdgroup.com/the-pros-and-cons-of-custom-software-vs-off-the-shelf-solutions/.

Chapter 6

Computerization in Health Informatics and Information Management

Learning Objectives

- Identify the information systems needed to support efficient operations in the health information management (HIM) department.
- Describe the role of health informatics in the delivery and evaluation of healthcare services.
- Explain the skills and knowledge needed to perform health analytics and other electronic functions in HIIM.
- Differentiate between the various software products used in the HIM department.
- Improve the quality of the data within the HIM systems.

Key Terms

Analytics (Data)
Automated codebook encoder
Birth certificate information system
Cancer registry
Cancer registry information system
Chart deficiency system
Chart locator system
Chart tracking system
Chief clinical informatics officer (CCIO)

Clinical documentation improvement (CDI) system
Computer-assisted coding (CAC) system
Data analytics
Dictation system
Disclosure of health information
Disclosure management system
Efficiency
Effectiveness

Encoder
Expander
Grouper
Health informatics
Healthcare quality indicator system
Natural language processing (NLP)
Rules-based encoder
Trauma registry software
Transcription system

Health information management (HIM) is an allied health profession that is responsible for ensuring the availability, accuracy, and protection of the clinical information that is needed to deliver healthcare services and to make appropriate healthcare-related decisions. A closely related field, **health informatics** is the scientific discipline that is concerned with the cognitive, information-processing, and communication tasks of healthcare practice, education, and research, including the information science and technology to support these tasks. Health informatics is an interprofessional specialty that exists at the confluence of three major domains: health, information science and technology, and social and behavioral science. As with all other health professions, health informatics is the practice of using data, information, and knowledge for clinical care, scientific inquiry, decision making, and problem solving to improve the health, safety, and effectiveness of those working and being cared for within the system of health care delivery (CAHIIM 2020).

Campbell, et al. 2018 states "Health informatics is a broad aspect of the development, implementation, and support of clinical information using various technologies". This collaboration between people, processes, and information technology help the healthcare industry utilize reliable and valid data to improve healthcare services. "Informatics" is a term that has been added to many HIM educational programs to indicate that more knowledge of information technology is being incorporated into the HIM curriculum while still maintaining the traditional focus of confidentiality, privacy and security of patient data and medical records, paper or electronic.

A relatively new title of "Health Informaticist" is emerging and that these professionals apply the principles of computer and information science to the advancement of life sciences research, health professions education, public health, and patient care. This multidisciplinary and integrative field focuses on health information technologies (HIT), and involves the computer, cognitive, and social sciences (AMIA 2020).

Specialty tracks within the field of informatics include, but are not limited to:

- Clinical informatics
- Dental informatics
- Nursing informatics
- Public health/population health informatics
- Consumer health informatics
- Pharmacy informatics
- Telemedicine and mobile computing informatics
- (Campbell 2018, AMIA 2020)

Analytics is the ability to use data and information to achieve its strategy, goals, and mission, or, in short, to realize the value of its information is critical to success with information governance. **Data analytics** (DA) is the science of examining raw data with the purpose of drawing conclusions about that information; it is a subset of informatics. It includes data mining, machine learning, development of models, and statistical measurements. Analytics can be descriptive, diagnostic, predictive, or prescriptive. Health Informaticists, through data analytics, provide value to the data by discerning the accurate, comprehensive, and relevant information from extraneous data in order for decision-makers to determine the most effective course of action. Chapter 3 includes more information on data analytics.

The entire culture of HIM is changing to accommodate the increasing use of technology, changing avenues of patient care, and consumer demands upon the healthcare field. As the data they manage are digitized, health information managers are becoming increasingly involved in information systems, automated systems that use computer hardware and software to record, manipulate, store, recover, and disseminate data (that is, an information system that receives and processes input and provides output). Many HIM skills have transferred to this digital environment, such as understanding the content of the health record, coding systems, documentation, and statistics. Other HIM skills have had to evolve, such as to the management of databases rather than the physical paper health record or managing the data dictionary rather than creating a form. It is important for the HIM profession to position itself as the central player in the EHR, data analysis, health information exchange, and other roles created by the digitizing of health information. The combination and depth of these skills make HIM professionals uniquely qualified for the roles discussed in this chapter and a valuable asset to the information technology staff, administration, medical professionals and providers, researchers, and others. As a result, HIM professionals frequently serve as liaisons between the technical information system staff (programmers, network administrators, and so forth), who are skilled in technology but may not understand healthcare, and the clinicians who provide excellent patient care but may not understand information and administrative technology.

As the traditional legal health record becomes more electronic, it is important that HIM professionals lead the transition, implementation, and evaluation of the EHR. The **legal health record (LHR)**, whether paper, electronic, or hybrid, comprises the documents and data elements that a healthcare provider may include in response to legally permissible requests for patient information. If the HIM professional is not involved in these processes, issues related to collection, retention, data quality, security, disclosure of health information, and other data management topics may be ignored or incorrectly implemented, thus increasing the risk of Health Insurance Portability and Accountability Act (HIPAA) violations, reimbursement denials, state licensing problems, lawsuits, and more. These changes are creating new career opportunities for HIM professionals. These opportunities are seen in the roles that HIM professionals are fulfilling today.

The HIM professional must have a broad range of skills in areas including data management, data analysis, system analysis, system implementation, health data structure, documentation requirements, data quality, information system management, privacy and security, coding, and reimbursement. There are other professions that require some of the same skills a HIM professional holds, but there is no other profession that requires the same mix, depth and breadth of these skills.

A recent study of HIM job postings found many of the job postings focused on "documentation, standards, data, health information technology and analytics" (Marc et al. 2017, 25). HIM professionals work in a number of different healthcare settings (hospitals, home health, long-term care facilities, and so forth), some of which are discussed in this chapter:

- Healthcare organizations
- Information system vendors
- Consulting firms
- Government agencies
- Standards developmental organizations
- Educational facilities

The importance and level of various information systems skills that a HIM professional needs depend on the setting in which he or she works. Later in the chapter, some specific HIM roles related to information systems in these settings are covered.

Traditional HIM Information Systems Job Titles and Descriptions

HIM professionals have been active in many information system roles for a number of years, although the variety of these roles is expanding with the evolution of technology and informatics. Many HIM positions are related to technology in one way or another. HIM professionals have long worked in information technology roles within healthcare organizations and vendor sites, including the more traditional information technology roles of systems analyst, system implementation, project manager, system development, technical support, training, and sales. A brief description of these HIM professionals' roles follows:

- Systems analyst—Identifies the stakeholders of an information system as well as the functionality required of a system. Tasks include data collection, data analysis, and developing data flow diagrams. The systems analyst would assist in the reengineering of business processes that would take advantage of the benefits of the system being implemented.
- System implementation—Assists in many aspects of the process, such as systems analysis, developing the request for proposal, selecting systems, setting configurations, training, reengineering, and other steps in the process.

- Project manager—Controls the budget, staff, and other resources allocated to ensure the goals of the system are met.

- System development—Adds value to the programming staff because they know the HIM functions and processes needed. HIM professionals are not computer programmers; however, they frequently help design the system that the programmers will create. For example, a HIM professional assisting in the development process would know that amendments to the EHR or other clinical information system must be documented as such, and the original information must be retained and available only with specific access rights. Their HIM knowledge allows them to determine if the needs of the healthcare organizations and regulatory and accreditation demands are being met.

- Technical support—Assists with technical problems that are encountered with an information system. They identify the source of the problems and take the necessary steps to resolve them. These problems could be inability to access an information system or a function that is not working.

- Information system trainer—Responsible for the development and implementation of the training plan.

- Vendor sales team member—Talks to the HIM purchasers of information systems with an understanding of the daily HIM issues.

Contemporary HIM Information Systems Job Titles

HIM professionals are going beyond the traditional information system roles they have occupied for years. They are now working in roles such as data integrity analyst, data analyst, and other new and evolving roles. Some of these roles include:

- The **chief clinical informatics officer (CCIO)** works with clinical providers, such as physicians and nurses, to lead them in the use of technology to improve quality of care, medical education, and healthcare research (AHIMA 2017a). The CCIO role is a "big picture" role in that the CCIO works to ensure that the technologies needed by the healthcare providers are identified and ultimately implemented.

- The **director of clinical informatics** is the leader in the implementation of the EHR as well as the post-implementation services. The director is the champion for the EHR and works with the implementation team to ensure they have the resources needed (AHIMA 2020).

- A **mapping specialist** creates maps between systems such as vocabularies and classification systems (AHIMA 2020). The mapping specialist must be an expert in both systems so that they can correctly create the maps. For example, in *International Classification of Diseases, Ninth Revision, Clinical Modification* the diagnosis code for pneumonia, unspecified is 486. The code for the same condition is J18.9 in *International Classification of Diseases, Tenth Revision, Clinical Modification*. Not only do the codes from both systems have to be correct when mapping, but also the rules of both systems have to be followed. These codes can be built into information systems facilitating the mapping and the use of the maps for reports, studies, and more.

- The **data integrity analyst** is responsible for ensuring the quality of the data in HIM information systems. Data integrity analysts must be able to apply data and content standards to data collection and data storage. They must be able to maintain the information systems, ensure compliance with legal and accreditation requirements, and be able to analyze data (AHIMA n.d.a).

- The **clinical informatics coordinator** requires knowledge of clinical information systems such as those described in chapter 8. They are experts in the data retrieval needed by healthcare providers while conducting patient care (AHIMA n.d.a).

- The **data analyst** applies his or her skills to manage, analyze, interpret, and transform health data into accurate, consistent, and timely information.
- The **content analyst** designs the clinical information system that will be implemented. Their work is directed by the needs of the users. They are also advocates in the usage of health information technology in healthcare (AHIMA n.d.a).
- The **chief technology officer (CTO)** assists in the development of the healthcare organization's strategic business plan in relation to information systems and technology. Their goal is to ensure the healthcare organization operates effectively and that they are competitive with other healthcare organizations within their community (AHIMA n.d.a).
- The **data quality manager** works with physicians and other healthcare providers to assist them in the achievement of the healthcare organization's data quality goals as needed for coding and reimbursement as well as general documentation throughout the healthcare organization. This role is responsible for the quality management functions at the organization (AHIMA n.d.a);
- The **chief security officer (CSO)** is responsible for protecting data from unauthorized access, alteration, and destruction. This role is responsible for
    - Developing and establishing a compliance program
    - Monitoring state, federal, and local laws as well as proposed regulations
    - Monitoring trends related to security and updating policies

New HIM graduates have learned many of the skills required for these roles in college and will learn more through on-the-job training. Current HIM professionals prepare for these roles in a number of ways, such as going back to school, on-the-job training, and in continuing education programs. A review of the AHIMA Career Map identifies many of these newer positions and their respective progression plans which identifies skills, knowledge, certifications, and experiences necessary (AHIMA 2020).

Roles for the HIM Professional in the Healthcare Arena

Regardless of the HIM professional's role in the delivery of healthcare services, two sets of skills are necessary for HIM professionals—hard skills and soft skills. Hard skills deal with basic areas of technology. These hard skills include:

- Informatics skills involve basic computer literacy; programming basics and languages (SQL and HL7); use of basic office application software including databases, graphics, and spreadsheets; and decision support systems
- Data analytic skills including healthcare statistics and research fundamentals; trend analysis and predictive modeling; financial data and budget analysis
- Data use skills encompass the application of secondary data; data visualization (display) techniques; and the ability to use any technology to collect, store, analyze, and report a wide variety of information

Soft skills refer to more subjective traits that involve perception and more analysis:

- Communication skills not only involve verbal and written forms but also interpersonal skills, collaboration, and understanding what was meant in addition to what was said
- Critical and creative thinking uses logic and reasoning to interpret situations and people, apply principles to processes, and creating new ideas, but also allowing for "thinking outside of the box" when coming up with innovative solutions
- Decision making and judgement aid the ability to choose the best options based upon some type of cost benefit analysis

- Empathy, to recognize and appreciate the emotions and experiences of another person, helps individuals better work with others with different cultural and social backgrounds, physical or emotional states, or socioeconomic status.

New graduates and HIM professionals must be assertive in trying to obtain the soft skills and strengthening their interpersonal skills as experience is the best teacher (Watzlaf 2019, Andriotis 2018).

CHECK YOUR UNDERSTANDING 6.1

1. Mary has become very proficient at identifying the best computers, software, and peripherals for many admitting physicians and their practices to help them improve the delivery of patient care. The best name for this area of expertise is termed:

   a. Data analytics
   b. Health informatics
   c. Clinical documentation improvement
   d. Database administration

2. Sam took many college courses in statistics in his HIM program and is very good at identifying and evaluating trends and patterns of patient care in his role in the Performance Improvement department at ABC Hospital. In what area is he specializing?

   a. Data analytics
   b. Health informatics
   c. Clinical documentation improvement
   d. Database administration

3. Claire works for a private healthcare analytics firm that provides research and support functions to healthcare providers who are implementing population health programs. She typically reviews the provider's data from the last 20 years. Her area of expertise is relating the old ICD-9-CM code(s) to their new respective ICD-10-CM code(s). An appropriate title for her would be:

   a. CDI coordinator
   b. Database administrator
   c. Mapping specialist
   d. Data quality manger

4. ABC Hospital has recently evaluated its information security protocols due to the recent increase in cybersecurity threats. They have developed a new position to oversee the development, implementation, training and enforcement of the cybersecurity department. This position would typically be called:

   a. CEO
   b. CFO
   c. CNO
   d. CSO

5. Identify a "hard skill" that the HIM professional should possess.

   a. Data analytics skills
   b. Critical thinking
   c. Communication
   d. Decision making

Health Information Management Systems Functions

Information systems are critical to the HIM department. Many of the HIM department's processes depend on information systems to function efficiently and effectively. Some of the information systems used by the HIM department staff, such as the master patient index and the financial information system, are available to authorized users throughout the organization. Efficiency and effectiveness are two buzzwords that are used frequently in healthcare. **Efficiency** is how the desired outcome is achieved or produced, particularly without wasting resources, such as time, personnel, and money; **effectiveness** is the degree to which stated outcomes are attained. For example, the proper use of an encoder would be an example of both concepts. It helps the coders assign codes faster and increase their productivity, thereby becoming more efficient coders. It also helps them to be more thorough in review of the documentation to assign more specific codes and/or assign more codes to better reflect the severity of illness of the patient, thereby becoming more effective. While encoder software may initially be expensive, the return on investment would be made up quickly since the coding is performed more efficiently and effectively usually increasing reimbursement due to higher paying MS-DRGs. This allows the billing personnel to submit claims sooner.

Other information systems are designed specifically for HIM functions, which may limit the usage to the HIM department only or for other departments to use to support the HIM department or the health record. Healthcare organizations vary in their organizational structure; as a result, some of these information systems may be used by staff in other departments but in support of HIM. For example, the birth certificate software may be solely used by the HIM department to create and report births occurring in the healthcare organization, whereas the dictation system may be purchased and managed by the HIM department but is used by physicians. All of these HIM information systems greatly improve the efficiency and effectiveness of the HIM department. The HIM information systems include the following:

- Disclosure of health information
- Encoder and grouper system
- Cancer and other registry systems
- Chart location system
- Birth certificate system
- Chart deficiency system
- Transcription system
- Healthcare quality indicators system
- Dictation system
- Computer-assisted coding (CAC) system
- Clinical documentation improvement (CDI) system

This chapter presents an overview of the information systems that support the HIM functions and their functionality, common data elements found in these systems, and reports.

Disclosure of Health Information Systems

The HIM department receives requests for copies of health records on a daily basis. These requests for copies of health records must be logged into the information system to allow for tracking of the status of the request. The **disclosure of information system**, also called release of information, is designed to manage the processing of requests for protected health information (PHI) received and processed by the HIM department. For more on PHI, refer to chapter 12. Use of the information system begins when a new request is entered into it. It continues to track the request as it is processed and acts as a historical database of all requests processed and ultimately used to generate reports.

It also tracks the disclosures made throughout the healthcare organization for reporting purposes. Disclosure is the release, transfer, provision of access to, or divulging in any manner of information outside the healthcare organization holding the information. This tracking is required by the Health Insurance Portability and Accountability Act (HIPAA). The covered entities (discussed in chapter 212) must provide the patient with an accounting of disclosures upon request. The disclosure management system may be part of the disclosure of health information system or it may be a separate information system used by HIM and non-HIM departments. In addition to disclosures, it may also track requests for amendments to PHI as well as restrictions to disclosures. Some disclosure of health information systems are built into the EHR but there are still standalone information systems. If a separate disclosure management system is used, it would also have a link to the hospital information system to populate basic patient demographic information. It would keep up with who received information, what information was provided, date of release, any charge for accounting of disclosures, and more.

Disclosure of Health Information System Functionality

The disclosure of health information system is a valuable tool for the HIM staff. Once the requests for copies of health records are entered into the disclosure of health information system, the data can be used for many different purposes to support the workflow.

The disclosure of health information staff also can use the information system to check on the status of requests. The staff will be able to determine where in the process the request is and to whom the request has been assigned. The patient's name or health record number can be entered and the appropriate request opened to identify status and the personnel responsible.

Throughout the release process, the status of a request must be updated and kept current by disclosure of health information staff at all times. The status can include details about issues encountered, a need for review by risk management, a need for a health record or microfilm to be pulled, or other action required. Once the health record has been copied (in hard-copy or electronically) or reports printed, the request should be marked as complete. Completed requests generally include an indicator showing that the request is in the complete status, the date processed, and specifically what has been sent. Individual reports and dates of reports would also be entered. Based on the number of copies and other activities, the disclosure of health information staff would also record any changes that were applied. See figure 6.1 for a workflow diagram of a typical disclosure of health information process.

The disclosure of health information system provides a number of reports and statistics for the HIM management team. Some of the data provided to the management team include the following:

- Requests that have not been processed
- Requests that have been processed
- Turnaround time of requests
- Revenue collected
- Accounts receivable
- Productivity by individual staff members
- Overall productivity
- List of frequent requesters
- Multiple customized letters

If the supervisor receives a complaint from a requester regarding the inability to obtain copies of health records, the disclosure of health information system would be the first place to start investigating the situation. The disclosure of health information system also can be used toward the healthcare organization's HIPAA compliance because it provides some of the information needed to respond to an accounting of disclosure request. This accounting report includes by whom and when request was made; the specific information requested; the process to release; when, how, and

Figure 6.1. Disclosure of health information process

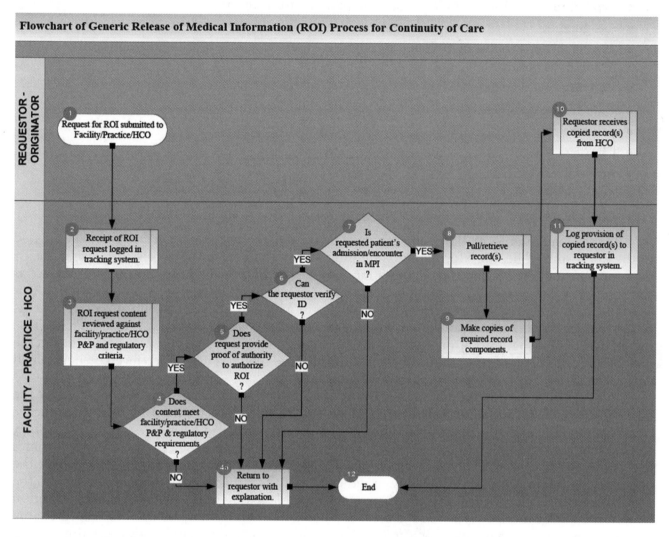

Source: Betz et al. p2013.

to whom information was transmitted; and more. The disclosure of health information system and the disclosure management system work together. Management may periodically archive old requests in the disclosure of health information system, but the completed requests should not be deleted until after retention requirements are met so that the disclosure management system can use the data to create reports. HIPAA requires accounting of disclosure information to be available to the patient for three years, so that is the minimum amount of time for the requests to be maintained.

Common data elements found in a disclosure of health information system are:

- Patient name
- Health record number
- Patient type
- Date request received
- Type of requester
- Name of requester
- Name of contact at requester

- Address of requester
- Type of request (for example, insurance, patient, attorney, or patient care)
- Assigned to
- Action taken (request completed, type of letter sent, records requested, valid authorization needed, and more)
- Date action taken
- Date request completed
- Information sent (specific documents and dates of reports)
- Charges
- Amount paid
- Amount due
- Comments

The basic patient information, such as name and health record number, are frequently populated in the disclosure of health information system by an interface from the admission, discharge, or transfer information system, thus eliminating the need to enter this information. An interface is the zone between different information systems across which users want to pass information (for example, a computer program written to exchange information between the information systems or the graphic display of an application program designed to make the program easier to use). This link between the two information systems improves data quality because there is consistency in the data and reduced risk of typographical error. Typically, the requests can be retrieved by items such as patient name, health record number, or requester name.

Tables are an important part of the disclosure of health information system. Some tables are the default within the information system while others can be set up and customized by the healthcare organization. For example, the user only has to enter the name and address of a requester once, thus managing time wisely. After the initial entry, the user is able to select the requester from a drop-down box or other graphical user interface tool. This customization function improves the efficiency of the processes making it easier and faster for the employee to complete the task. If the requester is from a large organization, there can be a table listing individuals in that organization so that the copies are forwarded to the correct person. Tables also may be used to record charge information, such as charge per copy, microfilm, certification, and other chargeable actions.

Another use of tables is identifying all of the individual forms or groups of forms that may be released. The table may list discharge summary, history and physical examination, operative report, pathology report, laboratory report, and other forms individually. The disclosure of health information system may feature requests for common groupings of reports, such as the entire health record or the discharge summary and history and physical examination. Tables help to save the user a significant amount of time because the user does not have to individually type each document released. Drop-down boxes or check boxes containing the individual documents or sets of documents also allow for consistent data entry.

The disclosure of health information system will allow disclosure of health information staff to pull up a work queue showing the requests that need to be processed. With the use of the electronic health record (EHR), more of the requests can be fulfilled without the need for the paper health record. disclosure of health information staff members just need to print, fax, or generate a CD (or other portable electronic storage media) of the requested documents from the appropriate information system. Once the number of pages and other chargeable actions are known, the disclosure of health information coordinator can post the charges into the information system and, once received, post payment.

The disclosure of health information software can perform many other tasks. For instance, the disclosure of health information system reminds the ROI staff of the need to perform maintenance tasks on the information system, which can include backups, deletion of old requests, or archiving of completed requests to speed processing.

Disclosure of Health Information Reporting

Reporting is an important part of a disclosure of health information system. Reports are used by disclosure of health information or HIM staff and to communicate with requesters. In a paper environment, the disclosure of health information coordinators can generate a list of health records to be pulled so that the appropriate contents of the record can be copied. This list can be sorted into terminal digit or other numeric or alphabetic order to facilitate the retrieval process. Depending on the structure of the department, the ROI or file area staff can use this list to retrieve the paper records.

Customized letters are critical to the disclosure of health information system. Customized letters and forms may be used to communicate with the requester for many purposes, including to:

- Notify requester that the healthcare organization does not have a record of the patient being treated at the healthcare organization or on that date
- Remind requesters that they have an outstanding balance for copies of health records
- Request that copies of health records be paid prior to their release
- Provide cover letter for health records being sent
- Notify requester that the authorization is invalid
- Notify requester that an authorization is needed
- Notify requester that there will be a delay in the release of the information
- Notify requester that the health records will be released as soon as the healthcare organization has received prepayment for copies
- Generate invoices for the copies of the health record
- Generate reminder invoices when payment is not received in a timely manner

HIM department managers monitor the efficiency of the disclosure of health information staff through a multitude of management reports. These reports provide information on various functions including turnaround times, productivity, backlogs, revenue, and accounts receivable, to name a few. Depending on the information contained in the report, the report can include requests by employee, by requester type, by specific requester, or all requests. For example, a report on the average turnaround time for all requests or for BlueCross BlueShield requests can be obtained. The manager also can track the turnaround times by employee, which can be used in performance evaluations and other management monitoring. Many of these reports come pre-packaged with the software, but many information systems allow users to develop and customize their own routine and ad hoc reports.

Encoder and Grouper

Healthcare organizations must assign diagnosis and procedure codes to every patient encounter. These codes are submitted to the insurance company on the bill. The **encoder** is specialty software used by coders to select the appropriate code for the diagnosis(es) and procedure(s) supported by the health record. There are two types of encoders. A **rules-based encoder** requires the user to type in the name or portion of the name of the diagnosis or procedure. This entry into the encoder generates a list of suggestions from which the coder selects. For example, if the coder types in pneu-, the encoder may suggest pneumonia and pneumonitis. From there the coder scrolls down until the proper code is selected. The **automated codebook encoder** lists diagnoses and procedures in alphabetic order much like the alphabetic index located in the *International Classification of Diseases, Tenth Revision, Clinical Modification* (ICD-10-CM) and *Current Procedural Terminology* (CPT) codebooks. This similarity eases the transition from the book to the encoder.

The **grouper** is a computer program that uses specific data elements to assign the diagnostic and procedural codes entered into the encoder into the appropriate Medicare severity diagnosis-related group (MS-DRG) or other diagnosis-related group (DRG). The grouper uses the appropriate grouping software for the insurer assigned to the patient. The most common groupers are the MS-DRG grouper and ambulatory payment classification (APC) grouper; however, other insurers, including some Medicaid programs, have developed their own groupers for use in determining payment to the healthcare organization. The MS-DRG or other DRG indicates the amount of reimbursement owed to the healthcare organization from the insurer. The grouper software is connected to the billing information system so it is important that the HIM staff have a strong relationship with the billing and finance personnel.

Coding quality and MS-DRG assignment are not ensured using an encoder because the code selected is only as good as the data entered into the information system. It is the responsibility of the coder to identify the correct diagnoses and procedures to be coded and entered into the encoder appropriately.

Encoder and Grouper System Functionality

One of the biggest advantages in the use of an encoder or grouper is prompts. For example, if a higher-paying MS-DRG can be assigned with the addition of a specific diagnosis, specific procedure, complication and comorbidity, or major complication and comorbidity, then the computer will ask the coder if any of them are present. The grouper allows the coder to re-sequence the principal diagnosis when more than one diagnosis meets the definition of the principal diagnosis. The coding guidelines allow the healthcare organization to choose any of the diagnoses as the principal as long as it qualifies. The encoder can assign the ICD-10-CM, ICD-10-PCS, CPT, and Healthcare Common Procedural Coding System (HCPCS) codes required on the patient claim. These assigned codes must be validated through the Medicare Code Editor, the National Correct Coding Initiative, and other edits. These edits will look for invalid codes, illogical codes, nonspecific codes, and other possible errors. For example, the coder cannot give a newborn code to an adult and cannot assign a hysterectomy code to a male. These edits are designed to catch errors before they can be submitted on a claim improperly and to improve the quality of the code assignment.

Coders are also permitted to manually enter codes into the information system rather than looking them up each time. For the more frequent diagnoses, such as diabetes or dehydration, this is a more efficient method. Once entered, the information system will then confirm and validate the code.

Common data elements in an encoder or grouper are:

- Admitting diagnosis
- Principal diagnosis
- Secondary diagnoses
- Principal procedure
- Secondary procedure
- Age of patient (or date of birth)
- Discharge disposition
- Gender
- Patient name
- Health record number
- Account number

The encoder and grouper are usually linked to the hospital's financial information system so that the codes can be automatically transferred to that information system for billing. Without this link, the coder would have to re-enter codes into the financial information system. This double entry leaves room for data entry errors, which would in turn cause problems with billing and reimbursement.

Encoder and Grouper System Reporting

The encoder or grouper does not contribute heavily to reporting. Rather, the encoder is more about assigning codes and MS-DRGs using edits to assist the coder in proper assignment of codes and other information transferred to the hospital financial system. However, if needed, the information system may be used to generate a report listing all of the codes and respective MS-DRGs or APCs assigned.

CHECK YOUR UNDERSTANDING 6.2

1. In order to improve the efficiency and accuracy of the coding staff, the Operations Manager and Coding Supervisor have decided to update the coding procedures. Identify the software programs they should consider using to assign the diagnosis and procedure codes.

   a. Registry
   b. Disclosure of health information
   c. Encoder
   d. Grouper

2. Todd, the Coding Supervisor, wants to make the transition to the new coding software easier for the staff. Since the majority of the coders have preferred to use their code books rather than an automated system. Identify the type of encoder that mimics a codebook.

   a. Rules-based encoder
   b. Disclosure of health information
   c. Automated codebook encoder   *Rules based*
   d. Disclosure management

3. The hospital's Billing Manager is evaluating the types of Medicare patients who are most frequently admitted through the Emergency Department and the economic impact that has on the facility. What software program is designed to place similar diagnoses codes into organized categories and calculate reimbursement depending on diagnoses and procedural codes is a(n) _____.

   a. Grouper
   b. Disclosure of health information
   c. Disclosure management
   d. Encoder

4. A new law firm started representing accident and medical clients earlier this year. Many of their requests for health records have been returned to them because of incompleteness due to lack of patient signatures on the forms or providing inaccurate dates of treatment or service. Which information system is used to notify this law firm of invalid authorization?

   a. Grouper
   b. Disclosure management
   c. Registry
   d. Encoder

5. A patient wants to know who has requested copies of their medical record. He has fired the first attorney he worked with and no longer them to have access to his health information. Identify the information system that would keep track of what health information was sent to authorized requesters?

   a. Grouper
   b. Registries
   c. Disclosure management
   d. Encoder

Cancer and Other Registries

There are many types of registries currently found in healthcare. A registry is a collection of care information related to a specific disease, condition, or procedure that makes health record information available for analysis and comparison. These registries track conditions such as cancer, diabetes, trauma, and transplants. Although registry software across these different diseases and situations has similarities, each has its own unique characteristics. All registries are designed to record data on patients who meet criteria for inclusion in the registry. These registries would generally require basic demographic information, reporting, treatment, description of condition, and frequently long-term patient tracking. Commonly found data elements across registries include:

- Patient name
- Health record number
- Dates of service
- Physician
- Date of birth
- Date of diagnosis

Two common registries will be discussed in more detail—cancer (tumor) and trauma registries.

Cancer (Tumor) Registry

The **cancer registry information system** tracks information about the patient's cancer from the time of diagnosis to the patient's death. The cancer registry information systems are extremely complex and track very detailed information regarding diagnosis and treatment. A **cancer registry** is a population-based dataset reporting to state and national agencies to track the epidemiology of the diseases and the treatment and outcomes of health and medical care of patients (CDC, 2019). Some of the common data elements unique to the cancer registry include:

- Site of cancer
- Type of cancer
- Treatment received
- Date of last contact
- TNM (tumor, node, metastasis) stage
- Number of lymph nodes involved
- Behavior type
- Date of death
- Grade of neoplasm
- Size of mass
- Physician name
- Accession number
- *International Classification of Diseases for Oncology* (ICD-O) codes (CDC 2017)

Cancer Registry Functionality

The cancer registry can electronically submit a file containing the data required for state cancer reporting. Once data on all the identified cancer cases for a designated time period are verified by the cancer registrar (or designee) of the healthcare organization, a programmed report is automatically generated and transmitted to the respective state-wide cancer registry normally housed in the state's Department of Health. As the patient's treatment and clinical follow-up progress, this information is entered into the registry so that it reflects the patient's current treatment and status of the cancer.

Figure 6.2 shows an information system that supports pathology analysis for staging the cancer to determine the severity of a diagnosis for a particular case.

Figure 6.2. Information system used for cancer staging

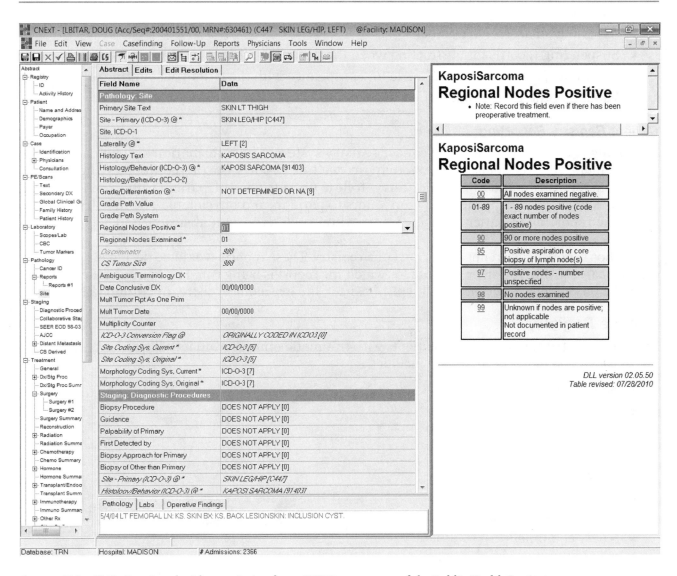

Source: CNet 2018. Reprinted with permission from CNET, a program of the Public Health Institute.

Edits assist the cancer registrar in the data entry and cancer staging. These edits, which vary widely, are key to ensuring the quality of the data in the registry. For example, an edit can notify the user that data, such as the discharge date, has been entered in an inappropriate format. It should be entered in MMDDYYYY format rather than MMDDYY. An edit may also verify that a code number is valid. Cancer registry software can also assist the registrar in the patient follow-up process. The software tracks the last contact date and manages letters and other activities related to the follow-up process.

Cancer registry software typically provides many functions for the registry staff. Some examples of this functionality are:

- Checking the Social Security Death Index to see if the patient died
- Transferring data to the state registry
- Performing edit checks on data entered

- Performing various cancer staging methods to determine severity of the illness
- Providing links to National Cancer Institute's (NCI) SEER (surveillance epidemiology and end results) manuals
- Referencing previous versions of staging systems such as Facility Oncology Registry Data Standards (FORDS)
- Assigning an accession number
- Suspending records for abstracting when the documentation is incomplete
- Providing a list of disclosures made for compliance with the HIPAA accounting of disclosure
- Validating the ICD-O code

Cancer Registry Reporting

Reporting is a key function of the cancer registry system. The information system can provide management reports such as productivity as well as reports on the content of the registry. Common reports include life expectancy, follow-up rate, list of patients due for follow-up, patients lost to follow-up, and follow-up letters to patients and physicians. The registry will also allow the reporting of patient-specific information such as patient abstracts and accounting of disclosures.

Ad hoc reporting is an important part of a registry. These reports would be designed specifically for a research project or other purpose for which the report is being run. For example, these reports could be based on site of cancer, cell type of cancer, life expectancy, or treatment modalities.

Trauma Registry

Trauma registry software tracks patients with traumatic injuries from initial trauma treatment to death. Data elements in this system include:

- Site of injury
- Type of injury
- How injury occurred
- Date of injury
- Time of injury
- Work-related injury
- ICD-10-CM and ICD-10-PCS codes
- Safety equipment
- Registry number
- Autopsy performed
- Emergency department arrival time (Florida Department of Health 2017a)

Trauma Registry Functionality

The trauma registry software also tracks care provided to the patient before and during hospitalization, as well as posthospital care. The trauma registry allows the registrar to code ICD-10-CM diagnosis codes to the injuries. This registry, like the cancer registry, requires follow-up of patients.

Trauma Registry Reporting

Trauma registry software packages generally include report writers for ad hoc reporting. The common reports for the trauma registry would be similar to those of the cancer registry, such as outcomes, follow-up rates, and best practices for patient care. The information system would provide statistics on cause of injuries, types of injuries, and other descriptive statistics.

Chart Locator System

The **chart locator system,** also called **chart tracking system**, is designed to identify the current location of the paper health record. This tracking is important because paper records are moved from place to place for patient care, quality reviews, coding, and many other purposes. The Joint Commission regulations require health records to be readily accessible for patient care. The chart locator supports that mandate. *Because of the transition to the EHR, the chart locator system will continue to become less important to the HIM department and will eventually be phased out as the paper record becomes obsolete.*

Chart Locator Functionality

The purpose of the chart locator is to provide the ability to track the location of the health record from one location to another. All of the functions of this information system support this objective. The chart locator is valuable to both HIM department staff and management. The data in the chart locator system identify where the record is currently physically located, how long it has been in that location, when the record is due for return to the HIM department, when a health record is overdue to be returned, and who checked out the health record. These data are used to generate a list of health records checked out to a location for auditing to ensure that the data in the chart locator system is accurate.

The emergency department and other locations may need 1 record or 50 records. When checking out multiple records to one location, the user only has to enter the location once and then enter all of the records being relocated. This entry of health records into the chart locator system is frequently supported by barcodes, which, at a minimum, contain the patient's health record number and volume number of the health record. Barcodes speed the data entry process and improve the quality of the data entered, thus improving the efficiency and effectiveness of checking in and out health records.

Common data elements in the chart locator are:

- Patient name
- Health record number
- Volume
- Location to which the health record is checked out
- Date record checked out
- Date health record returned
- Who checked out/checked in the record

The information system may provide the previous locations of the health record. This may be helpful in locating lost health records because it can help the user determine where in the process the health record has been and where it may have gone. Past locations may also be useful in privacy incident investigation or other risk management investigations to know who has had access to the health record. For example, if an employee has been accused of improperly disclosing a patient's PHI, it would be important to know if the record has been in a location to which that employee would have had access.

Data quality is important because a significant amount of time can be wasted looking for health records when the paper health record is not where the chart locator indicates. Tables, which are pre-programmed lists and options for a user to select from, can be used to save time and improve data quality. For example, only approved locations would be programmed into the "Locations" table. For example, all nursing units, emergency department, coding, and so forth. As a result, the user would choose the location desired from a drop-down box.

These tables are generally user defined during the implementation. The user can update the tables as needed to keep the content of the data current. To keep the chart location system accurate, routine audits should be conducted. These audits would confirm that records checked out to a location are actually at that location. It would also identify health records located outside the permanent file that had not been checked out at all.

Chart Locator Reporting

Management uses the chart locator reporting for multiple purposes, including identification of most user requests of health records, productivity tracking, identification of trends in the volume of health record retrievals, and identification of areas of the healthcare organization for which records are not returned in a timely manner.

Chart Deficiency System

Physicians and other clinicians have certain documentation requirements mandated by healthcare organization policy and medical staff rules and regulations. Documentation requirements are based on the accreditation regulations, state licensure regulations, federal requirements, and other standards or regulations that the healthcare organization is subject to. The specific documentation requirements mandate when reports such as the history and physical examination should be dictated or written. It should also mandate the content of the various reports analyzed and the deadline by which the entire health record should be complete. This deadline would include the presence of all required documents and the authentication of these documents. If the health record comes to the HIM department with a deficiency, then the documentation omission is recorded and tracked in the **chart deficiency system**. Deficiencies can be in paper, imaged, or electronic records depending on the information system used. With imaged or electronic records, the physician can complete the deficiency from his or her office, home, or other location. With paper records, the physician must come to the designated area in the healthcare organization. The chart deficiency system should be linked to the hospital information system so that patient name, discharge date, and other demographic information are maintained and automatically populated. With the implementation of the EHR, the need for a separate chart deficiency system is reduced or eliminated. The limited deficiency analysis needed in the future will be built into the EHR.

Chart Deficiency Functionality

The chart deficiency system is utilized by both staff and management. The chart deficiency system is used by staff to record what deficiencies a physician, or other clinician, has on specific health records. When these deficiencies are completed by the physician, the chart deficiency system is updated to reflect the change. The chart deficiency system will identify the incomplete records by physician so that the physician can be notified for completion. The following data elements are common:

- Patient name
- Health record number
- Discharge date
- Physician needing to complete deficiency
- Type of document with deficiency (for example, history and physical examination, discharge summary, or progress note)
- Type of deficiency (for example, sign or dictate)
- Date of surgery
- Comments
- Date physician last worked on records

When a patient is discharged from the hospital, the health record is automatically reviewed for deficiencies. When a deficiency is identified, the analyst is generally able to retrieve basic demographic information of the patient from the chart deficiency system. The analyst then enters other pertinent information, such as discharge date, physician, document type, type of deficiency, date of surgery, and any other information needed into the chart deficiency system. In a paper environment, sticky tabs or flags are frequently posted on the health record to indicate to the physician where a signature is needed. In an electronic environment, a work queue would route the deficiencies automatically to the assigned physician. The physician could then automatically complete all needed deficiencies from home, the office, or anywhere in the hospital.

When the physician dictates, signs, or completes the deficiency, the analyst is able to delete or update the status of the deficiency. An example of updating the deficiency would be to change the deficiency from dictated to transcribed or from transcribed to signed. Frequently there is an interface between the chart deficiency system and the transcription system to automatically update the transcription deficiency. There may also be a link between the dictation system and the chart deficiency system to automatically update the status when a report had been dictated or transcribed. This link would also help staff locate paper records for completion.

Data quality is critical to the chart deficiency system. Health records inappropriately entered into the system can also have a negative impact on the accreditation or state/federal regulatory statistics as well as customer service. To improve data quality, routine audits of the health records should be conducted to ensure that records are still incomplete and available to the physician.

Chart Deficiency System Reporting

Management uses the chart deficiency system to age the deficiencies for the Joint Commission tracking. The chart deficiency system can generate a report listing all physicians suspended for delinquent health records (an incomplete record not finished or made complete within the time frame determined by the medical staff of the healthcare organization), track when physicians are suspended (for use in medical staff credentialing), and monitor the volume of deficiencies by physician and service. A list of all health records in the information system can be printed out for use in auditing the quality of the data in the chart deficiency system.

The chart deficiency system also has customizable letters. These letters can be used for many purposes including notifying physicians that they have a deadline to complete health records, that they have been suspended for delinquent health records (or other penalty for noncompliance with medical staff rules and regulations), or to thank physicians for completing their health record(s).

CHECK YOUR UNDERSTANDING 6.3

1. Dr. Radcliffe wants to determine if there are health disparities in treatment protocols in her patients by comparing in-situ neoplasms and malignant neoplasms by using the assigned ICD-O codes. Identify the information system she would query to identify treatment outcomes.

   a. Trauma registry
   b. Chart locator
   c. Disclosure of health information
   d. Cancer registry

2. ABC Hospital wants to work with their state department of health to track diabetic patients to help monitor population health issues and develop comprehensive programs to improve patient's lives. Identify the software that tracks patients who meet criteria for inclusion such as a specific disease or treatment.

   a. Registry
   b. Chart deficiency
   c. Chart locator
   d. Disclosure of health information

(Continued)

CHECK YOUR UNDERSTANDING 6.3 (*Continued*)

3. XYZ University Hospital is involved in a myriad of medical research projects. Many interns are involved in gathering patient information from previous admissions, some dating back several decades. These reviews occur in the medical library of the hospital. The older records are paper-based. Identify the information system that tracks the location of the paper health record?

    a. Chart deficiency
    b. Chart locator
    c. Disclosure of health information
    d. Disclosure management

4. Dr. Smith wants to determine the percentage of patients who are diagnosed with metastatic colon cancer to evaluate the effectiveness of screening coloscopies. Identify the information system that she would use that collects the TNM stage.

    a. Chart locator
    b. Disclosure management
    c. Disclosure of health information
    d. Cancer registry software

5. Dr. Edmunds is working with local high schools to develop an educational program about distracted driving for high school students taking their driver's license exams. He wants to highlight the types of injuries young people typically experience because of car accidents. Identify the software that can identify all patients admitted in 20XX due to injuries resulting from motor vehicle accidents (MVAs).

    a. Trauma registry
    b. Disclosure management
    c. Disclosure of health information
    d. Cancer registry software

Birth Certificate System

For years, birth certificates were typed on a typewriter and manually sent to the local health department. Now, after the HIM staff interviews the mother or other parents or guardians and reviews the health record, the birth certificate data are entered into a state-approved **birth certificate information system**. This software reports births occurring in the healthcare organization to the state health agency. Birth certificate software will capture the minimum data set established by the National Center for Health Statistics (NCHS) and any state-required data. The most recent update for the content of US birth certificates was in 2003 (NCHS 2017). Figure 6.3 shows the standard content of a US birth certificate.

Birth Certificate System Functionality

Functionality common in birth certificate information systems includes:

- Collecting data mandated by NCHS
- Reporting standard information such as name of healthcare organization automatically
- Allowing users to choose from obstetrical physicians table

- Capturing demographic information from hospital information system to improve efficiency
- Preventing omissions of required data before birth certificate is sent to the state using mandatory fields and edit checks
- Submitting birth certificate data to the state or local health department
- Submitting parent's request for social security number to the Social Security Administration
- Printing out data captured for parent(s) to proof
- Creating birth log, eliminating need for paper log in labor and delivery
- Using drop-down boxes to improve data consistency
- Using edits to improve data quality
- Allowing parent(s) to order copy of birth certificate (Florida Department of Health 2017b)

Some electronic birth registration systems have incorporated the preparation of fetal death reports as well. Additionally, most information systems allow the healthcare organization to download the data on their births to a spreadsheet so that they can create their own reports.

Many birth certificate fields have check boxes for completion. For example, the field for infections present or treated during pregnancy lists gonorrhea, syphilis, chlamydia, hepatitis B, hepatitis C, and none of these.

The birth certificate coordinator would document all infections that apply. See figure 6.4 for an example of an intake screen for the information required for a birth certificate.

Birth Certificate System Reporting

The birth certificate systems used may be developed and provided to the healthcare organizations by the state or may be purchased from a vendor. State healthcare organization information systems are designed to focus on capturing and reporting birth certificate data. Vendor products may have more management and reporting tools than the state systems. These management tools may include reports such as productivity and turnaround times.

The birth certificate system may also generate statistical reports such as caesarean section rate or trending births rates. The key reporting capability, however, is the ability to report the births to the state in the approved format. The state may use the birth certificate data reported via the birth certificate system to feed other databases, such as immunization registry to enhance tracking of childhood immunizations.

Dictation and Transcription Systems

The **dictation system** is used by physicians to dictate various medical reports, such as history and physical examinations, discharge summaries, radiology reports, autopsy reports, catheterization reports, and other designated reports into the dictation system. The HIM department uses the dictation system to manage the dictated reports and to monitor the amount of transcription that is pending.

Dictating is the process of recording a physician's voice as he or she verbally describes a scenario, problem note, or some other type of report that is recorded electronically. The physician uses the dictation system to dictate, and the HIM department uses the system to transcribe the report.

Physicians and other appropriate clinical staff dictate into the healthcare organization's dictation system. The transcriptionist then types the actual report using the **transcription system**. Transcription is the process of deciphering the provider's recorded dictation and typing the medical document. The transcription system should be interfaced with the hospital information system so that the patient name, health record, and date of service are already populated within the information system. As voice recognition and the EHR are implemented throughout the healthcare organization, the dependence on this transcription system is reduced.

Figure 6.3. Content of US birth certificate of live birth

U.S. STANDARD CERTIFICATE OF LIVE BIRTH

LOCAL FILE NO.   BIRTH NUMBER:

C H I L D	1. CHILD'S NAME (First, Middle, Last, Suffix)		2. TIME OF BIRTH (24 hr)	3. SEX	4. DATE OF BIRTH (Mo/Day/Yr)
	5. FACILITY NAME (If not institution, give street and number)	6. CITY, TOWN, OR LOCATION OF BIRTH	7. COUNTY OF BIRTH		

M O T H E R	8a. MOTHER'S CURRENT LEGAL NAME (First, Middle, Last, Suffix)	8b. DATE OF BIRTH (Mo/Day/Yr)
	8c. MOTHER'S NAME PRIOR TO FIRST MARRIAGE (First, Middle, Last, Suffix)	8d. BIRTHPLACE (State, Territory, or Foreign Country)
	9a. RESIDENCE OF MOTHER-STATE 9b. COUNTY	9c. CITY, TOWN, OR LOCATION
	9d. STREET AND NUMBER	9e. APT. NO. 9f. ZIP CODE 9g. INSIDE CITY LIMITS? ☐ Yes ☐ No

F A T H E R	10a. FATHER'S CURRENT LEGAL NAME (First, Middle, Last, Suffix)	10b. DATE OF BIRTH (Mo/Day/Yr)	10c. BIRTHPLACE (State, Territory, or Foreign Country)

CERTIFIER	11. CERTIFIER'S NAME: _____ TITLE: ☐ MD ☐ DO ☐ HOSPITAL ADMIN. ☐ CNM/CM ☐ OTHER MIDWIFE ☐ OTHER (Specify)_____	12. DATE CERTIFIED ____/____/____ MM DD YYYY	13. DATE FILED BY REGISTRAR ____/____/____ MM DD YYYY

INFORMATION FOR ADMINISTRATIVE USE

M O T H E R	14. MOTHER'S MAILING ADDRESS: ☐ Same as residence, or: State: City, Town, or Location:
	Street & Number: Apartment No.: Zip Code:
	15. MOTHER MARRIED? (At birth, conception, or any time between) ☐ Yes ☐ No IF NO, HAS PATERNITY ACKNOWLEDGEMENT BEEN SIGNED IN THE HOSPITAL? ☐ Yes ☐ No	16. SOCIAL SECURITY NUMBER REQUESTED FOR CHILD? ☐ Yes ☐ No	17. FACILITY ID. (NPI)
	18. MOTHER'S SOCIAL SECURITY NUMBER:	19. FATHER'S SOCIAL SECURITY NUMBER:

INFORMATION FOR MEDICAL AND HEALTH PURPOSES ONLY

M O T H E R

20. MOTHER'S EDUCATION (Check the box that best describes the highest degree or level of school completed at the time of delivery)	21. MOTHER OF HISPANIC ORIGIN? (Check the box that best describes whether the mother is Spanish/Hispanic/Latina. Check the "No" box if mother is not Spanish/Hispanic/Latina)	22. MOTHER'S RACE (Check one or more races to indicate what the mother considers herself to be)
☐ 8th grade or less	☐ No, not Spanish/Hispanic/Latina	☐ White
☐ 9th - 12th grade, no diploma	☐ Yes, Mexican, Mexican American, Chicana	☐ Black or African American
☐ High school graduate or GED completed	☐ Yes, Puerto Rican	☐ American Indian or Alaska Native (Name of the enrolled or principal tribe)_____
☐ Some college credit but no degree	☐ Yes, Cuban	☐ Asian Indian
☐ Associate degree (e.g., AA, AS)	☐ Yes, other Spanish/Hispanic/Latina	☐ Chinese
☐ Bachelor's degree (e.g., BA, AB, BS)	(Specify)_____	☐ Filipino
☐ Master's degree (e.g., MA, MS, MEng, MEd, MSW, MBA)		☐ Japanese
☐ Doctorate (e.g., PhD, EdD) or Professional degree (e.g., MD, DDS, DVM, LLB, JD)		☐ Korean
		☐ Vietnamese
		☐ Other Asian (Specify)_____
		☐ Native Hawaiian
		☐ Guamanian or Chamorro
		☐ Samoan
		☐ Other Pacific Islander (Specify)_____
		☐ Other (Specify)_____

F A T H E R

23. FATHER'S EDUCATION (Check the box that best describes the highest degree or level of school completed at the time of delivery)	24. FATHER OF HISPANIC ORIGIN? (Check the box that best describes whether the father is Spanish/Hispanic/Latino. Check the "No" box if father is not Spanish/Hispanic/Latino)	25. FATHER'S RACE (Check one or more races to indicate what the father considers himself to be)
☐ 8th grade or less	☐ No, not Spanish/Hispanic/Latino	☐ White
☐ 9th - 12th grade, no diploma	☐ Yes, Mexican, Mexican American, Chicano	☐ Black or African American
☐ High school graduate or GED completed	☐ Yes, Puerto Rican	☐ American Indian or Alaska Native (Name of the enrolled or principal tribe)_____
☐ Some college credit but no degree	☐ Yes, Cuban	☐ Asian Indian
☐ Associate degree (e.g., AA, AS)	☐ Yes, other Spanish/Hispanic/Latino	☐ Chinese
☐ Bachelor's degree (e.g., BA, AB, BS)	(Specify)_____	☐ Filipino
☐ Master's degree (e.g., MA, MS, MEng, MEd, MSW, MBA)		☐ Japanese
☐ Doctorate (e.g., PhD, EdD) or Professional degree (e.g., MD, DDS, DVM, LLB, JD)		☐ Korean
		☐ Vietnamese
		☐ Other Asian (Specify)_____
		☐ Native Hawaiian
		☐ Guamanian or Chamorro
		☐ Samoan
		☐ Other Pacific Islander (Specify)_____
		☐ Other (Specify)_____

Mother's Name — Mother's Medical Record No.

26. PLACE WHERE BIRTH OCCURRED (Check one) ☐ Hospital ☐ Freestanding birthing center ☐ Home Birth: Planned to deliver at home? ☐ Yes ☐ No ☐ Clinic/Doctor's office ☐ Other (Specify)_____	27. ATTENDANT'S NAME, TITLE, AND NPI NAME: _____ NPI:_____ TITLE: ☐ MD ☐ DO ☐ CNM/CM ☐ OTHER MIDWIFE ☐ OTHER (Specify)_____	28. MOTHER TRANSFERRED FOR MATERNAL MEDICAL OR FETAL INDICATIONS FOR DELIVERY? ☐ Yes ☐ No IF YES, ENTER NAME OF FACILITY MOTHER TRANSFERRED FROM: _____

REV. 11/2003

MOTHER

29a. DATE OF FIRST PRENATAL CARE VISIT	29b. DATE OF LAST PRENATAL CARE VISIT	30. TOTAL NUMBER OF PRENATAL VISITS FOR THIS PREGNANCY
___/___/_____ □ No Prenatal Care M M D D YYYY	___/___/_____ M M D D YYYY	_____ (If none, enter A0".)

31. MOTHER'S HEIGHT ____ (feet/inches)	32. MOTHER'S PREPREGNANCY WEIGHT _____ (pounds)	33. MOTHER'S WEIGHT AT DELIVERY _____ (pounds)	34. DID MOTHER GET WIC FOOD FOR HERSELF DURING THIS PREGNANCY? □ Yes □ No

35. NUMBER OF PREVIOUS LIVE BIRTHS (Do not include this child)		36. NUMBER OF OTHER PREGNANCY OUTCOMES (spontaneous or induced losses or ectopic pregnancies)	37. CIGARETTE SMOKING BEFORE AND DURING PREGNANCY For each time period, enter either the number of cigarettes or the number of packs of cigarettes smoked. IF NONE, ENTER A0".	38. PRINCIPAL SOURCE OF PAYMENT FOR THIS DELIVERY
35a. Now Living Number ____ □ None	35b. Now Dead Number ____ □ None	36a. Other Outcomes Number ____ □ None	Average number of cigarettes or packs of cigarettes smoked per day. # of cigarettes # of packs Three Months Before Pregnancy _____ OR _____ First Three Months of Pregnancy _____ OR _____ Second Three Months of Pregnancy _____ OR _____ Third Trimester of Pregnancy _____ OR _____	□ Private Insurance □ Medicaid □ Self-pay □ Other (Specify) _____

35c. DATE OF LAST LIVE BIRTH ___/_____ MM Y Y Y Y	36b. DATE OF LAST OTHER PREGNANCY OUTCOME ___/_____ MM Y Y Y Y	39. DATE LAST NORMAL MENSES BEGAN ___/___/_____ M M D D YYYY	40. MOTHER'S MEDICAL RECORD NUMBER

MEDICAL AND HEALTH INFORMATION

41. RISK FACTORS IN THIS PREGNANCY
(Check all that apply)

Diabetes
- □ Prepregnancy (Diagnosis prior to this pregnancy)
- □ Gestational (Diagnosis in this pregnancy)

Hypertension
- □ Prepregnancy (Chronic)
- □ Gestational (PIH, preeclampsia)
- □ Eclampsia

- □ Previous preterm birth

- □ Other previous poor pregnancy outcome (Includes perinatal death, small-for-gestational age/intrauterine growth restricted birth)

- □ Pregnancy resulted from infertility treatment-If yes, check all that apply:
  - □ Fertility-enhancing drugs, Artificial insemination or Intrauterine insemination
  - □ Assisted reproductive technology (e.g., in vitro fertilization (IVF), gamete intrafallopian transfer (GIFT))

- □ Mother had a previous cesarean delivery
  If yes, how many _____

- □ None of the above

42. INFECTIONS PRESENT AND/OR TREATED DURING THIS PREGNANCY (Check all that apply)

- □ Gonorrhea
- □ Syphilis
- □ Chlamydia
- □ Hepatitis B
- □ Hepatitis C
- □ None of the above

43. OBSTETRIC PROCEDURES (Check all that apply)

- □ Cervical cerclage
- □ Tocolysis

External cephalic version:
- □ Successful
- □ Failed

- □ None of the above

44. ONSET OF LABOR (Check all that apply)

- □ Premature Rupture of the Membranes (prolonged, ∃12 hrs.)
- □ Precipitous Labor (<3 hrs.)
- □ Prolonged Labor (∃ 20 hrs.)
- □ None of the above

45. CHARACTERISTICS OF LABOR AND DELIVERY
(Check all that apply)

- □ Induction of labor
- □ Augmentation of labor
- □ Non-vertex presentation
- □ Steroids (glucocorticoids) for fetal lung maturation received by the mother prior to delivery
- □ Antibiotics received by the mother during labor
- □ Clinical chorioamnionitis diagnosed during labor or maternal temperature ≥38°C (100.4°F)
- □ Moderate/heavy meconium staining of the amniotic fluid
- □ Fetal intolerance of labor such that one or more of the following actions was taken: in-utero resuscitative measures, further fetal assessment, or operative delivery
- □ Epidural or spinal anesthesia during labor
- □ None of the above

46. METHOD OF DELIVERY

A. Was delivery with forceps attempted but unsuccessful?
- □ Yes □ No

B. Was delivery with vacuum extraction attempted but unsuccessful?
- □ Yes □ No

C. Fetal presentation at birth
- □ Cephalic
- □ Breech
- □ Other

D. Final route and method of delivery (Check one)
- □ Vaginal/Spontaneous
- □ Vaginal/Forceps
- □ Vaginal/Vacuum
- □ Cesarean
  If cesarean, was a trial of labor attempted?
  - □ Yes
  - □ No

47. MATERNAL MORBIDITY (Check all that apply)
(Complications associated with labor and delivery)

- □ Maternal transfusion
- □ Third or fourth degree perineal laceration
- □ Ruptured uterus
- □ Unplanned hysterectomy
- □ Admission to intensive care unit
- □ Unplanned operating room procedure following delivery
- □ None of the above

NEWBORN INFORMATION

NEWBORN

| Mother's Name   Mother's Medical Record No. _____ |

48. NEWBORN MEDICAL RECORD NUMBER

49. BIRTHWEIGHT (grams preferred, specify unit)
_____ 9 grams   9 lb/oz

50. OBSTETRIC ESTIMATE OF GESTATION:
_____ (completed weeks)

51. APGAR SCORE:
Score at 5 minutes: _____
If 5 minute score is less than 6,
Score at 10 minutes: _____

52. PLURALITY - Single, Twin, Triplet, etc.
(Specify) _____

53. IF NOT SINGLE BIRTH - Born First, Second, Third, etc. (Specify) _____

54. ABNORMAL CONDITIONS OF THE NEWBORN
(Check all that apply)

- □ Assisted ventilation required immediately following delivery
- □ Assisted ventilation required for more than six hours
- □ NICU admission
- □ Newborn given surfactant replacement therapy
- □ Antibiotics received by the newborn for suspected neonatal sepsis
- □ Seizure or serious neurologic dysfunction
- □ Significant birth injury (skeletal fracture(s), peripheral nerve injury, and/or soft tissue/solid organ hemorrhage which requires intervention)
- 9 None of the above

55. CONGENITAL ANOMALIES OF THE NEWBORN
(Check all that apply)

- □ Anencephaly
- □ Meningomyelocele/Spina bifida
- □ Cyanotic congenital heart disease
- □ Congenital diaphragmatic hernia
- □ Omphalocele
- □ Gastroschisis
- □ Limb reduction defect (excluding congenital amputation and dwarfing syndromes)
- □ Cleft Lip with or without Cleft Palate
- □ Cleft Palate alone
- □ Down Syndrome
  - □ Karyotype confirmed
  - □ Karyotype pending
- □ Suspected chromosomal disorder
  - □ Karyotype confirmed
  - □ Karyotype pending
- □ Hypospadias
- □ None of the anomalies listed above

56. WAS INFANT TRANSFERRED WITHIN 24 HOURS OF DELIVERY? 9 Yes 9 No IF YES, NAME OF FACILITY INFANT TRANSFERRED TO:_____	57. IS INFANT LIVING AT TIME OF REPORT? □ Yes □ No □ Infant transferred, status unknown	58. IS THE INFANT BEING BREASTFED AT DISCHARGE? □ Yes □ No

Rev. 11/2003
NOTE: This recommended standard birth certificate is the result of an extensive evaluation process. Information on the process and resulting recommendations as well as plans for future activities is available on the Internet at: http://www.cdc.gov/nchs/vital_certs_rev.htm.

Source: National Center for Health Statistics 2003.

Figure 6.4. Intake screen for necessary information for a birth certificate

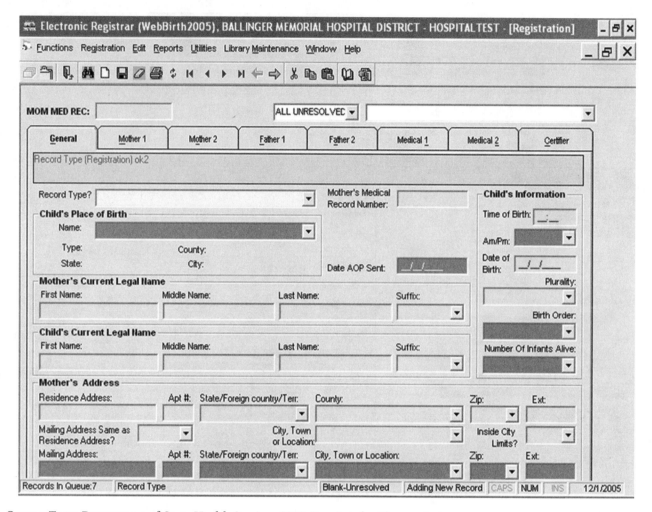

Source: Texas Department of State Health Services 2013. Reprinted with permission.

Most health information or EHR systems allow physicians to use dedicated dictation units or any telephone. However, voice and speech recognition technology is becoming more prevalent in EHR systems. Voice and speech recognition software translates the spoken word from the dictation to the written word or text in an electronic document. If the healthcare organization uses voice recognition, then the information system would be used by an editor, typically an HIM professional with transcription experience, to verify what has been translated into the written format rather than a transcriptionist to manually type what was dictated. The transcriptionist utilizes the transcription system to type the document. A document editor would use the appropriate documentation or transcription software to correct any errors that the information system made in the translation of voice to text. However, the physician or provider is ultimately responsible for the content of the transcribed report and must make corrections or changes accordingly, if necessary.

Dictation System Functionality and Reporting

When dictating the report, the physician is expected to enter the patient's health record number or encounter number as well as the document type. The physician also may indicate that the dictation should be transcribed immediately. The date and time of dictation is automatically captured by the dictation system. The transcriptionists utilize the dictation system to listen to the dictation for transcription. The dictation system will route priority reports to the transcriptionists ahead of other dictated reports in the work queue. Priority status may be assigned to the report by the physician because of patient transfer or other reasons. HIM managers use the dictation system to route dictated reports to the various transcriptionists. For example, the transcription supervisor may need to assign another transcriptionist to type history and physical examination information to meet a specific turnaround time (such as "within 24 hours of dictation"). The HIM manager also uses the dictation system to monitor backlogs and trends on volume.

The key reporting focus for the dictation system is on workload. The system is able to track the volume of work dictated and how much is remaining to be transcribed. This information can be used to determine transcription staffing levels, overtime workload justifications, and trends and patterns in dictation usage.

Transcription System Functionality and Reporting

The transcription system works much like any word processor in that the transcriptionist is able to type, edit, and spell-check a document, but there are many features in the transcription systems that are not found in the word processor. Basic information is collected about every document. This information can include:

- Patient name
- Health record number
- Date of admission
- Date of discharge
- Date of surgery
- Dictating physician
- Date of dictation
- Date of transcription
- Report type
- Name of transcriptionist

The transcription system typically has user-defined templates for each report type. The template prevents the transcriptionist from having to type headings (such as history of present illness or review of systems) every time a history and physical examination is dictated. The information system typically uses expanders, which may also be called macros. An **expander** allows transcriptionists to type an acronym such as "CHF" and the full phrase "congestive heart failure" will automatically be spelled out, thus saving keystrokes and time. The expanders can typically be controlled by the healthcare organization.

The spell-checking capabilities are able to handle both the common language as well as medical terminology. Medical terminology includes not only terms, such as esophagogastroduodenoscopy, but also surgical instruments, medications, and other terms specific to healthcare and medicine.

In the event of a request for information or error, the document may need to be retrieved. The transcription system allows the transcriptionist to search for the document by patient name, health record number, date of dictation, dictator, document type, document number, and transcriptionist.

The transcription software products in use today are designed to work seamlessly with dictation systems and voice recognition systems to promote efficiency in the entire process. These products also are designed for transcriptionists to work from home as appropriate.

Once a document is transcribed, the transcription system is able to route reports to a departmental printer, fax, or other location. The routing of the report is based on settings established in the transcription system. This routing enables reports to reach the physician or patient care area faster. The report may also be available in the EHR.

The transcription system is used by management for various purposes. One purpose is to track productivity, which is critical because transcriptionists usually are paid based on it. Another purpose would be for incentive pay. Many information systems can calculate incentive pay automatically based on criteria established by the healthcare organization. Incentive pay is a system of bonuses and rewards based on employee productivity and is often used in transcription areas of healthcare organizations. Management may also use reports to monitor overall volume by report type to help identify trends and needs.

Healthcare Quality Indicator System

The **healthcare quality indicator system** is an abstracting system that records information about the patient, the care provided to the patient, and the healthcare practitioner(s) involved in the care delivered. Abstracting is the process of extracting information from a document or data elements from a database to create a brief summary of a patient's illness, treatment, and outcome and entering the summary into an automated system. A quality indicator is a standard against which actual care may be measured to identify a level of performance for that standard. This software may be used by the HIM department or another department performing this function. HIM staff or nurses are the typical users of the healthcare quality indicator system; however, its use is limited. Users in the HIM department may be the coders or a separate group of employees with the necessary skills and qualifications to read, understand, and abstract information from the health record into the quality indicator system.

Abstracting and reporting are two critical aspects of the quality indicator systems. Information on the patient's care is entered into the information system to be in the healthcare organization quality improvement program. The data are then turned into information to evaluate the quality of care provided to the patient, patient safety, utilization review, and more. For example, the hospital could use information from the information system in the physician credentialing process. Problem areas would be identified and resources assigned in order to investigate and resolve the quality problems.

Healthcare Quality Indicator System Functionality

The healthcare quality indicator information system may be interfaced to the hospital information system to obtain demographic information. Data abstracting is the key functionality to the healthcare quality indicator system. Examples of data collected include:

- Units of blood
- Nosocomial infections
- Physician(s)
- Nursing unit
- Apgar score

The information abstracted can be used in reports and can be trended. The information can then be used to make changes in how care is provided. Some basic data are collected on all patients. Other fields required for data entry may change based on data entered previously. For example, the user may be required to enter estimated blood loss for a surgical patient, but would not be asked for this information when abstracting health patient data. Another example would be that an Apgar score is required for a newborn, but not for other patients.

Some of the data in the healthcare quality indicator system may be downloaded from other information systems used in the healthcare organization, saving time and improving data quality. These quality indicator systems could be the hospital information system's demographic information, the laboratory information system's laboratory results, and other clinical systems.

Healthcare Quality Indicator System Reporting

Because the data from this information system will be used in performance improvement, reporting is a key part of this information system. Reporting must be flexible so that the user is able to create the report needed for the study being conducted. The reports will include statistics and graphs to facilitate the identification of trends. Reports may include monitoring healthcare organization infection rate, number of deaths by physician, blood incompatibility, surgical errors, maternal deaths, and outcomes.

Computer-Assisted Coding System

The **computer-assisted coding (CAC)** system analyzes the clinical data found in an electronic health record. CAC is the process of extracting and translating dictated and then transcribed free-text data (or dictated and then computer-generated discrete data) into ICD-10-CM, ICD-10-PCS, and CPT procedural codes and evaluation and management codes for billing and coding purposes. It utilizes **natural language processing (NLP)** to analyze clinical data to identify diagnoses and procedures and to assign the appropriate ICD-10-CM, ICD-10-PCS, and CPT code to the CAC system. NLP is an artificial intelligence technology that converts human language (structured or unstructured) into data that can be translated then manipulated by information systems.

CAC may be done while the patient is still in the hospital and then updated after discharge. Doing so speeds up the coding turnaround time and improves efficiency because coding rules are applied consistently and error rates are reduced. Despite this, the coder must review the health record documentation to confirm the accuracy of the code.

CAC System Functionality

The CAC suggests codes to be assigned. The coder reviews the codes and either accepts or rejects them. There is a work queue of records that the coder needs to review. This work queue can be prioritized depending on the healthcare orgainzation's needs such as highest dollar or oldest unbilled claims.

CAC System Reporting

The CAC system generates productivity reports. It can also generate reports on the number of health records where the codes were changed from what the software originally recommended. These reports are important to evaluate the quality, accuracy, and completeness of the codes generated by the CAC system. This evaluation or review can be combined with the financial information to determine what impact this may be having on reimbursement claims and revenue cycle functions.

Clinical Documentation Improvement System

The **clinical documentation improvement (CDI) system** assists in identifying ways to improve clinical documentation in the health record. CDI is the process a healthcare entity undertakes that will improve clinical specificity and documentation that will allow coders to assign more concise disease and procedural classification codes. When documentation improves, the code assignment will be improved because codes can be more specific. Another benefit of improved clinical documentation is more accurate reimbursement.

CDI Software Functionality

The CDI information system assists HIM and CDI staff in the physician query process by facilitating communication between the coding professional and the physician (see figure 6.5). The software looks for missing information that is needed to improve documentation. For example, if a laboratory test identifies the organism causing pneumonia, but the organism is not documented by the physician, then the information system can notify the CDI coordinator and a physician query can be created using a query template that is programmed within the EHR. A work queue identifies what health records need to be reviewed by the CDI coordinator. The information system can also monitor what queries are pending so that the coder can work with the physician to receive a response to the query.

CDI Information System Reporting

Reports will provide the hospital with information on MS-DRG assignment, statistics on the number of queries written, productivity statistics, turnaround times, and more. These reports

Figure 6.5. Sample physician query

Dear (add provider(s) name)

Identify the opportunity was documented within the Reference document location(s)

Clinical Indicators: Signs and Symptoms: · Signs and Symptoms: · Risk Factors: ·

Treatment: · Treatment: · Other Indicators:

Based on the clinical indicators and your professional judgment Choose an item: ·
Please complete by selecting one of the options below.

- Click here to enter text:

- Click here to enter text:

- Other explanation of clinical findings Other Indicators:

- Unable to determine

- No further clarification needed

Source: Arrowood et al. 2016.

will help the HIM and performance improvement staff determine areas in need of upgrading and enhancements, correction processes, and best practices for populating the health record with thorough and complete information to better evaluate patient care and reimbursement protocols. Research regarding clinical or administrative functions and outcomes will improve as a result of more comprehensive and complete documentation available for analysis.

CHECK YOUR UNDERSTANDING 6.4

1. To avoid duplication in medical record numbers and charts, the HIIM and R-ADT departments are clarifying procedures to get the complete names of people being admitted. Additional fields are being added to capture the last names (particularly individuals who have married multiple times, people who have legally changed their surnames, or from persons from countries (Asian countries in particular) where the order of the names is different than the US. Identify the information system that would help build data granularity for multiple names, precision, clarity, and more detail in health information.

   a. Transcription
   b. Templates
   c. CDI
   d. Quality indicator monitoring

2. The Chief of the Medical Staff wants to improve the use and security of the physician's mobile devices to complete their medical records. When a physician speaks into their mobile phone and gives a summary of the patient's care, which is later transcribed. Identify the type of information system that the physician is using?

   a. Dictation
   b. Chart locator
   c. Chart deficiency
   d. Quality indicator monitoring

CHECK YOUR UNDERSTANDING 6.4 (*Continued*)

3. To monitor blood transfusion reactions, the Lab and Nursing departments have improved the documentation process for any patient receiving a transfusion. In order for a nurse to enter the number of units of blood that a patient received during a recent hospitalization, the nurse would use the _____ software.

   a. Dictation
   b. Chart locator
   c. Chart deficiency
   d. Healthcare quality indicator

4. A new Information Technician is being trained to interview new mothers in the Labor & Delivery department to gather comprehensive baby and parental information for the medical record. Identify the information system that one would use to enter data from the medical record to be used on a legal document for the newborn that is required by the NCHS?

   a. Birth certificate software
   b. Transcription
   c. Chart deficiency
   d. Quality indicator monitoring

5. To better meet the Joint Commission requirements for the use of abbreviations in ABC Hospital, the CDI and HIIM Departments will evaluate all abbreviations and acronyms used in their medical records. Several transcriptionists are helping to verify abbreviation usage in their system. Identify the information system that one would be using if one typed out the abbreviation CABG and the phrase coronary artery bypass graft was spelled out?

   a. Abstract
   b. Bar code
   c. Expander
   d. Template

Real-World Case 6.1

Certain members of the executive management team at ABC Hospital are interested in adding voice recognition software to their current EHR. As director of HIM, Cynthia is preparing an extensive report on the impact this would have on the department. She is proposing that a feasibility study and subsequent request for proposal be completed.

The report includes information on voice recognition such as the projected workload of voice recognition software and how it would be implemented in the daily EHR operations. This includes its usage for the standard transcribed reports, such as discharge summaries; histories and physical exams; operative, autopsy, and consultation reports; physician progress notes; nursing care documentation; and other therapy documentation. A review of historic and current transcription workload, number of staff with respective salary and benefits, supplies, and equipment is completed.

One of the objectives Cynthia has made is to interview HIM directors at other hospitals who use voice recognition. She wants feedback on how it changed the HIIM functions within the department and the hospital. In addition, she wants to know how this software affects the quality of the generated reports and how much time is invested in report editing by the staff. The physician query process is another area that she wants to scrutinize. The transcription supervisor is also trying to determine what criteria and updated skills will be needed in the retained employees.

The human resources department was consulted regarding the process of lay-offs for some of the staff whose positions are not upgraded.

Real-World Case 6.2

At ABC Hospital, as part of the Health Information Management Department's quality initiatives, a multidisciplinary approach is being established to ensure the quality of data management and it's use for organizational objectives. All activities need to emphasize one (or all) of these three areas: clinical aspects, administrative applications, and population health monitoring. Quality documentation management is essential for all of these endeavours and will be applied to the following.

Clinical documentation improvement (CDI) will address the clinical aspects with a team of nurses, ancillary staff (therapists, lab, radiology, etc.), physicians, and HIM coding staff. The increased need for clinical documentation specificity to meet ICD-10-CM/PCS requirements and quality reporting indicators for CMS, TJC, and other regulatory agencies makes this aspect to warrant more resources, time, and personnel to meet the quality objectives.

Computerized-assisted coding (CAC), working in conjunction with CDI, will help the Coding Staff better analyse documentation for more detailed ICD-10-CM/PCS and CPT code assignments in a more efficient manner. This, in turn, will facilitate the completion of grouping (inpatient and outpatient), getting the completed codes to the billing staff in an expedited manner, and statistical reporting of diagnoses and procedures as necessary.

Health information exchange (HIE) will assist in addressing population health monitoring. By strengthening the transmission of patient data to their outpatient care partners, ABC Hospital's goals are to increase the health of the community by offering additional services depending upon their needs. There has been an increase in the number of retirees who have relocated to the area, the African-American population is significantly higher than the national average due to a historically black university/college located within the county, and a fluctuating student/young-adult population due to four large universities and colleges within the city limits. Health services that address cardiovascular, cerebrovascular, endocrinology, emergency services, and family practice are being analysed and improved based on statistical trends.

REVIEW QUESTIONS

1. Robert is a high school junior who likes studying diseases and medicine but doesn't want to have direct patient contact. He's also very good at computer science and programming and wants to find a college major that combines his two interests. The phrase that describes the scientific discipline that is concerned with the cognitive, information-processing, and communication tasks of the healthcare practice, education, and research, including the information science and technology to support these tasks is:

   a. Health informatics
   b. Health information management
   c. Data analytics
   d. Epidemiology

2. The CIO and HIIM Director are developing an updated privacy and security strategic plan for the HIM department. Cybersecurity is a major area of discussion. The legislation that regulates the tracking of requests for and disclosure of health information is:

REVIEW QUESTIONS (*Continued*)

   a. ARRA
   b. HIPAA
   c. HITECH
   d. TEFRA

3. In order to meet the demands of the medical staff members to be notified when a malpractice request for medical records is processed, the HIIM Assistant Director has developed a specialty report with the pertinent information being requested. This report is presented at the monthly Medical Staff Committee meeting. The appropriate term used to indicate that reports and letters can be tailored and changed to meet the requirements of the request or the needs of the recipient within an disclosure of health information system is:

   a. Manipulation
   b. Conversion
   c. Customization
   d. Renovation

4. To better evaluate the denials of Medicare claims at ABC Hospital, Shelly (the Coding Manager) and Diane (the Fiscal Claims Manager) must work together to review documentation, ICD-10-CM/PCS code and MS-DRG assignment, and CMS denial reasons. In order to ensure an effective working environment to efficiently manage and produce MS-DRGs and the reimbursement claims, the _____ and the _____ departments should have a strong relationship.

   a. Medical staff and billing
   b. Finance and billing
   c. Disclosure of health information staff and coders
   d. HIM and billing staff

5. Dr. Roberts, the hospital pathologist, is presenting an education session to the coders about assessing the cancer severity in patients. He explains that oncologists used a specific method to determine how severe the cancer is by establishing the size of the tumor, the number of lymph nodes involved, and whether it has spread to other organs. Dr. Roberts refers to that method as:

   a. TNM
   b. HIM
   c. SEER
   d. FORDS

6. Dr. Simmons is giving an educational presentation on common birth defects that may be present in babies born at ABC Hospital. This information on congenital anomalies is important to note on the birth certificate. This presentation is given to the _____ department since their staff typically completes the birth certificate when a baby is born in the hospital.

   a. Local health department personnel
   b. NCHS staff
   c. HIM staff
   d. Registration—admission, discharge, transfer staff

(*Continued*)

REVIEW QUESTIONS (*Continued*)

7. Jonathon is comparing three different EHR systems. His hospital is looking to purchase a new system. He wants to make sure that each EHR system has the correct medical record content requirements before he makes a recommendation to Administration. All of the following organizations determine the requirements for the content of the hospital health record except: _____

   a. Joint Commission
   b. Medical staff rules and regulations
   c. State licensure and healthcare organization policies
   d. AHIMA

8. Tasha, the Transcription Coordinator, is compiling a list of new abbreviations that are being used more frequently by physicians. She needs to get these abbreviations approved by the Governing Board before officially adding them into the EHR system. She will then add them to the transcription software. The software programming that allows transcriptionists to use abbreviations and acronyms while the software types out the complete words of the abbreviation or acronym is referred to as:

   a. Expander
   b. Encoder
   c. Grouper
   d. Registry

9. Raul is evaluating the transcription productivity rates. The CFO wants a cost analysis comparing the transcription department versus new software. The information system that converts the spoken word into a documented word and may reduce the need to have human transcriptionists is referred to as:

   a. Registries
   b. Voice recognition
   c. MS-DRGs
   d. CDI

10. Raul is also evaluating the computerization of the coding functions as a cost saving measure for the hospital. The software that improves the efficiency of the coding process by using the translated dictation reports and NLP to analyze clinical data is referred to as:

    a. CDI
    b. TNM
    c. MS-DRGs
    d. CAC

Abbreviations/Acronyms Matching

COLUMN A	COLUMN B
1. SEER	A. an organizing system that better accounts for how sick a patient is and how much resources are used in treating the patient
2. NLP	B. preferred format for computer programming of a date
3. MS-DRG	C. disease reporting program for cancer registries
4. PHI	D. an artificial intelligence technology that converts human speech into electronic data that can be manipulated by computer systems

REVIEW QUESTIONS (*Continued*)

5. NCHS   E. medical data that is private and must be kept confidential

6. MMDDYYYY   F. federal agency responsible for collecting vital statistics of the US population

7. CTO   G. a coding scheme for cancer and oncology cases

8. ICD-O   H. an upper executive position that coordinates all technology necessary for an information systems

References

Agency for Healthcare Research and Quality. 2015. Quality Indicators. http://www.qualityindicators.ahrq.gov/Downloads/Modules/IQI/V50/IQI_Brochure.pdf.

American Health Information Management Association. n.d.a. Career Map. Accessed May 2, 2020. https://my.ahima.org/careermap

American Medical Informatics Association. 2020. What is Informatics? https://www.amia.org/fact-sheets/what-informatics

Andriotis, N. 2018. Learning Management Systems: Six Soft Skills To Teach Your Leaders. https://elearningindustry.com/six-leadership-soft-skills-training

Arrowood, D., L. Bailey-Woods, E. Barnette, T. Combs, M. Endicott, and J. Miller. 2016. Clinical Documentation Improvement Toolkit. http://bok.ahima.org/PdfView?oid=301829.

Betz, R., L. Bouma, M. Brodnik, S. Burgess, J. Courteville, E. Delahoussaye, R. Dunn, et al. 2013. Release of Information Toolkit: A Practical Guide for the Access, Use, and Disclosure of Protected Health Information. http://bok.ahima.org/PdfView?oid=106371

Campbell, Angela et al. "Beyond the Basics for Health Informatics Professionals" *Journal of AHIMA* 89, no. 8 (September 2018): 58–63.

CNet. 2018. Cancer registry pathology severity rating. http://www.askcnet.org/software/features/

Centers for Disease Control and Prevention. 2017. Program Manual: National Program of Cancer Registries Version 1.0. http://www.cdc.gov/cancer/npcr/.

Centers for Disease Control and Prevention. 2019. National Program for Cancer Registries. Accessed 5/27/2020. https://www.cdc.gov/cancer/npcr/index.htm

Commission on Accreditation of Health Informatics and Information Management (CAHIIM). 2020. HI and HIM Accreditation. https://www.cahiim.org/accreditation/hi-and-him-accreditation

Florida Department of Health. 2017a. Florida Trauma Registry Minimum Data Set Requirements. http://www.floridahealth.gov/certificates/trauma-registry/_documents/ftr-mds-list.pdf.

Florida Department of Health. 2017b. Florida commemorative birth certificate. http://www.floridahealth.gov/certificates/certificates/birth/Commemorative/index.html.

Marc, David; Robertson, Janet; Gordon, Leslie; Green-Lawson, Zakevia D; Gibbs, David; Dover, Kayce; Dougherty, Michelle. "What the Data Say About HIM Professional Trends" Journal of AHIMA 88, no. 5 (May 2017): 24–31.

National Center for Health Statistics (NCHS). 2017. U.S. Standard Certificate of Live Birth. https://www.cdc.gov/nchs/data/dvs/birth11-03final-ACC.pdf. Office of the National Coordinator for Health Information Technology (ONC). 2016. Health IT Curriculum Resources for Educators: What Is Health Information Management? https://www.healthit.gov/providers -professionals/health-it-curriculum-resources-educators.

Texas Department of State Health Services. 2013. Texas Electronic Registrar Birth Registration Facility User Guide. https://www.dshs.texas.gov/vs/handbooks/birth/terbirthmanual.shtm.

Watzlaf, Valerie. "Soft Skills and the Importance of Empathy in HIM." *Journal of AHIMA* 90, no. 5 (May 2019): 7.

Ch 7
Admn IS
HK

Decision Support
MPI
Registration
Scheduling

Money agment
Materials Mangmnt
Maternal Info. Sys
Facilities Mangmnt

Administrative Information Systems

Learning Objectives

- Determine what administrative information system is needed for a particular task.
- Compare and contrast the concepts of big data and business intelligence.
- Differentiate among the administrative information systems.
- Differentiate between a decision support system and an executive information system.
- Describe how administrative systems impact health information management practices.
- Explain the role of HIM in data stewardship.

Key Terms

Administrative information systems
Algorithm
Big data
Business intelligence (BI)
Chargemaster
Clinical documentation improvement (CDI)
Data stewardship
Decision support system (DSS)

Enterprise master patient index (EMPI)
Executive information system (EIS)
Facilities management systems
Financial information system
Hospital information system
Human resources information system (HRIS)

Master patient index (MPI)
Materials management system
Patient registration system
Practice management system
Registration-admission, discharge, transfer (R-ADT)
Revenue cycle
Revenue cycle management
Scheduling system
Soundex

Administrative information systems, which manage the business of healthcare, were the first information systems to be used in healthcare. The data collected in administrative information systems are mainly financial or business-oriented in nature, rather than clinical (patient care). The administrative information systems perform many tasks throughout healthcare organizations. Some administrative systems, such as the master patient index (MPI), are used by many departments and employees throughout the organization. Other administrative information systems, like the decision support system, are utilized only by a select group of authorized users. The **hospital information system,** the major information system used by a healthcare organization, is made up of many administrative systems, such as the financial information system and the MPI. The main administrative information systems are summarized in the following list. Each of these components will be discussed separately:

- The **financial information system** monitors and controls the financial aspects of the healthcare organization.
- The **human resources information system (HRIS)** tracks and manages all employees and other contracted personnel within the organization.
- The **decision support system (DSS)** gathers data from a variety of sources to assist management and staff in decision-making tasks associated with the nonroutine and nonrepetitive problems.
- The **master patient index (MPI)** provides a permanent record of patients treated at the healthcare organization.
- The **patient registration system** collects information on patients receiving treatment.
- The **scheduling system** allows the healthcare organization to make efficient use of resources such as operating rooms.
- The **practice management system** combines a number of applications required to manage a physician practice.
- The **materials management system** manages the supplies and equipment within the healthcare organization.
- The **facilities management system** allows physical plant operations to control the automated systems within the healthcare organization for patient safety and comfort—that is, heating and air systems, automated key control, and preventive maintenance tasks such as testing fire extinguishers, elevator inspections, and the care of various equipment used in the healthcare organization.

Financial Information System

The financial information system is critical to the fiscal health of the healthcare organization. The healthcare organization must receive accurate financial information in a timely manner to monitor and manage the finances of the healthcare organization. This information can be used to plan and control the expenses of the day-to-day operations, as well as long-term investments.

The management of the accounts receivable and the accounts payable on a daily basis by the healthcare organization is known as **revenue cycle management (RCM)**. The **revenue cycle** is a very complex process involving several departments and many employees who perform tasks of reviewing services provided for claims submitted as well as reviewing outstanding claims, returned claims, denials, missing accounts, bill holds, and other claims involving the revenue of the healthcare organization. Many health information management (HIM) professionals are involved in working with the revenue cycle in their healthcare organizations and some work for vendors who specialize in the area of revenue cycle management and clean-up as a business.

Financial Information System Functionality

The financial information system includes functions related to:

- Patient accounting
- Accounts receivable
- Accounts payable
- General ledger
- Investment management
- Contract management
- Payroll
- Billing and claims management

The patient accounting module collects all of the charges related to patient care. Some charges, such as the patient's room charge, are automatically generated, but others are created when nurses, respiratory therapists, and other staff enter charge information either through the financial information system or through a clinical information system that captures the information automatically and then shares it with the patient accounting system. These charges come from the chargemaster, shown in figure 7.1. A **chargemaster** is a financial management form or software that contains information about the healthcare organization's charges for the services it provides to patients (also called a charge description master [CDM]). The chargemaster automates the coding process for routine procedures such as laboratory tests and radiology examinations. Attached to each of these codes is the charge associated with the service. This amount and other charges recorded are used to determine the amount of money charged to the patient's account. For example, a healthcare organization may charge $100 for a chest x-ray. The information system then generates the bill and submits it to the third-party payer. The patient accounting system also generates the discharged not final billed report, which lists the patient accounts that have not been billed.

Figure 7.1. Example of a chargemaster

ABC Hospital Chargemaster					
Item Number	Description	Charge	HCPCS Code	Revenue Code	Department
110692	Chromosomal analysis	412.00	88285	172	Laboratory
128710	COVID antibody	225.00	81443	172	Laboratory
294558	Ultrasound, abdominal	361.00	93350	685	Radiology
312693	X-ray, renal cyst study	239.00	74470	685	Radiology
644338	Kidney stone removal	2,755.00	50080	407	Surgery
697021	Biopsy, breast	1,648.00	72776	407	Surgery

Source: ©AHIMA.

Because the chargemaster has such an impact on the healthcare organization, periodic updates are required. The classification system codes must be updated annually; HIM professionals must ensure that their respective chargemaster updates are completed annually by the healthcare organization's information systems (IS) department when the software updates are received. Otherwise, charges billed can mean a loss of revenue to the healthcare organization. Once the updates are performed on schedule, the healthcare organization is reimbursed the amount they are owed based on their particular geographic region of the country.

Accounts payable records what the healthcare organization owes to others. This amount may be a refund to a patient or an insurance company, or it may be payment to companies that provide supplies and equipment to the healthcare organization.

The general ledger records debits and credits to the various accounts managed by the financial information system. All of the financial transactions are recorded for the time frame. These transactions include receipt of payment, payroll, and disbursements.

Healthcare organization invest their excess cash. The investment management features of the financial information system track the investment accounts and analyze the return on the investments. Changes to the investment portfolio can be made according to the findings.

Healthcare organization sign many contracts, including those with software vendors, insurance companies, businesses that purchase healthcare services, and many other companies. The contract management portion of the financial information system can track particulars such as who the contract is with and expiration dates. The information that comes from the financial information system is used to negotiate managed care contracts and monitor the impact of the contract based on information such as the number of patients, amount of revenue, cost of care, and whether or not the organization is making money on the contract.

The last module of the financial information system to be discussed is the payroll functions. Payroll functions include tracking employees, salaries, taxes to be deducted, taxes to be paid, health insurance deductions, life insurance deductions, and direct deposits. The payroll functions would need to track salary increases and changes in deduction from one year to another.

The information is also used to generate financial reports that are needed by the healthcare organization's management staff. The financial information also provides the balance sheet, statement of revenue and expense, cost reports, and illustrates cash flow. These financial reports can assist in the pricing of services rendered, control inventory, analyses of productivity of staff, and other purposes.

Impact on HIM

The coding professional staff will populate the diagnosis and procedure codes either through direct data entry or from an interface to an encoder. HIM and coding staff have always played an integral part in the financial viability of the healthcare organization. This is particularly true with the completed transition to *International Classification of Diseases, Tenth Revision, Clinical Modification* (ICD-10-CM) and *International Classification of Diseases, Tenth Revision, Procedure Coding System* (ICD-10-PCS). Extensive and continuous training is required to maintain optimal skill in identifying the correct and appropriate diagnostic and procedural codes. With the massive increase in the number of codes due to increased specificity in ICD-10, coders must be thoroughly trained in anatomy and pathophysiology to assign the precise codes. However, codes can only be as accurate as the documentation allows, hence the need for **clinical documentation improvement (CDI)**. The ultimate goal of CDI is to provide comprehensive and unambiguous communication about a patient's medical condition, course of treatment, and care. Historically, CDI's initial focus was to provide clear documentation of diagnostic and procedural coding, but it has evolved to include the data governance (DG) aspects of availability and usability so that quality data and information can be used for any purpose within the healthcare organization. While there is still debate amongst many, a definition provided by AHIMA is that data governance is the overall management of the availability, usability, integrity, and security of the data employed in an organization or enterprise. HIM professionals are instrumental in devising the CDI plan for the healthcare organization.

Clinical documentation improvement (CDI) is the process an organization undertakes that will improve clinical specificity and documentation that will allow coding professionals to assign more concise disease and procedural classification codes. In addition to improving the coding process, CDI also improves and supports data quality, availability, and usability—all key aspects of data governance. The quality of this documentation is vital in order to properly evaluate patient care, meet all regulatory requirements, and obtain the appropriate amount of reimbursement. Because quality documentation, whether it be paper or electronic, is one of the cornerstones of the HIM profession, it is essential for the HIM and coding staff to be integral in all phases of CDI.

HIM professionals should also be involved in the development and management of the chargemaster. Services are added to and removed from the chargemaster as the services provided by the healthcare organization's change. Both ICD-10-CM and ICD-10-PCS (for diagnoses and procedures, respectively) and current procedural terminology (CPT) classification codes (for outpatient services) are updated on a regular basis. These changes must be implemented and verified within the healthcare organization's chargemaster. In addition, the monetary value associated with each code must also be confirmed. Updated ICD-10 codes must be implemented for the federal fiscal year which runs October 1st through September 30th (CMS 2020). Updated CPT codes are implemented each calendar fiscal year starting January 1st (AMA 2020).

Analysis of chargemaster data can indicate changes in billing time frames, productivity of coding submissions, reimbursement denials, diagnoses, and procedures that are most resource-intensive or cost-effective. The analysis of the billing and coding information and reports will help both HIM and finance departments to conduct performance improvement activities to become more efficient.

Human Resources Information System

A healthcare organization requires many staff members in order to operate. Many healthcare organizations operate 24 hours a day, 7 days a week. Because of staffing requirements, payroll expenses make up a large part of the operating budget. This large outlay of cash demands strong management of the human resources department within the healthcare organization.

Human Resource Information System Functionality

The HRIS tracks employees within the organization. This tracking includes promotions, transfers, terminations, performance appraisal due dates, and absenteeism. The individual data elements collected include:

- Employee name
- Employee number
- Department
- Title
- Salary
- Benefit information
- Hire date
- Results of performance appraisal
- Previous titles
- Termination date
- Certifications
- Disciplinary actions
- Eligibility for rehire

These elements and other data are used to create a permanent record for the healthcare organization. This information is used to manage current staff and to verify that past employees worked at the healthcare organization. The HRIS data will track the benefits that an employee has selected, such as family healthcare plan, dental insurance, long-term disability insurance, and retirement. The HRIS will be able to track the utilization of staff by department, job title, or other grouping. The human resources staff would have access to the records of all employees, whereas the various department directors should have access only to those employees reporting to that director.

Department managers may use an automated timekeeping system for their employees when staff members clock in and out. This HRIS tracks the hours per week worked by pay period. Human resources and managers can then use the HRIS to determine sick time, vacation time, and benefit time per employee.

The HRIS can also assist with the hiring process. For example, the HRIS can track résumés and applications submitted by potential employees. The information system can compare the skills and education of the candidate with those of the other applicants, thus speeding up the hiring process.

Reporting is important in the HRIS. Reporting features can be used to track items such as turnover rate, open positions, labor costs, benefits, budget, or overtime. The healthcare organization may also track employee satisfaction and report on the findings of the surveys. Many healthcare organizations offer in-house educational opportunities to employees and attendance at these events is tracked within the HRIS software. These might include optional educational seminars to advance managers with training and development skills. Other workshops might include cardiopulmonary resuscitation (CPR) training classes for staff. The HRIS software may also track mandated classes for all employees that require annual attendance such as fire and safety classes, OSHA standards, privacy and security training, and so forth. Department directors can then easily use the reporting function to assess the attendance within their own departments as well as results of these educational classes by their employees annually.

Impact on HIM

HIM department staff do not use the HRIS. However, the HIM director and the management staff may use HRIS to generate reports, perform queries, review applications, and perform other tasks related to the HIM department staff. Key positions within HIM (such as management, coding, cancer registry, etc.) require specific professional credentials or certifications. Varying amounts of continuing education is required to maintain these credentials. Tracking who needs training, checking credential expirations, how much training is needed, would be functions that management would need to perform. HRIS can assist in workforce scheduling since it takes into account the inpatient census levels and outpatient encounters of the healthcare organization. With a fluctuating census, there may need to be a reduction or increase in HIM staff due to the amount of work generated by the patient load. For example, if census is low for a long period of time, fewer health records (paper or hybrid) would need to be processed. The HIM department may need to decrease the staff temporarily for budgetary reasons. Conversely, if census remains very high, additional HIM staff may be necessary or overtime pay/schedules may need to be addressed.

CHECK YOUR UNDERSTANDING 7.1

1. Mary is evaluating the different types of surgeries performed on Medicare patients at the ambulatory surgery center. She is comparing the cost of supplies, personnel, and other resources to the reimbursement received from CMS. Identify the part of an administrative information system that she would use to identify which surgeries are most profitable for the healthcare organization.

   a. Encoder
   b. Decision support
   c. Financial management
   d. Practice management

2. The lead inpatient coder, Joe, is trying to determine which ICD-10-CM code to use to accurately code cholecystitis with calculus causing obstruction. The _____ information system would assist him in selecting the appropriate code.

   a. Encoder
   b. Decision support
   c. Chargemaster
   d. Practice management

3. Lucinda is completing a report for the CEO who wants to know why some departments have a much higher rate of employees leaving the organization. Identify the information

system that Lucinda would use to identify employee turnover rates in all departments within the healthcare organization.

a. Decision support
b. Revenue cycle
c. Human resources information system
d. Materials management

4. Margarite, one of the HIM Assistant Directors, is establishing her yearly calendar with all the dates for standing monthly committee meeting, weekly productivity reports, daily census tracking graphs, quarterly payroll accounts, etc. Identify the frequency Margarite would schedule the chargemaster software updates.

a. Annually
b. Quarterly
c. Monthly
d. Weekly

5. Alfred is tracking the amount of time it takes for physicians to respond to coding queries. He has found that these delays have caused a 30% increase in turn-around time for submitting the bills for reimbursement. The _____ system would assist him and the coders to have the necessary information to make timely coding assignment.

a. CDM
b. CPT
c. CDI
d. RCM

Decision Support System

Healthcare executives and managers are inundated with data and information from every angle. Efficient and effective use of all pertinent information available will assist in making appropriate decisions in a timely manner. The term **big data** is mentioned frequently when discussing data governance and business intelligence. IBM describes big data as

> *the use of advanced analytic techniques against very large, diverse data sets that include structured, semi-structured and unstructured data, from different sources, and in different sizes from terabytes to zettabytes. Big data is a term applied to data sets whose size or type is beyond the ability of traditional relational databases to capture, manage and process the data. For example, big data comes from sensors, devices, video/audio, networks, log files, transactional applications, web, and social media — much of it generated in real time and at a very large scale (IBM 2020).*

In order for healthcare organizations to effectively incorporate big data into their strategic and decision-making processes, sophisticated and cutting-edge technologies that address data storage, analytics, and visualization must be applied (Johns 2015, 229). The amount of data generated by the daily operations of just one healthcare organization is enormous because of the documentation requirements for administration and patient care. This big data is the foundation from which the business intelligence (BI) is created. Big data must be available, must be governed properly to provide quality information, and it must be secure—all of which are data governance (DG) responsibilities. Only then can it be turned into information from which BI is created.

Business intelligence (BI) is the broad category of applications and technologies for gathering, storing, analyzing, and providing access to data to help enterprise users make better business decisions (Johns 2020, 84). BI includes information technology and procedures to analyze all aspects of the healthcare organization's performance, including patient care and healthcare services delivery, personnel, clinical applications and outcomes, and all administrative functions (Johns 2015, 229). It requires quality data which is ensured and strengthened by data governance activities. The executive staff of the healthcare organization must develop the abilities to get quality data, transform that data into actionable information, and incorporate the received information into the healthcare organization's future processes and decisions. These are functions integral to supporting the healthcare organization's strategic mission and daily operations. For example, business intelligence would be used to determine where profits and losses occur and then analyze what contributed to the profit and loss. Administrators and managers, using the data and information generated by the healthcare organization's information systems, must also incorporate logic and reasoning, creative problem-solving, as well as self-awareness and emotional knowledge to successfully meet the challenges they face today and in the future. BI applications include dashboards. Refer to chapter 1.

For example, to address health disparities caused by systemic racism and sexism in disease outcome rates, hospital managers (both clinical and administrative) must perform population health statistical analyses to identify if, and if so, how much disparity there is between race and/or gender in the most prevalent diagnoses of the organization. After those numbers have been established, then a comparison review of the treatment protocols administered to the respective patients in each subgroup must be completed. Once differences in treatment protocols have been identified, suggestions for solutions are needed. One suggestion could incorporate the alert system within the EHR's clinical decision support system. If a patient did not receive an identified standard protocol, it would notify the medical team to investigate and justify why this particular step was not delivered. The tracking of these changes in treatment protocols can identify trends and patterns. These actions can then be evaluated and monitored to ensure fair and equitable treatment is given to all patients admitted to the hospital.

The **decision support system (DSS)**, as defined earlier, is an information system that gathers data from a variety of sources and assists in providing structure to the data by using various analytical models and visual tools in order to facilitate and improve the ultimate outcome in decision-making tasks associated with the nonroutine and nonrepetitive problems. It is also used to solve structured problems. This means that the DSS is not used to schedule staff, determine inventory levels, or perform other routine decisions, but rather to make decisions about whether to open a new women's health center or a geriatric center. Other decisions that may be candidates for the DSS are whether or not to add new examination rooms in the emergency department or to open new operating rooms. To make these decisions, the DSS utilizes the data in the data repositories and data warehouses. As mentioned in Chapter 3, the various types of analytics – descriptive, diagnostic, predictive, and prescriptive – are used extensively in DSS. The DSS uses models to run analyses such as "what if" (prescriptive analytics) to determine what would happen if certain decisions were made or to forecast the future. For example, the DSS would evaluate the profit or loss that would occur if a hospital added an extra patient room in the emergency department. It would take into consideration extra costs, extra patients, reduced wait times, extra staff, and more. For more on prescriptive analytics, refer to chapter 1.

Executive Information System

The **executive information system (EIS)** is a type of decision support system that is designed to be used by healthcare administrators. As such, it must be easy to use and have access to a wide range of data. With the EIS, a lot of graphs and charts generally are used as part of the results. Advantages of the EIS include:

- Improved competitiveness of the healthcare organization
- Knowledge of the healthcare organization

- Making information available to authorized users throughout the healthcare organization
- Assistance in making strategic decisions about the healthcare organization

The EIS assists the administrator and other top administration staff in making quick decisions. To generate the data manually that the EIS generates with a few clicks of the mouse would take days.

A dashboard report gives administration-structured information to make intelligent decisions for the future. The EIS can be programmed to monitor the status of key performance indicators (KPI), however defined by the healthcare organization. KPIs are critical measurable objectives that assess how well the healthcare organization is performing. Typical healthcare KPIs include bed occupancy rate (showing the volume of inpatients being treated daily), average length of stay (how long each inpatient stays in the hospital, which can be categorized by diagnosis), claims denial rate (how many reimbursement claims are rejected), training by department (total amount of training received by employees), and patient confidentiality breach rate (how often is protected patient information accessed or disclosed to unauthorized sources) (Mirkovic 2019).

In this example, administration can view the dashboard report and see from the diagnostic-related groups (DRGs) and the length of stay (LOS) what the healthcare organization was actually reimbursed and what it actually cost the healthcare organization to treat the patient. The last columns give administration an idea of the profit that was expected versus the actual profit made. This type of report is useful to administration in planning for the future to make decisions.

Figure 7.2 shows an example of an EIS dashboard report. Administrators can view detailed data by types of graphs that are selected, depending on the software used. For this example, several bar charts and graphics are used. Administrators can easily view an EIS dashboard report and see the practice performance activity of the physician highlighted. In this case, performance is evaluated by identifying patient load, wait times for the patients, satisfaction survey results, and general patient demographic information. The same measures can be used to evaluate and compare all the other physicians listed across the top of the screen. Administrators must focus on the fluctuating monthly patient load and the differences in monthly wait times for various physicians. The data from this EIS planning tool is a visual representation to administration of where the problem is greatest and where the priority should be focused. The HIM department may or may not use the DSS depending on the type of DSS and the data stored within it.

Master Patient Index

The MPI is part of the hospital information system. It is a patient-identifying directory, referencing all patients related to a healthcare organization, that also serves as a link to the patient health record or information, facilitates patient identification, and assists in maintaining a longitudinal patient record from birth to death. The MPI identifies every patient who has been admitted to the healthcare organization, and it is the key to locating all patient health records. The MPI lists patient names and health record numbers and cross-references them. An MPI is to be kept permanently as mandated by legal statutes. The information contained within the MPI was originally limited to demographics that could readily distinguish between any two patients as not having the same health record. These data include both demographic data and visit-specific information. The demographic information will include data such as the patient name. The visit information will include items such as discharge date. The data contained in the MPI include:

- Internal patient identification (that is, health record number)
- Person name (legal name with given name, surname, initial, suffixes, and prefixes)
- Date of birth
- Gender
- Race
- Ethnicity
- Address

Figure 7.2. EIS dashboard showing physician practice performance with bar charts

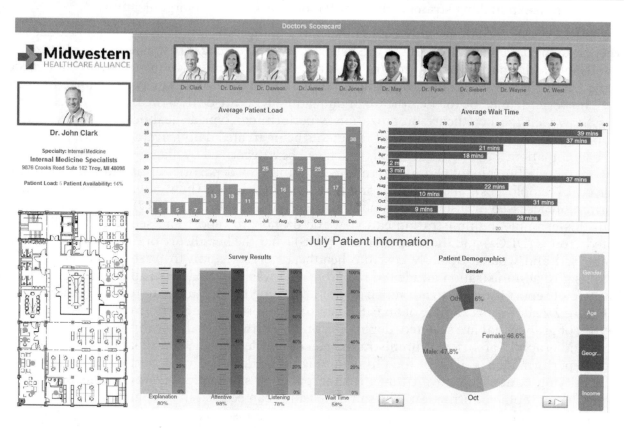

Source: iDashboards n.d. Reprinted with permission.

- Telephone number (where patient can be reached)
- Alias, previous, or maiden names
- Social security number
- Universal patient identifier (not yet established)
- Account or visit number
- Admission, encounter, or visit date
- Discharge or departure date
- Encounter or service type
- Encounter or service location
- Encounter primary physician
- Patient disposition (Reynolds and Sharp 2020, 133)

Other data may be collected depending on the needs of the healthcare organization.

The person who collects the data in the MPI is frequently an admissions staff member who interviews the patient upon entering the healthcare organization at the time of the visit encounter. Once data are entered into the MPI, data are easily transferable into other screens and other information systems within the software for other users.

Master Patient Index Functionality

Information about patients can generally be retrieved using many of the previously mentioned data elements. The most commonly used are patient name and health record number. The MPI usually has soundex capabilities, which allow the user to retrieve patients based on the sound of the name.

Soundex is a phonetic-based indexing system that is easily incorporated into computer software for searching surnames that sound alike but are spelled differently. The soundex search is useful when there are multiple ways to spell a last name, such as Burger, Burgur, Berger, and Burgher.

There are times when a patient is issued one or more duplicate health record numbers. When the duplication is identified, the MPI must have the capability to combine these health records under one health record number and keep a record of the health record number eliminated. The MPI must also be able to address overlays. Overlays occur when two patients are assigned the same health record number because of the incorrect assumption that they were the same patient. Duplicate numbers and overlays cause problems with data quality and ultimately can create a quality of care risk because either the patient's information is fragmented or two patients' records are intertwined.

As mentioned earlier, the MPI is the data storehouse of patient information, which by legal statutes must be maintained permanently. The information stored in the MPI is also vital to the administrative functions of the healthcare organization's database system. When a patient is admitted, discharged, or transferred, the **registration—admission, discharge, transfer (R-ADT)** application is updated with the demographic information and serves as the foundation for the MPI. This is particularly important since it relates to the assignment of the patient's health record number. If a patient has never visited the healthcare organization before, the R-ADT system generates a new health record number. If an established patient is treated again, then R-ADT system connects all records under the previously assigned health record number. A health record number stays the same throughout the life of the patient. A new billing number is generated for each admission, encounter, or service provided to distinguish between episodes of care.

Enterprise Master Patient Index

Integrated delivery systems (IDSs) typically have an **enterprise master patient index (EMPI),** which provides access to multiple repositories of information from overlapping patient populations that are maintained in separate information systems and databases. An IDS is an organizational arrangement of a network of health providers that may include hospitals, physicians, and health maintenance organizations (HMOs) that provide coordinated services along the continuum of care from ambulatory, acute, and long-term care and may extend across a geographical region.

An EMPI allows all of the components of the IDS to share information about the patient. The health record number assigned may be the same for all hospitals, ambulatory settings, and other components of the healthcare system. There may also be an enterprise health record number, with each component issuing its own health record number to the patient. The EMPI would identify all patient visits to the IDS and the data stored would include the healthcare organization that the patient visited.

Impact on HIM

The HIM department is a key user of the MPI. The HIM staff is responsible for the data quality of the MPI, so they perform the various tasks to maintain quality, such as combining duplicate health records and correcting overlays, along with other data quality issues. The HIM staff also uses the MPI to:

- Look up health record numbers
- Identify discharge dates
- Confirm that the health record contains all patient visits
- Look up when the patient was last seen in the healthcare organization
- Merge duplicate health record numbers
- Correct errors in data entry
- Unmerge overlays when one patient's record is overwritten by another patient health record; these records must then be separated into their original files (Reynolds and Sharp 2016, 130)

Even though this is not a comprehensive list of activities, the amount of time HIM staff spend using the MPI is significant. For example, the disclosure of information staff must look up the health record number on every authorization to release information that comes into the department. Depending on the number of requests, this could take hours.

An MPI can link to other databases within the healthcare organization and, as a result, duplicate health record numbers can easily be assigned by other departments such as admissions, clinics, and the emergency department. It is extremely important that the MPI be routinely maintained and updated for accuracy and data control.

Patient Registration (Registration—Admission, Discharge, Transfer)

Patient registration systems are frequently known as R-ADT. The R-ADT is defined as a type of administrative information system that stores demographic information and performs functionality related to registration, admission, discharge, and transfer of patients within the organization. The data collected include:

- Basic demographic information such as name, address, and gender
- Insurance information such as insurance company, policy number, and group number
- Information about the stay such as the admission date, discharge date, and attending physician

Functionality

The information collected in the R-ADT is transferred to other information systems. This transfer of data ensures that the demographic information is consistent and prevents data from being entered over and over again. If a patient needs multiple tests or services performed on the same day, such as laboratory, physical therapy, and x-ray, the registration system should be able to schedule all of these tests with one phone call. The R-ADT system issues the health record number assignment to the patient folder.

Because the MPI and R-ADT systems are both parts of the hospital information system, sophisticated algorithms can be used to help prevent duplicate health record numbers when admitting a patient. **Algorithms** are relatively short computer programs of rules or procedures containing conditional logic for solving a problem or accomplishing a task. When the user enters a patient's name and other identifying information into the R-ADT and there is a patient with the same or similar information, the R-ADT notifies the user. Essentially, the R-ADT asks the user if the patient being admitted is one of the patients listed. If so, duplication of the health record number can be avoided. Not only can algorithms identify exact matches based on name, social security number, and other identifying information, but they can also identify patients whose information is nearly identical, such as a patient whose social security number or date of birth is one digit off from an existing entry or whose last name has changed because of marriage or divorce since the last visit. Many MPIs utilize a ranking system to identify the amount of confidence that the MPI system has in the match. Exact information would receive the maximum score. A potential match with almost everything identical would be a high score but would not be perfect. A potential match with very little, if anything, matching will be a low score.

The R-ADT system generates some key reports used by many departments within the healthcare organization. These include the daily admission list, discharge list, census report, transfer list, and bed utilization reports. The healthcare organization may also generate monthly, quarterly, yearly, and ad hoc reports to show type of patient treated, number of discharges, number of admissions, occupancy rates, and other information needed. The R-ADT system may also print out routine documents, such as general consent form, notice of privacy practices acknowledgment, and advance directives that the patient needs to sign.

Impact on HIM

Although the HIM department does not generally register patients, the HIM department utilizes the reports that come from the R-ADT. For example, the discharge list is often used to confirm that all discharged health records arrive in the HIM department after discharge.

CHECK YOUR UNDERSTANDING 7.2

1. Sam is performing the quarterly data scrubbing of the MPI to eliminate redundancy and verify accuracy of newly assigned medical record identifiers. The only thing Sam would not be doing in this process is:

   a. Merging duplicate health record numbers
   b. Identifying discharge dates
   c. Printing out patient general consent forms
   d. Looking up health record numbers

2. Amanda, the CIO, wants to give administrators structured information in a variety of graphs, tables, and other visual illustrations so that they are better able to evaluate and implement their operational plans for each respective department. The tool that Amanda is recommending for the department administrators to use is the:

   a. EMPI
   b. IDS
   c. R-ADT
   d. EIS Dashboard

3. Sam is analyzing HIM software to identify why some individual patients have more than one medical record number. Identify the software that uses algorithms to match duplicate patients.

   a. Decision support system
   b. Executive information system
   c. Master patient index
   d. Enterprise master patient index

4. Cheryl, the CIO, is developing a 10-year strategic plan for the information needs of the hospital. Identify the type of information system that would be beneficial to her when developing strategic plans for the healthcare organization.

   a. Decision support system
   b. Executive information system
   c. Master patient index
   d. Enterprise master patient index

5. Elena is the case manager for Mr. Jones who had a hip replacement at ABC Hospital. Elena schedules Mr. Jones for a two-week admission to ABC's sister facility, a comprehensive rehabilitation institution. Mr. Jones will then be discharged home and followed by ABC's Home health/Outpatient physical therapists for approximately four weeks. Each of these organizations have access to ABC's EHR system to document his care and progress. Explain the IDS.

   a. A network of coordinated healthcare providers under the umbrella of a single HCO
   b. A database of all patients who have received services at an HCO
   c. A short computer program of rules and procedures to solve problems
   d. A type of decision support used by executive management in an HCO

Scheduling System

Scheduling systems are used to control the use of resources throughout the healthcare organization. These resources can include staff, equipment, rooms, and more. Scheduling systems may be centralized or independent. Centralized scheduling allows the scheduling of all services of the healthcare organization so that one call can make multiple appointments. The decentralized system utilizes the scheduling features of individual systems in use in each department, so calls would have to be made to more than one location to schedule multiple tests.

Functionality

Healthcare organizations need to keep expensive equipment and other resources generating revenue rather than allowing them to remain idle. The scheduling system can help with this by scheduling tests, beds, operating rooms, staff, and other resources wisely. For example, a subsystem of the main scheduler is used for scheduling surgeries. If Dr. Smith needs to perform an appendectomy on a patient, the scheduling system knows what operating rooms are available, how long the operating room will be needed, the staff required, and what equipment will be required. This scheduling of the patient and resources ensures that everything is available when needed, thus preventing unnecessary cancellation of surgeries.

To schedule a patient for admission, tests, or other services, the physician office may call the hospital or other healthcare organization to make the necessary reservations or the information system may be available for direct access by the healthcare provider.

In a typical appointment book scheduling system, a patient appointment can be made by the month and date by clicking on the month and date that is desired for the next appointment follow-up.

The patient's name is then entered into the timeline of the hour that the appointment time is made. Physician offices use these types of appointment books for routine patient visits in their offices. Clinics and ambulatory surgical facilities may also use these software applications. In some cases, the patient is able to log in and schedule routine tests, such as an annual mammogram.

The scheduling system can assist with many management functions. The reporting capabilities of the scheduling system can track cancellations, resource utilization, patient volume, and other topics important to management. The reservations can also be used as part of the preadmission process to collect data such as insurance information and precertification.

Impact on HIM

The HIM department does not use the scheduling system.

Practice Management

Practice management systems are used by physician practices. Scheduling, patient accounting, patient collections, claims submission, appointment scheduling, human resources, and other functions all are built into this single information system.

Functionality

The practice management system may be fully functional information systems, or the physician practices can select from a variety of modules as needed by the practice.

The practice management system can automate prescription renewals and other routine tasks. The practice management system may also connect to administrative information systems at the healthcare organization. One of the major functions of the practice management system is billing. The practice management system will capture the necessary data, review the claim to determine if all the necessary data are available, and then submit the data either to the insurance company or to a healthcare clearinghouse. The practice management system is able to generate reports. Sample reports include number of patients, profit or loss, most common services, and much more.

Impact on HIM

The HIM professional who works in the physician office manager role will utilize the practice management information system in many of the same ways as the financial information system, master patient index, and other administrative systems. These tasks include chargemaster management, entering codes for billing, reporting, and tracking patient visits.

Materials Management System

Healthcare organizations must manage a large amount of equipment and supplies. The typical materials management system automates the:

- Purchasing process
- Inventory control
- Menu planning
- Food service

Materials management personnel would work with the dietary or food service personnel to order and track various food stuffs and supplies for patients and staff. The materials management staff would work with clinical personnel to track and order bandages, blood pressure cuffs, thermometers, and other patient-centered resources.

Functionality

The materials management system can create requisitions, which use workflow in order to gain the necessary approvals for the purchases. Part of the process can be comparing the purchase to the budget to ensure that the necessary funds are available.

This functionality helps control costs in the healthcare organization. The materials management system can be set up to automatically order supplies and equipment based on predetermined thresholds for inventory supplies, allowing for just-in-time inventory controls. For example, if the healthcare organization wants to keep at least 200 suture kits in stock, the materials management system automatically triggers an order for suture kits with the preferred vendor when the inventory drops to 250 suture kits. The materials management system can notify the financial information system when the supplies arrive so that the vendor can be paid, thus increasing the efficiency of the healthcare organization.

The materials management system can generate bar codes to be applied toward supplies to be used and charged to the patient correctly. The use of materials management systems includes cost savings through improved efficiencies, better knowledge of the supplies in stock, reductions in the amount of supplies retained in inventory, and reduced lost charges.

The dietary component of the materials management system tracks the patient's dietary needs, the healthcare organization's food inventory, and food costs. A number of menus can be entered into the information system from which the dietary management and dietitians can work. The materials management system should have a variety of menus available from which to choose.

Impact on HIM

The HIM department is not a frequent user of the materials management system however some employees might use it to create purchase requisitions to order office supplies and other supplies for the HIM departments. This is dependent on the setup of the materials management and ordering system of each healthcare organization.

Facilities Management

The physical plant will require maintenance and upgrades over the years. The physical plant refers to the building structure, surrounding grounds, parking lots or decks, and various building equipment such as elevators. A facilities management system is used by a healthcare organization to manage the physical plant. A facilities management system will track routine maintenance such as elevator inspections, fire extinguisher inspections, and equipment preventive maintenance. Preventive maintenance will enable the equipment to last longer, so tasks such as filter changes, inspection of electrical cables, and other tasks will save the healthcare organization money. The facilities management system will track the preventive maintenance tasks and other inspections that can be used in risk management investigations as well as inspections from outside sources, such as accreditation and state licensing. With the focus by the Joint Commission on patient safety, the physical plant is focused on providing equipment and a healthcare environment that is vital to the well-being of the guests, staff, and ultimately the patients within the healthcare organization.

Functionality

The facilities management software can control various features of the healthcare organization, such as the thermostat, automatic locks, and key cards. For example, the temperature provided by the air conditioner and heating systems can be controlled, making the healthcare organization more energy efficient. Doors can be locked and unlocked automatically at a prescheduled time, and employees can be given access to or denied access to restricted areas.

Facilities management software can also track preventive management tasks, such as testing fire extinguishers, elevator inspections, and the care of various equipment used in the healthcare organization. It keeps track of when repairs and maintenance are performed, such as when a roof was put on a building or when filters are changed in the air conditioning system.

From time to time, major renovations or new construction is necessary. The facilities management system can track and plan the project through the use of project management tools such as project evaluation and review technique (PERT) charts and Gantt charts (refer to chapter 4).

Impact on HIM

The HIM department is not a direct user of the facility management information system. Indirectly, the HIM department may use key cards for entry into locked areas or doorways or use the automated HVAC (heating, ventilation, and air conditioning) system from the physical plant. The HVAC system is set by the physical plant staff, usually in zones for larger buildings, to run at set temperatures during various seasons to make operating costs of heating and cooling more economical.

CHECK YOUR UNDERSTANDING 7.3

1. Julio must coordinate the schedules of five physicians and seven nurse practitioners based upon the needs of the patients within an increasingly busy internal medicine group practice. The current information system is not able to handle the workload efficiently. Julio discusses this issue with the Clinical Manager who agrees with him. At the next monthly staff meeting, Julio wants to discuss the _____ software.

   a. Materials management
   b. Practice management
   c. Facilities management
   d. Scheduling

2. Jared is tracking staffing levels of the HIM department. He is looking for trends and patterns in admissions and discharges to help plan the schedules for staffing the department. Identify the information system that Jared would access for daily, weekly, monthly, and annual numbers of admissions and discharges to help him in this project.

CHECK YOUR UNDERSTANDING 7.3 (*Continued*)

    a. Materials management
    b. Registration
    c. Facilities management
    d. Scheduling

3. Based on the increased use of newer technology, surgeons are able to perform many surgeries in shorter periods of time. The surgeons at QRS Surgi-Center want to investigate how to more efficiently plan for surgeries. To help with this process, the OR Nurse manager would use the scheduling system to determine the:

    a. Amount of time needed to perform colonoscopy
    b. Physicians who are up for reappointment to the medical staff
    c. Census report
    d. The latest version of the notice of privacy practice

4. Given the increase in litigation at ABC Hospital, the Risk Manager wants to establish a list of departments to prioritize for a safety review. He decides that the area most closely aligned with meeting the Joint Commission's focus on patient safety should be first. This department would be _____.

    a. Facilities management
    b. Practice management
    c. Registration
    d. Scheduling

5. The Record Processing Supervisor, Henry, investigates why there is an increase in redundant health record numbers for patients being admitted through the Emergency Department. He talked with the Emergency Department Manager, Eve, and they decide an electronic audit needs to be performed to identify what the specific issue is causing this problem. Identify the information system that Henry and Eve will review that typically assigns the patient's health record number to the patient.

    a. Scheduling
    b. Materials management
    c. Facilities management
    d. Registration

Real-World Case 7.1

The cardiology department of Smithville Community Hospital wants to expand the cardiovascular lab to include additional procedure rooms and equipment. Several cardiologists have mentioned that there seems to be an increase in the number of patients and number of cardiac procedures performed. The hospital CIO was asked to evaluate the request and provide an initial report to the Board of Directors. The CIO worked with the VP of clinical operations to write the report. Using the physician and procedure indices within EHR, the CIO and VP completed a 10-year historical analysis of all cardiac patients and procedures. They identified inpatient and outpatient procedures, documented the number of outpatients who were also cardiac inpatients at some point, and reviewed wait times for scheduling of procedures. Four years of historical data was available in the current EHR for wait-time analysis. The previous system was not able to track wait times for scheduling.

The CIO and VP identified financial data, including cost analysis of each procedure, how reimbursement of procedure varied by type of insurance, average length of stay (if inpatient), profit margins of each procedure, and MS-DRG analysis performed on inpatient cases. They performed physician profiles to identify which and how many procedures were performed by each cardiologist. Using external data provided by the city government and local economic development council, the CIO and VP made population projections for the next 20 years and found an increase in the local population of the over-50 age group. They generated anticipated cardiac services and procedures using predictive statistical modeling.

Based on the information the CIO and VP collected, they projected how many additional staff members and physicians might be needed and made space allocations for the increased number of procedure rooms. They are currently investigating the cost of additional equipment needed and completing a renovation budget and timeline. They expect to present their findings to the board by the end of the first quarter, and a final decision should be reached by the end of July.

Real-World Case 7.2

Members of the executive staff of ABC Hospital are anticipating another pandemic, much like COVID-19, within the next 10 years. After discussions with local and state epidemiologists, it was determined that a comprehensive plan was essential to mitigate the impact of another outbreak, pandemic, or other disaster on their community.

With the help of the hospital's EIS, the hospital's executive staff are reviewing community population projections, economic and financial projections for the community and the hospital, technology growth and needs (both clinical and administrative), and personnel needs (again, both clinical and administrative). They have developed a task force with the community emergency management, local health department, and other elected officials. Each group is using their respective information systems to run statistical scenarios and prospective community plans. Subsequent meetings will address the various projections and determine priorities and budget restrictions.

At a future point in time, they will seek more community input from various civic, political, and religious groups so that there is more buy-in and support for this all-hazard mitigation plan from the community at large.

REVIEW QUESTIONS

1. Ronald is interviewing at a large orthopaedic clinic for a job that includes the duties of submitting claims for reimbursement, reviewing denials, settling billing matters, applying general accounting principles, and dealing with any other issues or follow-up on claims. Identify the area in which Ronald will be working.

   a. Deterministic algorithm
   b. Revenue cycle
   c. R-ADT
   d. Chargemaster

2. Antoinette is reviewing the financial management software that contains information about the healthcare organization's charges for the services it provides to patients for any errors or updates that need to be added. Identify the software that Antoinette is evaluating.

   a. Deterministic algorithm
   b. Revenue cycle
   c. R-ADT
   d. Chargemaster

3. In order to maintain accreditation, Samantha, the Clinic Manager, must keep track of all the credentialed status for the occupational and physical therapists, registered nurses, and certified nursing assistant for the ABC Rehab Hospital. She is working with Harold from the Personnel department using the _____ software.

   a. DSS
   b. R-ADT
   c. HRIS
   d. EIS

4. There are several hospitals in Smithville. They are constantly competing with each other about retaining specialty/credentialed staffing positions. Identify the information system that the HIM director can use to determine salaries, assist in hiring new staff, evaluate turnover rates, and track training sessions.

   a. Practice management
   b. Materials management
   c. Facilities management
   d. Human resources

5. Dr. Smith treats highly unusual medical cases requiring many laboratory, radiology, and other diagnostic tests. Hospital administration wants to determine if additional facilities, personnel, and equipment are needed to meet current and future community demands. The _____ information system would be helpful in this scenario.

   a. DSS
   b. R-ADT
   c. HRIS
   d. EIS

6. Every October, the CEO and other members of the upper administrative staff have strategic planning meetings to address the upcoming year's goals and objectives. The _____ information system would assist them in this process.

   a. DSS
   b. R-ADT
   c. HRIS
   d. EIS

7. During a disaster, the _____ information system would help track the patients' movements through the hospital as they go through triage, surgery, intensive care unit (ICU), regular patient care floor, and finally discharge to a rehabilitation organization.

   a. DSS
   b. R-ADT
   c. HRIS
   d. EIS

8. The _____ information system is the gateway into a healthcare organization to identify if a patient has been treated there, contains demographic information to confirm patient identity, and shows if the patient has been treated at other facilities within an IDS.

(*Continued*)

REVIEW QUESTIONS (*Continued*)

    a. EMPI
    b. EIS
    c. HRIS
    d. R-ADT

9. If the CFO wanted to evaluate the supply shipping schedule, storage costs for supplies and equipment, timeframes for ordering supplies, and the distribution of equipment and supplies to the correct departments, identify the information system that would facilitate this process.

    a. Materials management
    b. Practice management
    c. Facilities management
    d. EIS

10. If the medical office manager wanted to compare the amount of time it takes for a patient to be seen by a physician versus a nurse practitioner, identify the information system that would be helpful in this analysis.

    a. Materials management
    b. Practice management
    c. Facilities management
    d. EIS

11. Identify the abbreviation that is used to describe the process an organization undertakes that will improve clinical specificity and documentation that will allow coding professionals to assign more concise disease classification codes.

    a. IG
    b. CDI
    c. ITG
    d. DG

Abbreviations/Acronyms Matching *May not be in this order.*

1. HRIS   A. a patient-identifying dataset of every patient seen at a healthcare organization that links it to the patient's health record

2. MPI   B. software used by C-suite managers to help make administrative decisions

3. RCM   C. another term to describe the dataset of CPT codes and their respective charges

4. BI   D. alphanumeric coding scheme for diagnoses and inpatient billing

5. CDM   E. software that tracks the movement of patients in to, out of, and around the healthcare organization

6. ICD-10-CM   F. the continuous financial and billing processes performed by businesses

7. R-ADT   G. numeric outpatient coding scheme used for billing of provider services

8. EIS   H. the end result of using all information and tools available in a healthcare organization to analyze and improve its performance

9. CPT   I. software that tracks personnel, salary, and employee issues within an organization

References

American Medical Association. 2020. AMA Releases 2020 CPT® code set. Accessed June 20, 2020. https://www.ama-assn.org/press-center/press-releases/ama-releases-2020-cpt-code-set

Centers for Medicare and Medicaid Services (CMS). 2020. 2021 ICD-10-PCS. Accessed June 20, 2020. https://www.cms.gov/medicare/icd-10/2021-icd-10-pcs

Downing, K. 2016. Importance of Data Stewards in Information Governance. http://bok.ahima.org/doc?oid=301584#.WnPf7ainFRY.

IBM. n. d. What is Big Data Analytics? Accessed June 20, 2020. https://www.ibm.com/analytics/hadoop/big-data-analytics.

iDashboards. n.d. Healthcare—Doctor's Scorecard. Accessed February 10, 2018. https://www.idashboards.com/dashboard-examples/healthcare-dashboards-doctors-scorecard/.

Johns, M. 2020. Governing Data and Information Assets. Chapter 3 in *Health Information Management: Concepts, Principles, and Practice*, 6th ed. Edited by P. Oachs and A. Watters. Chicago: AHIMA Press.

Johns, M. 2015. *Enterprise Health Information Management and Data Governance*. Chicago, IL: AHIMA.

Mirkovic, M. 2019. Healthcare KPIs - 12 KPIs You Should Be Tracking. Accessed 9/13/2020. https://www.executestrategy.net/blog/healthcare-kpis

Pilato, J. 2013. Charging vs. coding: Untangling the relationship for ICD-10. *Journal of AHIMA* 84(2):58–60. http://library.ahima.org/doc?oid=106071#.Wn271KinFRY.

Reynolds, R. B. and A. Morey. 2020. Health Record Content and Documentation. Chapter 4 in *Health Information Management: Concepts, Principles, and Practice*, 6th ed. Edited by P. Oachs and A. Watters. Chicago: AHIMA.

Chapter 8

Clinical Information Systems

Learning Objectives

- Differentiate between the various clinical information systems.
- Define clinical information system.
- Compare and contrast executive decision support tools with a clinical decision support system.
- Determine what clinical information system is needed to meet the needs of the healthcare organization.
- Explain the importance of clinical information systems to value-based healthcare.
- Make recommendations on the use and implementation of document management systems.

Key Terms

Anesthesia information system
Annotation
Artificial intelligence (AI)
Backscanning
Barcode
Clinical decision support tools (CDS)
Clinical documentation
Clinical information system (CISs)
Cloud computing
Document management system (DMS)
Emergency department system (EDS)
Interdisciplinary charting system

Laboratory information system (LIS)
Logical Observation Identifiers, Names and Codes (LOINC)
Nursing information system (NIS)
Optical character recognition (OCR)
Patient monitoring system
Pharmacy information system (PIS)
Picture archival communication system (PACS)
Radiology information system (RIS)

Remote patient monitoring (RPM)
RxNorm
Scanner
Scanning workstation
Smart card
Storage area networks (SAN)
Symbiology
Target sheet
Telehealth
Telemedicine
Teleradiology
Telesurgery

A **clinical information system (CIS)** collects and stores medical, nursing, clinical ancillary areas (such as radiology and laboratory), and therapy department information related to patient care. Data contained within the various information systems are patient identifiable and are therefore protected by the Health Insurance Portability and Accountability Act (HIPAA). The clinical data stored in the CIS are used to diagnose a patient's condition, make treatment decisions, monitor the current condition, and manage overall care. The CISs discussed in this chapter are:

- Clinical decision support tools
- Document management system (DMS)
- Radiology information system (RIS)
- Laboratory information system (LIS)
- Nursing information system (NIS)
- Pharmacy information system (PIS)
- Interdisciplinary charting system
- Emergency department system
- Anesthesia information system
- Patient monitoring system
- Telehealth
- Smart cards

Other CISs include computerized provider order entry (CPOE) and electronic medication administration system. These systems are discussed in chapter 9. CISs are frequently source systems for the electronic health record (EHR) because they populate the database that serves as the foundation for the EHR.

Demographic information is collected in the administrative or hospital information system which includes registration—admission, discharge, and transfer (R-ADT); see chapter 7 for more information on administrative information systems. The demographic information is passed on to the CIS, eliminating the need for duplicate data entry, which saves time and improves the quality of the data. Some of the data elements generally passed from the hospital information system to the CIS include:

- Last name
- First name
- Middle initial
- Date of birth
- Health record number
- Social security number

The CIS interface may be designed so that any changes to demographic information in the CIS are fed back to the hospital information system to keep demographic information in all information systems consistent. See figure 8.1 for an example of how individual departmental information systems feed into the main hospital information system.

Clinical information systems are used to support patient care throughout the healthcare organization in many areas. The information provided within the information system offers healthcare providers timely access to clinical data and complete data regarding the patient's care.

Clinical Decision Support

There is an avalanche of medical and health information published every day. No healthcare provider could reasonably be able to keep up with this amount of data. But what if there was a tool that would help physicians and providers make better decisions based updated information and newly published best practices that helped save lives, improve outcomes, increase productivity,

Figure 8.1. Health information systems

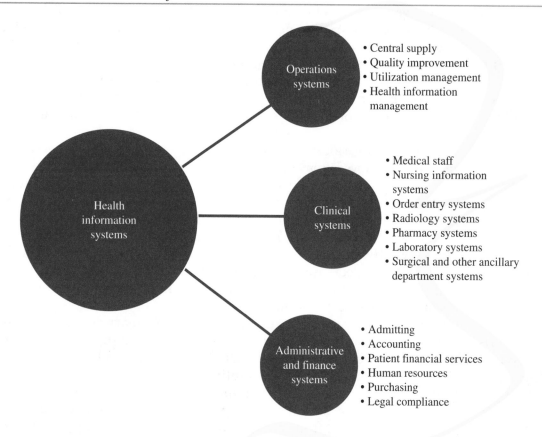

and decrease costs? This software tool is referred to as clinical decision support. The Office of the National Coordinator (ONC) defines clinical decision support as:

> Clinical decision support (CDS) provides clinicians, staff, patients or other individuals with knowledge and person-specific information, intelligently filtered or presented at appropriate times, to enhance health and health care. CDS encompasses a variety of tools to enhance decision-making in the clinical workflow. These tools include computerized alerts and reminders to care providers and patients; clinical guidelines; condition-specific order sets; focused patient data reports and summaries; documentation templates; diagnostic support, and contextually relevant reference information, among other tools (ONC 2018).

A recent survey by the American Hospital Association (AHA) indicated that 92% of all hospitals are using clinical decision support and that more than half of them have more than one CDS platform (AHA 2017, Spitzer 2018). Another study showed that over 40% percent of hospitals had advanced CDS (Sutton 2020). The usual areas where hospitals are using CDS are orders for medications, lab, and medical imaging, and clinical practice alerts (Spitzer 2018).

The ONC says that **CDS** can encompass "computerized alerts and reminders to care providers and patients; clinical guidelines; condition-specific order sets; focused patient data reports and summaries; documentation templates; diagnostic support, and contextually relevant reference information, among other tools" (Bresnick 2017). The purpose is to include:

- the **right information** (evidence-based guidance, response to clinical need)
- to the **right people** (entire care team – including the patient)
- through the **right channels** (e.g., EHR, mobile device, patient portal)
- in the **right intervention formats** (e.g., order sets, flow-sheets, dashboards, patient lists)
- at the **right points in workflow** (for decision making or action) (Bresnick 2017)

Something that is assisting both the executive and clinical information systems decision making processes is artificial intelligence. **Artificial intelligence (AI)** is "the theory and development of computer systems able to perform tasks that normally require human intelligence, such as visual perception, speech recognition, decision-making and translation between languages" (Monga 2017). Combining AI with machine learning can be powerful tools helping make better and more impactful decisions for patients. AI is having a positive impact in the delivery of healthcare services. It is being used to study the genome and improve cancer diagnoses, developing new treatments and medications, improve efficiency of patient experiences, and mining and manging medical data (Daley 2020).

There is ample evidence from various studies that CDS is very effective in decreasing sepsis mortality rates, improving cardiovascular disease prevention results, decreasing medication interactions, evaluating severity of head injuries, and increasing productivity of nurses' phone screenings (Bresnick 2017, CDC 2020, Sutton 2020). Studies have also shown that CDS improves the adherence to established clinical guidelines. The further use of CDS on clinical guideline applications can lead the way to decreasing health disparities in a variety of subpopulations (Sutton 2020). As with many software applications it can be costly initially. However, studies have shown that the use of CDS helps decrease the average length of stay, offer cheaper medication recommendations, improve clinical documentation leading to improved coding and billing, and decreases duplications of diagnostic tests (Sutton 2020).

However, alert/alarm fatigue is a very real issue in healthcare. Primary care physicians average at least 77 alerts per day, some physicians spend more looking at a computer screen than their patients, and physician burnout due to inefficient EHR technology and practice situations is at epidemic proportions (Bresnick 2017). Administration and practice managers must try and balance use of CDS technology with physician/patient interaction lessening frustrations and excess time in front of a computer monitor. To improve CDS acceptance, workflow evaluations prior to implementing CDS is critical; input from all clinical, nursing and therapy staff is essential; obtaining clear feedback; and monitor productivity are critical (Bresnick 2017).

Document Management System

A **document management system (DMS)** is an electronic method of capturing and managing documents. The DMS is used primarily by health information management (HIM) departments and other departments to handle documents regarding patient care. These documents can be scanned or obtained electronically from other information systems. One of the advantages to the DMS is the use of workflow. The workflow processes identified with the DMS include health record completion, disclosure of health information, and routing documents for review. The DMS can be a standalone information system or a component of the EHR. A DMS can also be used in other areas of the healthcare organization besides the HIM department, such as human resources, patient financial services, purchasing, registration, and the business office.

Automated forms processing technology allows the user to type data directly into the computer, eliminating the need to manually complete a paper form and then scan it into the DMS. By entering the data directly into the information system, the data are available for manipulation. Electronic signature, document annotation, and editing are critical to the DMS because physicians and other users can electronically sign the documentation entered into the information system from anywhere. The user also should be able to add notes to existing documentation and to edit documents when errors are identified. Because the health record is a legal document, the original documentation must be retained so that the differences between the two documents are shown.

Document capture is much more than scanning paper images into the DMS. Voice, video, electronic transactions, and other forms of technology may be used to capture data. One example is **optical character recognition (OCR)**. OCR is defined as a method of encoding text from analog paper into bitmapped images and translating the images into a form that is computer readable.

With OCR, a text can be scanned, and the content can be edited. Document indexing, barcoding, and character and form recognition are ways to link documents to a particular patient, thus allowing for retrieval. An index is an organized (usually alphabetical) list of specific data that serves to guide, indicate, or otherwise facilitate reference to the data. These indexing tools allow the user to locate and retrieve a specific patient's health record, a specific encounter, and even a specific document through the use of indexing by entering search criteria into one or more of the index fields. The user is then able to view the desired document as well as print, fax, or use another method of transmission. The purpose of the DMS is not to eliminate paper, but rather to manage documents. To manage these documents, the healthcare facility needs to use the DMS for more than document imaging. It should also use character recognition along with imaging to manage all documents for the healthcare facility and not just the health record. The DMS also uses workflow in order to facilitate the business process of the healthcare facility. The DMS includes multimedia technologies and moving documents from one information system to another without printing the document on paper.

Document Management System Versus Electronic Health Record

The DMS is not the same as the EHR. The EHR is an electronic record of health-related information on an individual that conforms to nationally recognized interoperability standards and that can be created, managed, and consulted by authorized clinicians and staff across more than one healthcare organization. Based on this definition, document imaging does not qualify as an EHR because the healthcare providers do not create the data within the DMS. If employees' expectations are not managed and they believe that a DMS is an EHR, they are often disappointed in the information system when it is implemented. Employees will soon recognize that the DMS will not be able to perform the functionality of the EHR. For example, unless OCR has been used, the DMS will not be able to perform searches on the content of the health records because the images are pictures of the paper documents. The DMS also will not assist in clinical decision support.

With the DMS, the image can be retrieved by any authorized user from any location. Multiple users can also view the same image at the same time, enhancing communication between care providers. The image of the scanned document cannot be searched, edited, or changed unless OCR is used. Although document imaging is not an EHR, it is a valuable tool to healthcare organizations that do not have the space needed to store paper records and that do not want to use microfilm. Many of the healthcare organizations that elect to implement a DMS use it as a component of the EHR.

Components of a Document Management System

A DMS is made of many components, including a scanner, magnetic storage, and file server. All of the components work together to scan, store, and retrieve the health record documents.

Scanner

The **scanner** is the hardware that is used to transform the paper document into a digital image. Scanners are rated based on the number of pages per minute (PPM) the scanner can process. High-powered scanners used to accomplish high-volume scanning, usually found in HIM departments, resemble a copier with an automatic document feeder. Departments with only light scanning needs may use a flatbed scanner. A flatbed scanner can only scan one page at a time because each page must be manually placed on the screen, scanned, and then manually removed before the next page is manually placed on the scanning bed. A high-powered scanner can scan a pile of documents in a short period of time because each page is automatically fed through the imaging bed of the scanner.

The scanner chosen should be fast enough to accommodate the volume of scanning that needs to be accomplished. Generally, the larger the healthcare facility, the faster the scanner needed. The scanner should be able to adjust the density and contrast of the scanning automatically based on the type of form being scanned. Contrast refers to the difference between the lightness or darkness of a letter, word, or diagram and the background color of the document. Density refers to how much content is on a document; a form that has many blank spaces is less dense than a full page of text. The need to adjust for density and contrast automatically comes from the fact that some forms or their documentation are lighter or darker than others; thus, they will need to be scanned darker or lighter accordingly—just as when a document is copied on a copy machine. The scanner is able to identify the type of form and make needed adjustments because of barcodes on either the form or the target sheets. **Target sheets** are pages that contain only a barcode that tells the scanner and, ultimately, the computer the content of the pages that follow. The barcode may contain the form name, the patient name, or some other piece of information. If the scanner cannot scan both sides of a two-sided document, the operator must scan the other side manually.

Because of the movement of the scanner and the dust that collects from the paper movement through the scanner, scanners must undergo frequent preventive maintenance. There will be times that even with preventive maintenance, the information system will become inoperable. This must be considered when selecting the number of scanners and PPM ratings needed.

Scanning Workstation

The **scanning workstation** is the desktop computer or tablet that controls the scanner. Once a document is scanned, either by optically scanning equipment or digitally transferred, it can be upload into the EHR or other digital storage depending on the needs of the organization. Each file is indexed which identifies the patient (name and medical record number usually), the type of form, and each page that has been scanned (Reynolds 2020). The healthcare organization determines the data elements to be indexed based on its needs. During the quality control process, the technician views every image to check for the quality of the image and verifies that indexing is accurate and patient demographics are correct.

Because the amount of data, images, and scanned material has increased dramatically in healthcare, storage management has become a significant issue. Storage management is the process of determining on what type of media to store data, how rapidly data must be accessible, arranging for replication of storage for back up and disaster recovery, and where storage systems should be maintained. Many healthcare organizations have dedicated personnel, usually within the IT department, who are solely responsible storage management functions and operations so that multiple users are able to access crucial information whenever necessary (Lee-Eichenwald 2020, 382). **Storage area networks (SAN)** can be local to the healthcare organization or remote and use cloud computing. These SANs are able to retrieve health data acquired by the organization from any storage location. **Cloud computing** is the use of computer services over the Internet, typically by a vendor, to store data or provide other computing resources and functions (Amatayakul 2020, 345). Individuals and organizations pay for the type and amount of storage they need. Two popular examples of cloud computing are Amazon Web Services and Microsoft Azure (Knorr 2018). Some of the benefits to cloud computing include:

- cost savings: the healthcare organization does not need to invest in additional hardware, software, or personnel
- scalable: the healthcare organization contracts for only the amount of storage it needs; and can be increased at a later point in time
- reliability: the healthcare organization is provided with backup, disaster recovery services, and contingency plans mitigating the impact of negative event (Microsoft 2020).

Printers

The healthcare organization will need to determine who has the rights to print reports from the DMS. The size of the printer will be based on the volume of printing performed by that area. For example, in the typical HIM department a high-quality, high-speed laser printer is needed in order to print large volumes of information. The print server controls the location where documents are printed and controls the work queue or order in which a document prints. The fastest way to print is to use a print file server to control and facilitate the printing process. There must be an computerized print tracking log, similar to an audit log, that indicates who requested or submitted the print order, where the printing occurred (which printer was used and in what area of the healthcare organization), date and time of printing, what forms or reports were printed, and any other pertinent information the healthcare organization deems appropriate.

Annotation

One of the functions of a DMS is the ability to annotate the images. **Annotation** is the ability to add to the image in some way. Because the image may be a legal document, the image itself cannot be altered; however, an overlay to the document will show the annotation. These annotations are useful to call attention to some data on the form and to enhance viewing. There are several ways to annotate a document:

- Note—The note tool will allow the physician or other user to add a note to the image. This may be useful if additional data have become available and the physician wants to call it to the reader's attention.
- Highlighting—The highlighting tool emphasizes important sections of text, much like a highlighter pen on paper. The purpose is to call the reader's attention to specific test results or other documentation.
- Drawing—The drawing tool can be used to draw circles, arrows, or other markings. This is another way to bring the reader's attention to specific data or, in the case of radiology imaging, the anomaly.
- Zoom and reduction—The zoom and reduction tool enlarge or reduces the size of the image to enhance viewing. This is helpful if the writing is small or there is a lot of writing on the page that is difficult to read. It is very helpful in the interpretation of radiology reports because the radiologist can enlarge portions of the image to better see any anomalies.
- Rotate—The rotate tool allows the user to flip an image. This is useful if a document has been scanned upside down or sideways.

Advantages and Disadvantages

There are many advantages and disadvantages to the DMS. Some healthcare organizations choose to focus on the advantages and implement the DMS in their progression toward the EHR; others choose to skip this step and go directly to the EHR. Some advantages are space savings, productivity gains, and immediate access to patient information. Disadvantages include lack of manipulation and reporting capabilities and fear of change to work processes.

Space Savings

Space savings is a definite advantage of the DMS because paper health records take up a lot of space. Space in a healthcare organization is a valuable commodity, and healthcare organizations are always looking for ways to improve space utilization. To realize the space savings, many healthcare organizations destroy the paper health records after a predetermined period of time. This practice ultimately eliminates the need for the long-term file area, opening the space for other needs, such as expansion of the HIM department or reallocation to other departments. The elimination of the file room may take several years as health records are destroyed, scanned, or microfilmed.

Retrieval of Large Number of Records

The HIM department is constantly pulling large numbers of health records for audits, research, and other purposes. HIM staff must pull the health records for review and later refile them once the review is complete. This process takes up a lot of time and space because the health records have to be stored during the review process and space has to be allocated for the reviewers to work. With a DMS, health records are stored electronically. If a researcher or auditor needs to access large numbers of health records, these records can be placed in a work queue. The reviewer can view the health record from any location as long as proper authorization is provided, thus eliminating the need to pull, manage, and refile the health records.

Productivity Gains

Through the use of DMS and workflow technology, employee productivity is improved because they no longer have to look for health records or move them from one location to another. A DMS eliminates health record retrieval and assembly and many other routine paper-based traditional health record functions. Other functions, such as coding, analysis, and qualitative and quantitative analysis, can be done electronically. With the DMS, patient care providers have 24-hour access to patient information without the need for around-the-clock staff. Another productivity gain comes from the elimination of lost or misplaced health records. Hours spent looking for health records could be better spent on other tasks such as eliminating duplicate health record numbers, documentation improvement, compliance audits, and privacy audits.

Online Availability of Information

When it comes to emergency patient care, minutes count. The availability of the patient's past medical history can be the difference between life and death. For example, if the patient has an allergy and the physician does not know, an inappropriate medication could be prescribed to the patient, thus resulting in harm to the patient and possibly death. The ability to access critical information in seconds—not minutes or hours—improves the quality of the care to patients and can prevent unnecessary or duplicate testing. Another benefit to the online availability of information is that multiple users view the same health record simultaneously, even the same document at the same time. This accessibility improves user satisfaction and ultimately improves patient care through improved communication and accessibility.

System Security and Control

With access controls, audit trails, and other security measures, the security of the health record is improved over that of the traditional paper health record. With the paper health record, there is only one point of access, but there is no way to know who viewed the health record and what they looked at. With proper security measures, only authorized individuals will be able to view what they have a need to know and there will be a record of not only the health record viewed but also the specific documents.

Database Retrieval

The DMS allows for searches based on indexed data. For example, a search could retrieve all patients who were discharged from the healthcare organization on December 1, 20XX, or all of Dr. Smith's patients, or John Brown's health record. This function is great for research and saves time from having to identify patients and then retrieve their data individually. The searching is limited to the data elements captured during indexing.

Lack of Manipulation or Reporting

Because the images are pictures of the health record document and not entries into the EHR, the user is unable to manipulate the data to show trends or other views. Likewise, the user cannot generate reports related to the images rather than entered data.

Fear of Change

People are inherently afraid of change. Research on DMS implementations has shown that, at least initially, the number of employees needed increases because the HIM department is still managing the paper health record in addition to the EHR. Because of this, management must let the employees know the status of their positions. Usually, staff members will maintain their current jobs, but some jobs may change or even be eliminated. Instead of filing reports in the health record, they may be scanning documents. Keeping employees informed of the changes will keep their fear manageable and may prevent the department from losing good employees. Fear can develop not only in staff but also within management. Fears such as the risk of not being able to access information because of technology failure, power outages, bad media, or other reasons add to the responsibility and accountability expected of management.

Implementation

Healthcare organizations must manage the existing paper health records when a DMS is implemented. The healthcare organization has to decide if these existing records will be scanned into the information system and, if so, how many. Healthcare organization's decisions on this matter vary widely. Some scan only health records with a discharge date on or after the DMS implementation date. Other healthcare facilities choose to backscan some or all existing health records to provide *Hint* users electronic access to the old health records. **Backscanning** is the process of scanning past health records into the DMS so there is an existing database of patient information, making the DMS valuable to the user from the first day of implementation. Although this methodology provides an immediate database of health records in the DMS on the first day of the go-live, it also gives the healthcare organization a long backlog of information to be scanned, preferably before implementation. Many patients may never come back to the healthcare organization, so it will not realize any benefit from many records scanned into the DMS. The healthcare organization should choose how far back to go with the scanning, such as six months or two years. Healthcare facilities that choose to backscan documents typically participate in medical research and have high readmission rates to the healthcare organization. An example of this research could be a pediatric longitudinal study that looks at patient care or treatment protocols over a number of years or decades, such as in the case of babies born with certain birth defects. Other healthcare organizations choose to backscan on a patient-by-patient basis upon future admittance. The decision should be based on the needs of the healthcare organization, cost, filing space, and other resources. The decision should balance the needs of the user and the resources available. Many healthcare organizations only provide the HIM department access to the DMS initially if they decided not to backscan. The logic behind this decision is to prevent users from going to the DMS and not locating health records on a patient, which can lead to assumptions that records do not exist or frustration with the DMS. Once there is a strong repository of data, access should be rolled out throughout the healthcare organization. Record scanning can be performed by the healthcare organization HIM or other designated staff or it can be outsourced to a vendor. If the healthcare organization decides to scan the health records themselves, additional staff would be needed to manage the current workload and to add backscanning to their tasks. Many healthcare organizations overcome this need by hiring temporary employees to cover the difference in workload. Healthcare organizations that choose vendors to scan (because of their high productivity and experienced staff) enable the scanning to be completed more quickly. The vendor usually charges by the number of images scanned and the actual tasks performed. These tasks may include preparation of the health record for scanning, indexing, and quality control.

Many hospitals begin implementation of the DMS by scanning the current emergency department patient records and gradually working up to inpatient records. Emergency department records are smaller, more controllable, and easier to manage than the inpatient records. An inpatient health record can have 75 to 100 pages or more for a three- to four-day stay on a regular nursing unit, whereas an emergency department record may be 5 to 15 pages.

Scanning may be performed in either a centralized or a decentralized approach. In the centralized approach, all scanning is performed in one location, generally the HIM department. In the decentralized approach, scanning is performed throughout the healthcare organization—wherever the documentation is created. These locations include admissions, nursing units, emergency department, and many more.

Justification of Cost

Healthcare organizations justify the cost of DMS with the savings that occur from decreasing the operating costs of the HIM department and the healthcare organization as a whole. The savings come from reductions in clerical staff, improvement in accounts receivable as health records are no longer misplaced and are therefore able to be coded, and increased revenue due to decreased expenses. Although staffing may increase at first while both the existing paper health record and the DMS are managed, over time staffing can be reduced below original levels. Additionally, operating cost reductions of the HIM department can be achieved, including elimination of file folders and other supplies related to processing the paper health record.

Because costs may actually go up in the short term, the return on investment for a DMS may be calculated over a 5- to 10-year period. When the file area is eliminated, the healthcare organization can reallocate that space to a revenue-generating department. Productivity is also increased, thus offsetting the cost of staffing. For example, the disclosure of health information coordinator no longer has to stand in front of a copy machine and the coder does not have to wait for health records to be assembled and analyzed in order to code them.

Forms

Forms management is a key implementation issue that must be addressed. At least six months prior to implementation of the DMS, forms should be evaluated and redesigned to facilitate the scanning process. The weight of the paper used should be appropriate for use in a scanner. Paper that is too heavy or too light may jam the automatic feeder. White paper is recommended for all forms because the color of the document is scanned along with the content of the form. This significantly increases the size of the computer file and the quality of the printed document. The forms should be standardized to 8.5 by 11 inch dimensions where possible. The redesign should include the addition of barcodes to each form. The **barcode** makes indexing more efficient because the barcode can enter metadata automatically. Standards for the use of barcodes must be established to facilitate scanning. These standards should include the size of the barcode, the standardized location of the barcode, and the amount of white space between the barcode and any text. The new forms with the barcode should be in use at the time of implementation. The recommended barcode **symbiology**, or format, is Code 39, also known as Code 3 of 9. These barcodes should be placed on the form in a standardized location.

Staffing Changes

With the transition of employees from filing paper to scanning, indexing, and quality control, new job titles and job descriptions will be required, and staffing needs may be reduced. For example, the file clerk role could be replaced by a clerk who performs both scanning and quality control for the scanning process. These tasks require additional technology skills, which may elevate the clerk's pay grade. However, since the workload is electronic, fewer pages would need to be filed within a paper health record, reducing the time and, thus, the personnel required to complete the task. Test results and other documents would be entered into the EHR automatically, without the need of human assistance. Over time, fewer paper documents would need to be scanned and incorporated, further decreasing the workload. However, there would still be a need for quality control measures, including both electronic precautions and physical monitoring procedures performed by the staff, to ensure that the information incorporated would go to the appropriate health record.

Changes in job titles and job descriptions must be in place at the time of the DMS implementation and would be decided after discussions with administration and the human resources department. The HIM department and other affected staff must be trained on the DMS prior to implementation to prevent backlogs from occurring, which would impact user satisfaction.

Process Redesign

The implementation of a DMS will have a tremendous impact on the workflow of an HIM department. As a result, the HIM department will have to reengineer workflows to adapt to an electronic environment and review and update policies and procedures, among many other tasks, to aid in the transition. The HIM department will no longer have to assemble the health record; they will prepare the health record for scanning instead. The way the traditional discharge processing, such as coding and health record analysis, is done will also drastically change. For instance:

- Analysis is done online.
- Physician completion of records can be completed from any location.
- Electronic signatures are used.

When to Scan the Health Record

Ideally, scanning should be performed as documents are created to allow immediate online access to orders, progress notes, and other written documentation. In practice, however, the health record is not usually scanned until after discharge. Some healthcare organizations scan the record immediately following discharge and use workflow technology to facilitate the record discharge processing. Other healthcare facilities complete the health record, obtaining all necessary documents and signatures, and then scan it.

Immediately Following Discharge

Many healthcare facilities scan the health record immediately following the patient's discharge from the hospital. There are a number of advantages to scanning the health record at this point. This timing allows coding and analysis to be performed remotely if the healthcare facility so chooses. It also allows immediate access to the health record for patient care, coding, analysis, and other healthcare operations. In the traditional paper environment, the discharge processing of the health record is a linear process. One step has to be completed before the next because only one employee can access the health record at a time. With DMS and workflow technology, coders, analysts, and other users no longer must wait for other steps in the discharge process to be complete before accessing the health record because imaging allows concurrent access. This speeds up the discharge processing function. Many patients are readmitted to the healthcare facility immediately after discharge, so having the recent discharged health record scanned and available to the emergency department or other patient care areas improves the quality of care provided.

There are also disadvantages to scanning immediately after discharge. Not only do staff members have to be trained to use the DMS as part of their discharge processing, but physicians must also be trained on how to complete health records online. In addition to retrieval of images, the physician would need to know how to use the annotation tools discussed earlier in this chapter and how to sign the documents electronically. The physician would also need to know how to complete forms electronically and to dictate discharge summaries and other documents.

The healthcare organization must have sufficient staff and equipment in place to ensure that the scanning is performed quickly so that the records are available to HIM staff, physicians, and other users in a timely manner. If scanning is not done promptly, health record users quickly become disillusioned with the DMS and not want to use it. It is especially important to have records available in the appropriate time period in the early days of the DMS, when everyone is getting used to it and learning about its benefits.

Scanning Upon Completion

Some healthcare organizations choose to scan the health record after the completion of the health record discharge processing. This method does not impact physician health record completion, and it does not allow coding and analysis to be performed remotely. Those who need access to the health record in the immediate discharge period still must wait for it to be processed in the traditional linear method—that is, the process in which the health record goes from the first step in discharge processing (usually putting all pages in the correct sequence) to each subsequent step and is completed when the final deficiency analysis is complete. The health record is scanned once all final paperwork (such as lab results) is received, all forms signed by the appropriate medical/nursing personnel, and transcribed reports are incorporated.

There are expenses related to the management of the paper record during the discharge process, such as the cost of folders and space for health record completion.

Retrieval of Images

To retrieve and view document images stored in the DMS, one must be an authorized user with the proper permissions. A user enters one or more of the indexed fields, such as a patient's health record number, to retrieve the appropriate health record and its associated document images for review.

Future of Document Management System

It is unlikely that imaging itself will be outdated anytime soon because there continue to be paper documents brought by the patient or from an outside source that will need to be scanned into the appropriate health record in the EHR. Upwards of 85 percent of office-based physicians use an EHR system (CDC 2017). More than 95 percent of hospitals use an EHR. Much of these statistics are influenced by location and financial status of the healthcare provider, with rural, critical access, and non-profit healthcare organizations lagging behind their counterparts (Parasrampuria 2019). However, not all of these healthcare organizations are completely electronic. Many are still not using all components of their respective EHR systems completely. The hybrid paper/electronic medical record will be with us for some time to come.

CHECK YOUR UNDERSTANDING 8.1

1. Sarah, the Scanner Technician, is preparing documents to scan into the EHR system. In order to differentiate between the various documents, she must a place a page that has a specialized barcode on it that contains identifying information about the following document in between each document. Pages that tell the scanner information about the page(s) that follow are called _____.

   a. Target sheets
   b. Automatic forms processing
   c. Barcodes
   d. Indexing

2. For each set of patient documents, Sarah must also create a record of the names, dates, contents, and types of documents therein contained to help catalog this information. The process that Sarah is performing of getting and listing specific information about a document so that it can be retrieved easily from a DMS is referred to as

   a. Scanning
   b. Target sheets
   c. Indexing
   d. Routing

3. It has come to Anne's (the HIM Assistant Director) attention that a large amount of printer paper is being sent to the Nursing floors. She's heard that nurses are printing patient documents to make notes on while working with patients. The pages are thrown away after the nurse inputs the appropriate notes into the EHR, a significant violation of HIPAA. What is the best tool Anne would use to help identify who, where, when, and how often this occurs?

   a. Provider authentication
   b. Password protection
   c. Print tracking log
   d. Biometric authentication

4. Dr. Randolph, the chief radiologist, has asked that any radiologic or imaging scans being input into the DMS be enlarged to twice the normal size. The older radiology system doesn't enlarge the images as clearly as the DMS. You instruct Sarah to do which of the following to oblige Dr. Randolph's request? _____.

CHECK YOUR UNDERSTANDING 8.1 (*Continued*)

    a. Annotation
    b. Abstracting
    c. Analytics
    d. Auditing

5. Dr. Smith receives an alert that the antibiotic that she is trying to prescribe for Mr. James is contraindicated since he is allergic to it as noted in his medical history of three years ago. In addition to the alert, the computer system provides a list of different antibiotics that would be more appropriate for his care. It asks which one she would choose to order for the patient. This is an example of:

    a. CDI
    b. DMS
    c. Value-based healthcare
    d. CDS   *Clinical decision Support*

Radiology Information System

A **radiology information system (RIS)** is used to collect, store, and provide information on radiological tests such as x-rays, ultrasound, magnetic resonance imaging (MRI), computed tomography (CT), and positron emission tomography (PET). The RIS also supports other radiological procedures performed in radiology such as ultrasound-guided biopsies and upper and lower gastrointestinal series. A RIS is designed to assist the technician by identifying the steps required to prepare for each test or procedure. The RIS can also assist the technician with taking x-rays and other radiological examinations by controlling radiation exposure, positioning of the patient, and image quality. Ultimately, the RIS provides patients with follow-up instructions to take home after the procedure.

The RIS can be used to assist in the management of the radiology department as well as document patient care. A RIS can perform many administrative tasks:

- Schedule patient examinations and procedures
- Report charges to the financial information system
- Generate management reports
- Generate radiology reports
- Track nuclear materials
- Transcribe documents
- Retrieve test results
- Fax radiology reports to the ordering physician
- Monitor supply inventory

Some of the management reports generated by the RIS include number of tests performed, types of tests or procedures performed, productivity by technicians, utilization of the various radiology machines, and productivity levels for each radiologist.

A RIS frequently has a **picture archival communication system (PACS)**. A PACS is an integrated information system that obtains, stores, retrieves, and displays digital images. In a PACS, x-ray films, MRIs, mammograms, and other radiological examinations (such as cardiac catheterization films and ultrasounds) are stored digitally, thus eliminating the need to store and manage the physical film. The digital image is immediately available for patient care, which is especially important in emergency department and intensive care situations. The filmless radiology saves the healthcare facility money and physical space by eliminating steps such as making copies for patients or purchasing folders for storage. As a result, radiology departments are able to provide improved (more efficient) customer service because there is no waiting for films to be pulled and copied. In addition, the PACS eliminates lost files.

The ability to view radiology images from any location by the radiologist and other users is called **teleradiology**. The images can even be viewed at multiple locations at the same time. A radiologist can read images from home in the middle of the night, from another city, or even from other countries. Teleradiology is also used frequently for consultations between radiologists who are in distant locations.

Because radiology images must have high resolution to be of diagnostic quality, the image must be compressed as it is transported across the network or Internet and then decompressed in a lossless manner to maintain its original form. PACS provides this capability.

A PACS affords the radiologist many conveniences. He or she can easily compare previous films to current ones, zoom in on suspicious areas, enhance an image, relocate or reposition an image, and apply pointers to identify problem areas. Once the images are pulled up in the PACS, the radiologist is able to magnify, rotate, measure, and use many other tools to view the images. When an image is read, the radiologist is able to dictate the report for transcription or use voice recognition software to create the report from within the information system.

Laboratory Information System   *LOINC - Lab only*

The **laboratory information system (LIS)** collects, stores, and manages laboratory tests and their respective results. LISs can be both internal within a healthcare organization or externally with a contracted laboratory providing the necessary services. The LIS can speed up access to test results through improved efficiency from various locations, including anywhere in the hospital, the physician's office, or even the clinician's home. The LIS has the necessary functionality to be used in all areas of the laboratory, including blood chemistry, blood banks, microbiology, virology, and pathology. Currently, LISs involve many interfaces because they are still typically standalone information systems, separate from the EHR. Interfaces are software that works between two or more systems to enable the two systems to share data. It is important for these interfaces to work seamlessly with the specified EHR system to ensure integration with the clinical and communications needs of the healthcare organization (Biedermann and Dolezel 2017, 84). The healthcare organization must get assurances from the EHR vendor that the interfaces between the new EHR and the existing information systems are complete and sustainable to avoid issues with transmission of the data. **Logical Observation Identifiers, Names and Codes (LOINC)** is a clinical terminology with more than 93,000 terms, for laboratory and clinical functions and provides electronic exchange standards for lab results. As with many terminologies and standards, LOINC programming and codes provide standardized communication between entities when transmitting results (Palkie 2020). For example, the code 94500-6 (*SARS coronavirus 2 RNA [Presence] in Respiratory specimen by NAA with probe detection*), should be used if a patient's upper or lower respiratory tract is being tested for COVID-19 (LOINC 2020).

The physician order for a laboratory test is generally received from a CPOE or other order entry system. The CPOE identifies what tests need to be run, schedules them, and creates a list that indicates where the patient is located and if the test is routine or urgent. Test results can be entered into the LIS manually or collected automatically from the instruments running the test. The LIS can also print out various laboratory reports needed, such as all of the tests performed on a single day or during a patient's entire hospitalization. Other functions include:

- Identifying normal ranges for each laboratory test
- Generating laboratory reports

CPOE - Computerized Physician Order Entry

- Marking laboratory values as high, low, or panic
- Notifying laboratory staff and physicians of panic (very high or low) values via alerts (such as an audible ping or alarm, results highlighted in a different color, or a note sent to the "to-do list")
- Printing barcode labels to track specimens
- Recording quality control activities
- Generating management reports
- Submitting charges to the financial information system

The LIS can assist management in running the laboratory department through the management reporting capabilities. It should be able to generate reports such as the number of tests run per month, the tests ran, turnaround time, and productivity reports on individual laboratory technicians. The LIS also assists in public health reporting for state departments of health requirements. Many states have lists of conditions or diseases where "immediately" or "suspect immediately" reporting is mandated (FDOH 2016). This is particularly important during disease outbreaks. Cyclical outbreaks such as influenza are relatively predictable since they occur yearly but can fluctuate in intensity and/or volume. Unusual or unanticipated outbreaks, such as measles, Zika virus, or COVID-19, can wreak havoc on local and state health resources. The state can use the data from hospitals' LIS to plan and determine courses of actions, adjust supply routing, and healthcare personnel distribution.

CHECK YOUR UNDERSTANDING 8.2

1. Now that the Radiology Department has gone completely digital, Dr. Randolph has asked for your assistance. He wants to know what to do with the filing shelves that are no longer necessary. They are no longer needed because Radiology no longer needs the space to store which of the following?

    a. Coding
    b. Certification
    c. Invoices
    d. Film

2. One of the Processing Techs asks you why she is not able to find hemoglobin results when she accesses the RIS. You inform her that an RIS has results for all of the follow scans except _____ since those results would be found in the LIS.

    a. PET
    b. MRI
    c. CT
    d. Complete blood count

3. A radiologist specializing in cardiac structure abnormalities is located in a different city 400 miles away. She is consulted to review a series of echocardiograms on an pediatric patient. She discusses the results with the parents and their pediatrician and does not recommend surgery at this time. The term used to describe viewing images from a remote location is _____.

(Continued)

CHECK YOUR UNDERSTANDING 8.2 (Continued)

    a. PACS
    b. Teleradiology
    c. RIS
    d. Symbiology

4. Dr. Singh, who has a new gastroenterology practice in town, comes to you because of several error messages he receives from the RIS when accessing the contrast media scans of his patients. You contact Jeremy in IT to help identify the issue. Jeremy finds that Dr. Singh's EHR communicate with the RIS as smoothly as it should. Jeremy states he can write a software program that would fix this issue. The type computer program that Jeremy talked about that allows two different information systems to communicate with each other is referred to as an _____.

    a. Interface
    b. Interchange
    c. Integration
    d. Annotation

5. Jerome is investigating why there is such a significantly higher number of CBC diff tests run in the past week even though there was no increase in the number of patients seen. He's discovered that the bar code labels attached to each vial of blood to identify which tests should be run were incorrectly printed. Which system is Jerome using to evaluate this issue?
    a. LIS
    b. RIS
    c. NIS
    d. CIS

Nursing Information System

A **nursing information system (NIS)** assists in the planning and monitoring of overall patient care. A NIS will document the nursing care provided to a patient. **Clinical documentation** is any manual or electronic notation or recording made by a physician or other healthcare clinician related to a patient's medical condition or treatment. There may be different NISs available for the emergency department, intensive care areas, and other nursing areas because of the differing needs of each specialization. The capabilities of a strong nursing information system are flexible to accommodate the needs of the nurse. Conveniences such as efficient and quality documentation practices as well as easy access to quick reference guides are important. Advantages to NIS include:

- Reduction in costs of providing nursing care
- Improved patient care
- Immediate access to information on services rendered by the nursing staff
- Immediate notification of results from laboratory, radiology, or other ancillary departments
- Reduction in lost charges
- Reduced average length of stay
- Submitting charges to the financial information system

Many of these advantages result from the documentation of information at the time of care.

An NIS must be designed to support and promote quality documentation and practices through the use of protocols and vocabularies. Based on information entered into the NIS, such as the patient's diagnosis or procedure, the appropriate nursing protocol is selected.

The nurse plans the patient's nursing care needs based on this protocol. Nursing documentation traditionally includes:

- Admission assessment
- Nursing activities
- Intake and output
- Graphic information
- Activities of daily living
- Nursing care plans
- Nurses' notes
- Medication administration record

The NIS can also assist in the administrative management and daily operations of the nursing department by:

- Monitoring staffing allocation
- Scheduling nursing staff
- Generating performance improvement reports

Pharmacy Information System

A **pharmacy information system (PIS)** assists providers in ordering, allocating, and administering medication. With a focus on patient safety issues, especially medication errors, the PIS is a key tool in providing optimal patient care. The PIS stores the patient's demographic information, allergies, medication history, diagnoses, laboratory results, and other key information. Much like an LIS, the PIS can be internal within a healthcare organization or external using contracted pharmacy services.

Data contained within the hospital information system and the functions of the PIS help providers reduce medication errors by using the hospital information system, the EHR, and the PIS, combined with information from medical databases and drug formularies. For example, a patient may have indicated an allergy in her history and physical exam, which may have been performed many days or weeks ago. If the physician attempts to prescribe a medication that is contraindicated by the documented allergy, the PIS would alert the physician to this contraindication and suggest another medication. **RxNorm** is the standardized nomenclature of drugs and medications providing unambiguous and consistent information regarding chemical composition, dosages, and forms (pill, injection, etc.). Like LOINC, this standardization helps with the interoperability between systems for smooth electronic exchange of health information (Palkie 2020).

The PIS can stand alone or be integrated with other systems in the healthcare organization such as CPOE. The greatest benefits come from the integration of data. For example, CPOE can record the medication order in the pharmacy system, which, in turn, can automatically update inventory levels—thus, automatically charging the patient.

PISs are used in hospitals, drugstores, and other healthcare settings. Functions vary according to the needs of the setting and facility. For example, a drugstore might need to track the number of refills remaining on a prescription, whereas this function would not be as important to a hospital.

PISs check for drug interactions, food and drug interactions, and other contraindications. When problems are identified, the PIS alerts the pharmacist or end user. It should also determine whether or not the dosage and administration method is appropriate for the size and age of the patient. The PIS can also manage the inventory of drugs in the pharmacy. This includes:

- Ordering drugs
- Inventory control
- Managing the formulary
- Tracking the costs of drugs
- Reporting on the usage of controlled medications

The pharmacy can analyze data stored within the information system, such as looking for patterns of drug usage and signs of abuse. These patterns may identify potential abuse by patients or physicians. The use of PIS within an EHR assists pharmacy, clinical, and administrative personnel with quality improvement activities and research of pharmacy usage and applications.

PISs can assist in the dispensing of medications in the pharmacy, which can help the nursing units in a number of ways:

- Creating individual dosages
- Use of secure storage systems
- Robotics
- Secure access to medications
- Documentation of medications administered, including when and by whom
- Barcodes

Interdisciplinary Charting System

An **interdisciplinary charting system** can be used by any healthcare professional to collect and store patient assessments, progress notes, and care plans. Examples of these healthcare professionals include physicians, nurses, physical therapists, respiratory therapists, pharmacists, dietitians, and the like. The information system can also collect data, such as vital signs and input and output, automatically. Handheld devices such as tablets are frequently used to allow for documentation at the bedside.

Emergency Department System

The **emergency department system (EDS)** is designed to meet the unique needs of the emergency department, including tracking patients from triage to discharge. The EIS is also able to record test results and other clinical information. Demographic information is obtained from the hospital information system. The emergency department system can also assist in the department's workflow and generate management reports such as turnaround times, patient wait times, and more. This information system has become increasingly important in population health reporting.

There is a need to notify state health authorities regarding diagnoses of newly emerging diseases, such as Zika virus infection or multidrug-resistant tuberculosis; injuries due to mass casualty events, such as terrorist bombings or train derailments; and injuries due to natural disasters, such as tornadoes and hurricanes.

Anesthesia Information System

An **anesthesia information system** collects information on preoperative, operative, and postoperative anesthesia-related clinical information. This system follows the patient through the surgical process. The information system collects information on risk factors, vital signs, type of anesthesia, anesthetic agents used, dosage of anesthetic agents, and much more. The information system uses the information that is captured to create charges for billing purposes.

As with other clinical information systems, the demographic information comes from the hospital information system. The data captured can also be used for quality improvement. Management reports can be created to provide statistics on a number of operations, frequency of anesthetic agents, and such.

Patient Monitoring System

The **patient monitoring system** automatically collects and stores patient data from various information systems used in healthcare. Data collected include fetal monitoring, vital signs, and oxygen saturation rates. Patient monitoring systems are typically utilized in the intensive care units and other specialty areas such as the operating and recovery rooms.

A patient monitoring system must be able to capture the desired data automatically. The nurse or other user should be able to monitor a patient's condition from the nursing unit, physician office, or other remote location if necessary. This may require the use of the Internet to access the information system. A nurse or other user must be able to create notes if needed to document and report variations in results, such as if the fetal monitor slipped out of position. Vital signs and other data collected must be also reviewed and approved by the user regularly to ensure proper system functioning.

Telehealth

Telehealth has two aspects:

- Professional services given to a patient through an interactive telecommunications system by a practitioner at a distant site
- A telecommunications system that links healthcare organizations and patients from diverse geographic locations and transmits text and images for (medical) consultation and treatment

These locations can be across town, in rural areas, or in another country. Most specialists are located in urban areas, leaving patients in rural areas without easy access to them. Telehealth allows a physician to examine and treat a patient remotely. Telehealth can utilize video telephone, computers, smart phones, and other medical devices with wireless capabilities, such as cardiac pacemakers, glucose monitors and insulin pumps, or neuromonitors that can be checked remotely. Access to the patient or the device through the healthcare organization's EHR is also feasible. A nurse may be required to interact directly with the patient in order to support the physician's evaluation and treatment.

Benefits of telehealth include:

- Improved access to healthcare, such as specialty consultations, biomedical monitoring, and second opinions
- Improved continuity of care, patient education, and timely treatment—follow-up visits for chronically ill patients, reduced travel time for all involved, increased care to underserved areas
- Cost efficiency—managing chronically ill patients more efficiently decreases admissions and shortens length of stay
- Improved access to health records and patient information with online health information available for learning, peer support groups, research information
- Improved training and education for medical/clinical personnel as well as patients, clinical trial research, improved interactions with medical personnel for disease management (Villines 2020)

Physicians find clinical telehealth a benefit in giving patients medical consultations and monitoring those living in rural areas or those who are homebound. Telemonitoring is used at the

Remote Pt Monitoring — RPM

patient's home to monitor cardiac rhythms, blood sugar, blood pressure, and other values to be submitted to the care provider. This type of monitoring can be performed through the use of the telephone or the computer. The data collected at the patient's home are digitally submitted into a CIS and thus made a part of the EHR.

Telehealth is a very sophisticated technology. Technology used includes virtual reality and robotics, which may be used to assist with the examination or treatment of a patient. The use of robotics to perform surgery is called **telesurgery**. This allows surgery to be performed on a patient in a different location.

Issues that healthcare facilities need to consider when developing or using **telemedicine**—a subset of telehealth that focuses on the provision of care whereas telehealth includes administrative uses and education—programs:

- Privacy, confidentiality, and security must be ensured during the telemedicine event.
  - Safeguard patients' privacy
  - Network security among hospitals, clinics, practitioners
  - Contract specialties, such as radiology and mental health, with private networks with point-to-point connections
- Liability is usually shared between referring provider and consulting provider, but for telemedicine vendors and technical staff there is no legal precedent yet.
- Licensure and accreditation rules differ by states for both licensure and accreditation; there is no federal legislation for telemedicine at this time.
- Fraud—vendor services, billing for healthcare services provided, and contracts need clear legal analysis.
- Policies and procedures must be developed and agreed to by all parties.
- Documentation requirement for patient information and services is provided (Johnson and Warner 2013).

Telehealth provides many advantages, such as improved access to care, treatment provided via communication tools, and home monitoring. The problem is that the infrastructure is expensive, and because physicians are licensed to practice medicine by state, the geographic range in which the physician can consult is limited. Remote patient monitoring (RPM) is an example of homecare telehealth that use smart phones and various mobile medical devices to collect patient-generated health data (PGHD). This is particularly relevant for patients with chronic conditions, who are high-risk, or require senior care. This not only benefits the practitioners by providing timely and pertinent health information on the patient's condition, but benefits the patient by increasing their participation, support, and engagement in the healthcare decision making process (Rouse 2019).

Telehealth records must be managed as with any other patient care encounter. There are no differences in the documentation requirements between patient care provided remotely or at bedside, so the current documentation practices and forms are adequate. The American Health Information Management Association (AHIMA) recommends the following minimum information:

- Patient name
- Identification number
- Date of service
- Referring physician
- Consulting physician
- Provider facility

- Type of evaluation performed
- Informed consent
- Evaluation results
- Diagnosis and impression
- Recommendations for further treatment (Johnson and Warner 2013)

The HIM professional must take the necessary steps to ensure that the privacy and security of patient's health information is protected according to HIPAA requirements and any applicable state laws. For example, procedures in the administrative, technical, or physical safeguards domains may require revision to remain HIPAA-compliant while accommodating telehealth. This may involve providing a secure area where physicians can consult with the patient, ensuring additional security and encryption capabilities on the HIS, and established procedures and training for conducting telehealth sessions. The HIM professional may also be involved in the medical staff credentialing process to ensure physicians are indeed licensed and qualified to practice within the state. Finally, specific attention must be paid to the varying state laws and regulations to ensure compliance with them. More information on telehealth can be found in chapter 10.

Smart Card

A **smart card** is a plastic card, similar in appearance to a credit card, with a computer chip embedded in it. Smart cards have been widely adopted for use in banking, retail, government, and other applications. Three uses of smart cards in healthcare are emergency treatment, reducing fraud and abuse, and reducing administrative costs (Secure Technology Alliance 2017a).

Smart cards enable portable storage of health and insurance information. They are relatively inexpensive and are able to protect the information stored within them from unauthorized access. In an emergency situation, smart cards can provide a physician with the critical information needed for proper care and treatment of a patient such as allergies, significant conditions like diabetes mellitus, and more. There are two categories of smart cards: contact and contactless. The contact smart cards require a scanner through which the card is scanned in order to read it. The contactless card only has to be close to the scanner (Secure Technology Alliance 2017b).

Although smart cards are useful tools, the patient must manage and maintain the accuracy of information on the card. Some smart cards require a password or a personal identification number that the patient must remember for access. Another concern is privacy of the information on the card in the event that it is stolen.

Impact of Clinical Information Systems on HIM

The HIM professional is typically not a direct user of the various CISs discussed throughout this chapter, although the HIM professional accesses the information through either the CIS or the EHR. However, the HIM professional is the expert on the management of health records, and input from this individual is important to ensure that accreditation, regulatory, and other requirements are met. The same is true for privacy and security issues. HIM professionals are highly recommended to be a part of the information system implementation team to ensure that all HIM-related concerns such as quality documentation, confidentiality practices, and retention schedules are addressed up front. As each CIS submits charges to the financial information system, the HIM professional may be involved in developing the charges, similar to the involvement in the facility's chargemaster. Lastly, remember that every clinical information system can populate the EHR with information that is ultimately managed and maintained by HIM professionals.

CHECK YOUR UNDERSTANDING 8.3

1. Due to a diagnosis of sepsis, Mr. Walters, is given IV antibiotics and is monitored closely for fever. His temperature is checked every two hours along with other vital signs. The EHR places these readings on charts and graphs so it is easy to see any fluctuations over time. Data such as graphic information and activities of daily living would be typically found within the _____ information system?

   a. Telehealth
   b. Pharmacy information system
   c. Nursing information system
   d. Telemedicine

2. Interfaces are important between systems so that communication flows smoothly. When Dr. Neal prescribes antibiotics using the CPOE and her patient is able to pick it up on her way home from the appointment, it's beneficial for all involved. Identify the clinical information systems that easily operates with the CPOE.

   a. Telehealth
   b. Pharmacy information system
   c. Nursing information system
   d. Telemedicine

3. When Edward was hired at his new firm, the local HMO providing services issued him a new health ID card. It looks much like his driver's licence with his picture, insurance information, and health plan number. Once he establishes a relationship with a physician, basic health information will be added to the chip that is embedded in it. A portable method of storage of health data is known as _____.

   a. E-medicine
   b. Smart card
   c. E-health
   d. E-care

4. Another term used interchangeably with telehealth is _____.

   a. Teleconference
   b. E-health
   c. Teleradiology
   d. Telemedicine   *Quality Improvement*

5. Amanda, one of your QI techs, had to request permission from you to access the hospital formulary for a current research project. Additional permission is necessary due to HIPAA security protocols limiting employees' access to areas of the EHR that are not in their normal daily routine. Identify the personnel that typically do not use the clinical information systems directly in their daily tasks?

   a. Radiology
   b. Nursing
   c. Pharmacy
   d. HIM

Real-World Case 8.1

Due to the tropical nature of most of the state of Florida and the large influx of travelers from the southern Atlantic islands, and Central and South America, the spread of the Zika virus is a very real concern. The sudden increase in cases of coronavirus 2019 (COVID-19) has made Florida one of the epicenters of the pandemic. The Florida Department of Health (FDOH) can receive real-time electronic notification from a Florida healthcare organization's CIS of any suspected or confirmed diagnoses of Zika or COVID-19.

Using the patient demographic information received from the hospitals' LIS public health reporting systems, FDOH uses a geographic information system (GIS) to map and track the spread of the Zika and corona virus anywhere in the state. Based on the tracking information, mosquito eradication, patient testing, tracking, tracing protocols, and hospital bed utilization efforts can be coordinated and focused on the most at-risk locations. The respective local government officials, county health departments, and hospital administrations can then provide additional and more aggressive screenings and initiate earlier treatment on the identified at-risk populations.

Real-World Case 8.2

Due to the COVID-19 pandemic, the ABC Internal Medicine Group (IMG), a large group practice of internal medicine and cardiology specialists, has instituted new procedures regarding telehealth appointments for a majority of their patients. One example is the use of remote monitoring of all cardiac patients who have a pacemaker. Each patient was sent a simple-to-use remote monitoring device (so they did not have to come to their doctor's office) to be used in their home. This device looks much like a computer mouse. At regularly scheduled intervals, the patient places the mouse-like device directly above the location of their pacemaker. The device uploads all the monitoring history stored in the pacemaker and then sends the information electronically to the IMG clinical information system. The patient's respective cardiologist then reviews the patient information that was downloaded to the CIS system. Providers can make recommendations for additional diagnostic activities and/or treatments, changes in medication, or just maintain the established treatment protocols. Follow-up discussions between the patients and cardiologists can be performed over the patient's personal computer or given the option to come to IMG. Patients have been very receptive to this model of care since they do not have to leave their homes in the midst of a quarantine and put themselves at additional risk for being exposed to COVID-19.

REVIEW QUESTIONS

1. Rene is a new Processing Technician. You are explaining where she would find specific information in the EHR for her various work duties. Since one of her areas is R-ADT productivity, she will have access to the MPI and DSS but not the CIS. Identify the function that does not fall under the CIS.

   a. Quality improvement
   b. Surgery
   c. Nursing
   d. Pharmacy

2. Dr. Olsen wants to know more about the differences between an EHR and a DMS. He thinks he'll be able to update the old documents once they have been scanned into the system. Identify a disadvantage of a DMS.

(Continued)

  a. Space saving
  b. Retrieval of a large number of records
  c. Lack of ability to manipulate data
  d. Multiple users can access data at one time

3. As HIM Director, you explain to the CEO that clinicians need patient information on the go-live date for the new EHR. You discuss with her the importance of having the old health records input into the new system at least 6 months prior to the go-live date. Your productivity calculations show that you will need four clerical positions to complete this task in the allotted time. The term _____, is used for the processing of scanning past health records into the information system so there is an existing database of patient information, making the information system valuable to the user from the first day of implementation.

  a. CPOE
  b. OCR
  c. Backscanning
  d. Barcoding

4. The CFO wants to know which patient charts will be scanned first. You explain that the records with fewer pages per encounter would have the most productive impact. Typically, the health record that is smaller, more controllable, and easiest to manage and that should be scanned first when implementing a DMS is the:

  a. Inpatient
  b. Outpatient surgery
  c. Newborns
  d. Emergency department

5. During the discussion of the DMS with the CFO, he asks about the high initial personnel costs of implementing such a system. You explain once all the old records are backscanned, the costs go down significantly. You explain that the return on investment for a DMS is usually calculated using _____ time period?

  a. 5–10 years
  b. 6–12 months
  c. 1–3 years
  d. 1–3 months

6. The CFO wants to know what methods the HIM personnel are using to increase productivity and accuracy of the data when scanning old records into the DMS. The use of _____ makes the indexing of scanned health record more efficient because it can enter metadata automatically.

  a. Barcodes
  b. Backscanning
  c. OCR
  d. CPOE

7. Jennifer is the HIM Operations Manager. She is evaluating the conversion workflow of paper documents received from external providers into her hospital's EHR system. Identify the component that Jennifer will not be reviewing within the DMS.

REVIEW QUESTIONS (*Continued*)

    a. Scanner
    b. LIS
    c. File server
    d. Workstations

8. Identify the diagnostic test that is not completed within a RIS.

    a. MRI
    b. PET
    c. CPOE
    d. CT

9. Within the RIS, the _____ software obtains, stores, retrieves, and displays digital images.

    a. CPOE
    b. OCR
    c. PIS
    d. PACS

10. Where would you typically find robotics performing specific and complex tasks?

    a. Telehealth
    b. Telesurgery
    c. EDS
    d. Telemedicine

11. Edna is told that she needs to wear a Holter monitor for 72 hours to check her heart rate during this time. There is an app she downloads on to her smartphone so that this cardiac information is sent to her doctor's office for evaluation every 24 hours. She does not have to go to the doctor's office everyday and only needs to wait until her doctor checks the information to determine if Edna needs to see a specialist. Identify the activity that Edna is participating in.

    a. RPM
    b. Telesurgery
    c. EDS
    d. PACS

12. You are working with the IT and Radiology Managers to develop a list of all the radiological images that would be included in the EHR. Your group is developing an inventory for the data dictionary. Which of the following data or documents would not be used in a PACS?

    a. CT scan
    b. Ultrasound
    c. Discharge summary
    d. X-ray

Abbreviations/Acronyms Matching

1. EDS   A.   software that coordinates the ordering of all tests, scans, and other diagnostic activities for the patient

(*Continued*)

REVIEW QUESTIONS (*Continued*)

2. DMS   B. a method to evaluate the speed and capability of a scanner

3. CDS   C. software that converts images to digital format eliminating the need for films

4. PPM   D. helps patients who live far away to send information and status updates of their health and medical devices to their healthcare providers

5. NIS   E. IS that is important in tracking outbreaks due to monitoring activity of patients seeking emergency care for symptoms

6. PACS   F. software that incorporates paper and external documents into the provider's EHR system

7. CPOE   G. software that documents the overall nursing care of the patient

8. CIS   H. makes text scannable and readable in order to be inputted into a DMS and EHR

9. OCR   I. software that helps medical professionals determine the best course of action for their patients

10. RPM   J. software that collects, stores, and manages all health and medical information on a patient

References

Amatayakul, M. 2020. Health Information Systems. *Health Information Management Technology, An Applied Approach.* 6th ed. Chicago: AHIMA.

American Hospital Association (AHA). 2018. Improving Patient Safety and Health Care Quality through Health Information Technology. Accessed June 24, 2020. https://www.aha.org/system/files/2018-07/18-07-trendwatch-issue-brief3-patient-safety-quality-health-it.pdf.

Biedermann, S. and D. Dolezel. 2017. *Introduction to Healthcare Informatics,* 2nd ed. Chicago: AHIMA.

Bresnick, J. 2017. Understanding the Basics of Clinical Decision Support Systems. Accessed 7/12/202. https://healthitanalytics.com/features/understanding-the-basics-of-clinical-decision-support-systems.

Campbell, Angela et al. "Beyond the Basics for Health Informatics Professionals" Journal of AHIMA 89, no. 8 (September 2018): 58–63.

Centers of Disease Control and Prevention (CDC). 2020. Implementing Clinical Decision Support Systems. Accessed 7/15/2020. https://www.cdc.gov/dhdsp/pubs/guides/best-practices/clinical-decision-support.htm

Centers of Disease Control and Prevention (CDC). 2017. Electronic Medical Records/Electronic Health Records (EMRs/EHRs). https://www.cdc.gov/nchs/data/nehrs/2017_NEHRS_Web_Table_EHR_State.pdf

Daley, S. 2020. 32 examples of ai in healthcare that will make you feel better about the future. https://builtin.com/artificial-intelligence/artificial-intelligence-healthcare. July 29, 2020.

Florida Department of Health (FDOH). 2016. Laboratory Reporting Guidelines for Reportable Diseases and Conditions in Florida. Accessed 717/2020. http://www.floridahealth.gov/diseases-and-conditions/disease-reporting-and-management/_documents/guidelines-laboratories.pdf

Johnson, M. L. and D. Warner. 2013. Practice Brief: Telemedicine services and the health record (2013 update). http://bok.ahima.org/doc?oid=300269#.Wduo3GhSxRa.

Knorr, E. 2018. What is cloud computing? Everything you need to know now. https://www.infoworld.com/article/2683784/what-is-cloud-computing.html

Lee-Eichenwald, S. 2020. Health Information Technologies. *Health Information Management, Concepts, Principles, and Practice*, 6th ed. Chicago: AHIMA.

Logical Observation Identifiers Names and Codes(LOINC). 2020. Guidance for mapping to SARS-CoV-2 LOINC terms. https://loinc.org/sars-coronavirus-2/

Microsoft. 2020. What is cloud computing. Accessed 9/23/2020. https://azure.microsoft.com/en-us/overview/what-is-cloud-computing/#benefits

Miliard, M. 2012. Healthcare IT News. Bringing the ED to the C-suite. http://www.healthcareitnews.com/news/bringing-ed-c-suite.

Monga, Kapila. "Mining Medical Records: A Case for Artificial Intelligence in Health Systems" Journal of AHIMA 88, no. 10 (October 2017): 54–56.

New England Journal of Medicine (NEJM). 2017. What Is Value-Based Healthcare? NEJM Catalyst. Accessed June 24, 2020. https://catalyst.nejm.org/doi/full/10.1056/CAT.17.0558

Office of the National Coordinator. 2018. What is clinical decision support (CDS)? Accessed June 24, 2020. https://www.healthit.gov/topic/safety/clinical-decision-support

Parasrampuria, S. and Henry, J. (2019). Hospitals' Use of Electronic Health Records Data, 2015-2017. ONC Data Brief, no. 46. https://www.healthit.gov/sites/default/files/page/2019-04/AHAEHRUseDataBrief.pdf

Park, A. 2019. Machines Treating Patients? It's Already Happening. Time magazine. March 21, 2019. Accessed June 26, 2020. https://time.com/5556339/artificial-intelligence-robots-medicine/

Palkie, B. 2020. Clinical Classifications, Vocabularies, Terminologies, and Standards. *Health Information Management, Concepts, Principles, and Practice*, 6th ed. Chicago: AHIMA.

Reynolds, R. and Morey, A. 2020. Health Record Content and Documentation. *Health Information Management, Concepts, Principles, and Practice*, 6th ed. Chicago: AHIMA.

Rouse, M. 2019. Remote patient monitoring. Accessed June 24, 2020. https://searchhealthit.techtarget.com/definition/remote-patient-monitoring-RPM

Secure Technology Alliance. 2017a. Smart Card Applications in the U.S. Healthcare Industry. http://www.smartcardalliance.org/smart-cards-applications-healthcare/.

Secure Technology Alliance. 2017b. Smart Card Primer. http://www.smartcardalliance.org/smart-cards-intro-primer/.

Spitzer, J. 2018. Here's where hospitals are using clinical decision support. Accessed June 24, 2020. https://www.beckershospitalreview.com/healthcare-information-technology/report-here-s-where-hospitals-are-using-clinical-decision-support.html

Sutton, R.T., Pincock, D., Baumgart, D.C. *et al.* An overview of clinical decision support systems: benefits, risks, and strategies for success. *npj Digit. Med.* 3, 17 (2020). https://doi.org/10.1038/s41746-020-0221-y

Villines, Z. 2020. Telemedicine benefits: For patients and professionals. Accessed 7/18/2020. https://www.medicalnewstoday.com/articles/telemedicine-benefits

Electronic Health Record

Learning Objectives

- Create a development and implementation plan for an electronic health record (EHR).
- Explain the role of clinical vocabularies in the EHR.
- Support the need for and address issues related to the EHR.
- Educate the provider on benefits of the EHR.
- Identify the need for the multiple information systems required to support the EHR.
- Support the need for the personal health record.

Key Terms

Audit log
Barcode medication
  administration record
  (BC-MAR)
Certified EHR technology
Clinical decision support
  (CDS) system
Clinical messaging
Computerized provider order
  entry (CPOE)
Continuity of care record
  (CCR)
Core data set
Digital signature
Digitized signature
Document management
  system (DMS)
Electronic medical
  record (EMR)
Electronic medication
  administration record
  (EMAR)

Electronic signature
General equivalence mapping
  (GEM)
Health information blocking
Health information
  technology (HIT)
Health Level Seven
  International (HL7)
Hybrid record
Interoperability
Longitudinal health record
Merit-based Incentive
  Payment System (MIPS)
National Voluntary
  Laboratory Accreditation
  Program (NVLAP)
Office of the National
  Coordinator for Health
  Information Technology
  (ONC)
ONC–Approved Accreditor
  (ONC-AA)

ONC–Authorized Certification
  Bodies (ONC-ACBs)
Order entry and results
  reporting
Patient-provider portal
Personal health record
  (PHR)
Population health
Quality Payment
  Program (QPP)
Radiofrequency identification
  devices (RFIDs)
Reminders
Source systems
Standards
Structured data
Template-based entry
Unstructured data

As defined in chapter 1, an EHR is an electronic record of health-related information on an individual that conforms to nationally recognized interoperability standards and that authorized clinicians and staff across more than one healthcare organization can create, manage, and consult. With its seminal publication, *To Err Is Human: Building a Safer Health System*, the Institute of Medicine, now the National Academy of Medicine (NAM), advocated for the use of **health information technology (HIT)** to help prevent many of the mistakes that regularly occur in the delivery of healthcare and that lead to the injuries and deaths of tens of thousands of patients (NAM 2000, 1). HIT includes the hardware, software, integrated technologies or related licenses, intellectual property, upgrades, or packaged solutions sold as services that are designed for or support the use by healthcare entities or patients for the electronic creation, maintenance, access, or exchange of health information. Included under the umbrella of HIT is the EHR. Among its many recommendations, the NAM promotes the EHR to include the following:

(1) longitudinal collection of electronic health information for and about persons, where health information is defined as information pertaining to the health of an individual or health care provided to an individual; (2) immediate electronic access to person- and population-level information by authorized, and only authorized, users; (3) provision of knowledge and decision-support that enhance the quality, safety, and efficiency of patient care; and (4) support of efficient processes for health care delivery (IOM 2003, 1).

A **longitudinal health record** is a permanent record of significant information listed in chronological order and maintained across time, ideally from birth to death. Access to the EHR should not be limited to the healthcare organization, but rather be accessible remotely for providers as well as the consumer.

The EHR should not be confused with an **electronic medical record (EMR)**. An EMR is an electronic collection of all the patient's health information and clinical care that is stored, managed, and referred to by authorized members of one healthcare entity, much like the actual paper health record only in digital or electronic form. An EHR includes everything in an EMR, but is much more comprehensive in terms of the patient's overall health, the care and services provided to the patient, and all healthcare providers participating in the patient care. In addition to the clinical sources of patient information, such as lab, radiology, and intensive care units, the EHR also includes administrative sources such as registration, patient financial services, quality improvement applications, and reporting and analytics. The EHR provides the "big picture" of the patient's encounter for health services, not just the medical information generated from the encounter.

The EHR must meet national standards for interoperability set by the Office of the National Coordinator for Health Information Technology (ONC). **Interoperability** is the ability of different information technology systems and software applications to communicate; to exchange data accurately, effectively, and consistently; and to use the information that has been exchanged. Additionally, an EHR is an information system in which the clinical information is utilized for the following purposes:

- Reimbursement, diagnostic and procedural coding, claims processing
- Computerized provider order entry (CPOE) and results reporting for laboratory, radiology, and other diagnostic tests
- E-prescriptions sent to the patient's pharmacy
- Medication management
- Population health reporting
- Quality improvement activities
- Clinical decision support
- Healthcare organization administrative reports and analytics
- Other additional authorized activities (Lee-Eichenwald 2020, 371)

The EHR is designed to not only be used by the originating healthcare entity but be able to be referred to and transmitted to authorized and authenticated users at other healthcare entities (Amatayakul 2017, 9).

According to the Healthcare Information and Management Systems Society (HIMSS), there are four levels of interoperability:

- Foundational (Level 1): Establishes the inter-connectivity requirements needed for one system or application to securely communicate data to and receive data from another
- Structural (Level 2): Defines the format, syntax and organization of data exchange including at the data field level for interpretation
- Semantic (Level 3): Provides for common underlying models and codification of the data including the use of data elements with standardized definitions from publicly available value sets and coding vocabularies, providing shared understanding and meaning to the user
- Organizational (Level 4): Includes governance, policy, social, legal, and organizational considerations to facilitate the secure, seamless and timely communication and use of data both within and between organizations, entities and individuals. These components enable shared consent, trust and integrated end-user processes and workflows (HIMSS 2020).

Health information management professionals can be found and involved in any of the levels of interoperability due to their education and training computer literacy, database management, and information systems applications.

Purpose and Components of the Electronic Health Record

The EHR is not like a software program that can be bought, loaded on a server, and used immediately. It can take years to properly implement an EHR because of the number and complexity of the system components. The EHR is a collection of multiple technologies and information systems that work together. **Source systems** are information systems that capture and feed data into the EHR. Source systems include the electronic medication administration record (EMAR), laboratory information system, radiology information system, hospital information system, nursing information systems, and more. Source systems are not just clinical systems, but also include administrative and financial systems (Lee-Eichenwald 2020, 3374). The technology includes patient monitoring equipment, dispensing devices and robotics, and supporting infrastructure of networks, cloud-based storage, and telehealth technologies. See Figure 9.5 for a schematic of source systems. More information about source systems is presented later in this chapter. To realize the full benefits of the EHR, data should be captured at the point of care or data origination. Data can be captured in a multitude of ways, which can include personal computers, handheld devices, voice recognition, handwriting recognition, and other methods of data entry.

The healthcare organization must have the necessary infrastructure, the underlying framework and features of an information system, to integrate data. Much of the infrastructure for the EHR is the same as that for any information system—computers, monitors, network, printers, operating system, and application software. The EHR infrastructure may also include a clinical data repository to centralize the data from the source systems. Another component of the EHR infrastructure is clinical decision support that controls alerts, reminders, order sets, and protocols (Amatayakul 2017, 14). The EHR should have access to knowledge-based resources such as MEDLINE, electronic drug references, and research databases. An example of this would be a recommendation from the CDS for an improved diagnostic method or more effective medication to treat a patient's condition.

EHRs include a **continuity of care record (CCR)** and a personal health record. The CCR is a **core data set,** which is the most relevant administrative, demographic, and clinical information about a patient's healthcare, covering one or more healthcare encounters. The CCR is *not* the minimum dataset for the EHR; it is information that is deemed most important for the continued care of the patient who is transferred to or seen by another healthcare practitioner (Amatayakul 2017, 302). It provides a means for one healthcare practitioner, system, or setting to aggregate all of the pertinent data about a patient and forward it to another practitioner, system, or setting to support the continuity of care. ASTM International, a standards development organization, has established a core data set defining the minimum requirements for the CCR. In addition to these minimum requirements, the CCR core data set has some optional data elements. Data contained in the CCR (shown in figure 9.1) can be provided to care providers in electronic format using extensible mark-up language (XML) or Health Level 7 International formats as well as traditional paper format. **Health Level Seven International (HL7)** is a not-for-profit, American National Standards Institute–accredited standards-developing organization dedicated to providing a comprehensive framework and related standards for the exchange, integration, sharing, and retrieval of electronic

Figure 9.1. Core data set for CCR

1. CCR identifying information

   a. Referring ("from") practitioner
   b. Referral ("to") practitioner
   c. Date
   d. Purpose or reason for CCR

2. Patient identifying information—required information to uniquely identify the subject patient; not a centralized system or national patient identifier but a federated or distributed system identifier

3. Patient insurance or financial information—basic information from which eligibility for insurance benefits may be determined for the patient

4. Advance directives—indicators that resuscitation efforts are to be either unrestricted or limited in some way; includes what is commonly known as the Do Not Resuscitate status of the patient as addressed in such documents as living wills, healthcare proxies, and powers of attorney

5. Patient health status

   a. Conditions, diagnoses, problems
   b. Family history
   c. Adverse reactions, allergies, clinical warnings, and alerts
   d. Social history and health risk factors
   e. Medications
   f. Immunizations
   g. Vital signs and physiologic measurements
   h. Laboratory results and observations
   i. Procedures and imaging (this section may be expanded in extensions for clinical specialty-specific information regarding the patient.)

6. Care documentation—details of the patient—practitioner encounter history, such as:

   a. Dates and purposes of recent pertinent visits
   b. Names of practitioners seen (this section may be significantly expanded in future extensions)

7. Care plan recommendation—includes planned or scheduled tests, procedures, or regimens of care for the patient

8. Practitioners—information about those healthcare practitioners who are participants in the patient's care; links as appropriate to 5a (conditions, diagnoses, problems) and 6 (care documentation) encounters

Source: ONC 2013, 38.

health information that supports clinical practice and the management, delivery, and evaluation of health services (HL7 2018). HL7 is an important standards development organization most focused on data exchange standards across health information systems (Amatayakul 2017, 401). HL7 has recently released the newest adaptation of health information exchange standards called Fast Healthcare Interoperability Resources (**FHIR**, pronounced FIRE). This includes clinical as well as administrative, public health, and research data for both human and veterinary medicine. It encompasses the care provided in acute inpatient, ambulatory and outpatient, long-term, community, and allied health settings (HL7 2019).

The **personal health record (PHR)** is an electronic or paper health record maintained and updated by individuals that can be used to collect, track, and share past and current information about their health or the health of someone in their care. PHR information includes a wide range of data including allergies, diagnoses, medications, health status tracking (such as diet, nutrition, and fitness activities; blood pressure or glucose monitoring), healthcare provider contact information, and social and family history. There are apps for smart phones and other mobile technology that can assist the individual keep this information up to date and allow easy access to their information.

A personal health record that is tied to and EHR system is referred to as a patient portal. In most patient portals, the patient or caregiver can add information. Now that many providers are providing patient portals, it is not necessary for individuals to maintain a separate PHR (Mayo Clinic 2020). See Chapter 10 for more information on PHRs and patient portals.

There are many benefits in having an EHR. Healthcare is facing many changes with reductions in reimbursement, the focus on reducing medical errors, increased use of technology, escalating healthcare costs, and a need to coordinate care of the patient. The traditional paper health record is not meeting the needs of patients or healthcare professionals because of the fragmentation of the health record, difficulty in analyzing data in a paper environment, and frequent accessibility issues because of missing information or lost health records. EHRs can help to improve efficiency and quality of care throughout a healthcare organization. For example, alerts built into the EHR can prevent a medication error before the prescription is executed and the EHR can eliminate issues encountered with handwriting and illegibility. Also, health record accessibility will not be lost or delayed, thus preventing treatment errors such as removing the wrong kidney. **Reminders** can notify physicians of screenings that should be performed based on the patient's age and gender. For example, the physician would be reminded that the patient needs an annual mammogram or a colonoscopy.

Healthcare today can be complicated depending on care and treatment needed. It may require patients to go to multiple physicians and possibly multiple hospitals. The fragmentation of the health record that results from these patient visits results in a lack of consistency and completeness of the health information, which impacts the quality of care provided to the patient. For example, a patient may be placed on medications that his or her primary care physician is not aware of. The primary care physician may also be unaware of past serious medical or surgical conditions, restricting the thoroughness and accurateness of the patient care rendered. The EHR allows for patient information to be complete and accurate because the information system can be programmed to require that key data elements be entered before a user can proceed to the next screen, ultimately improving the quality of the documentation captured. Patients can also receive individually designed and detailed patient instructions.

In 2016, the United States spent 3.3 trillion dollars on healthcare expenditures, which makes up about 17.9 percent of the Gross Domestic Product (CMS 2018). This percentage continues to escalate. A large percentage of these expenses are a result of performing administrative tasks, and the EHR is designed to help reduce these tasks to save time and money (ONC 2018a). For example, e-prescribing decreases turnaround time for patient prescriptions; laboratory and diagnostic tests are received faster; coding, billing, and claims management are more efficient; improved documentation provides for higher-compensating codes; and streamlined communication improves care coordination (ONC 2018).

CHECK YOUR UNDERSTANDING 9.1

1. One of the older cardiologists expressed dissatisfaction with using an EHR, stating that he doesn't understand why it's necessary. Sandy, as the EHR Clinical Coordinator, talks about his work as the first physician at ABC Hospital to use computerized technology for cardiac patients and how cardiac diagnosis outcomes improved. She relates to him that the EHR will have the same impact and that the best reason to implement an EHR is to _____.

   a. Determine the cost of care
   b. Improve patient care
   c. Eliminate medical errors
   d. Meet Joint Commission mandate for the EHR

2. Dr. Wilson asks you, the EHR Manager, to explain the difference between an alert and a reminder. You explain that reminders are typically used for things that can be scheduled or that occur on a regular basis. An example of a reminder that would be given to Dr. Wilson would be:

   a. Use of anticoagulant is contraindicated.
   b. Patient is due for MMR immunization.
   c. Patient is allergic to sulfa drugs.
   d. Drug does not come in this format.

3. A new nurse is being trained in discharge planning. She asks how does ABC Hospital know what to send to the new care team at XYZ Rehab Clinic in another city. You explain that the EHR has continuity built into its subsystems to improve the transition of care for patients. The subsystem that includes the relevant patient information from both the patient, his treatment, and the healthcare provider is called the _____.

   a. CCR *Continuity of Care Record*
   b. PHR
   c. source system
   d. Mini-EHR

4. XYZ Hospital is embarking on an ambitious plan to acquire as much of the patient's previous medical history as possible. Every time a patient is admitted, EHR Technicians start a trace of all previous providers and treatment the patient received throughout their lifetime regardless of geographic location in order to improve the comprehensiveness of the EHR system. A health record that contains all health information on a patient from birth to death is referred to as _____.

   a. CCR
   b. PHR
   c. EHR
   d. Longitudinal

5. The HIIM Manager frequently does educational presentations to local civic groups explaining the importance of the EHR and the PHR. She likes to emphasizes the benefits for patients when speaking to these groups. Identify a benefit of the PHR.

   a. It is maintained by the patient.
   b. It can be used in clinical decision support processes.
   c. Orders for lab tests and x-rays can be entered and results are reported back.
   d. Medication prescriptions can be sent electronically to the patient's pharmacy.

Status of EHR Adoption

Prior to the 2004 Presidential Directive for the development and implementation of HIT and EHRs, many healthcare organization had been slow to implement the EHR for reasons such as financial constraints, concerns about the technology, privacy and security, a lack of standards, lack of resources, and conflicting standards. Many of these issues have been addressed by Congress, federal agencies, and independent organizations. The Office of the National Coordinator for Health Information Technology (ONC) is the lead federal agency spearheading this national effort to improve patient safety and health outcomes. ONC is responsible for advising the secretary of the Department of Health and Human Services (HHS) and for establishing guidelines and requirements for the adoption of HIT and to coordinate all efforts to develop and implement the nationwide health information exchange and its infrastructure to help improve healthcare in the United States. In 2011 with the implementation of ARRA and HITECH legislation, CMS created the Meaningful Use (MU) program as a way to spur the acceptance and adoption of HIT and EHR usage in healthcare. The ONC developed the criteria for the certification of EHRs to ensure consistency, interoperability, and quality of this technology. Approved EHR systems that meet these criteria are deemed "CEHRT" – certified electronic health record technology (CMS 2020b). Certified EHR technology is used to improve quality, safety, and efficiency; reduce health disparities; engage patients and family; improve care coordination and population and public health; and maintain privacy and security of patient health information.

In 2018, MU was replaced by the **Merit-based Incentive Payment System (MIPS)**. CMS created *MIPS* the **Quality Payment Program (QPP)** to improve patient care and outcomes while managing the costs of services patients receive (CMS 2020a). The QPP gives monetarily rewards providers for improved value and patient outcomes. MIPS consolidates multiple quality programs into a single program to improve quality care. Provider performance is evaluated in four criteria and a weighted score is calculated:

1. Quality: the quality of care delivered by the clinician based on specific performance measures; 45%
2. Promoting Interoperability: this replaces the MU program; this portion focuses on patient engagement and the electronic exchange of health information using CEHRT; 25%
3. Improvement activities: evaluates how providers improve their care processes, enhance patient engagement in care, and increase access to care. Allows providers to choose activities appropriate to the practice from established categories; 15%
4. Cost: cost of care provided will be calculated by CMS based on the provider's Medicare claims. MIPS uses cost measures to gauge the total cost of care during the year or during a hospital stay; 15%

This data is reported annually to CMS. The clinician's final score determines what their payment adjustment will be (CMS 2020a).

According to the 2017 National Electronic Health Records Survey, 79.7% of office-based physicians use a certified EHR system (Myrick 2019). Hospitals faired somewhat better with 99% of larger organizations having a certified EHR, but only 93% of rural and critical access hospitals adopted one. See Figure 9.2 showing the percentage of CEHRT being used by various-sized hospitals. Certified EHR technology (CEHRT) is a complete EHR that meets the requirements included in the definition of a qualified EHR and has been tested and certified in accordance with the certification program established by the ONC. While the actual EHRs are being used, the health information exchange among providers still lags behind. Almost 75 percent of hospitals have exchanged health information electronically with other providers, but physician practices lag behind at only 26 percent. It is encouraging that health information exchange has improved public health reporting. For example, almost 90 percent of healthcare providers participating in the MU program had reported immunization information to local or state public health departments. Patients are also showing interest in using the EHR, also referred to as patient engagement. Approximately, 52 percent of individuals have been offered online access to their medical record by a health provider or insurer. Over half of those who were offered online access viewed their record within the past year; this represents 28 percent of individuals nationwide (ONC 2018c).

Figure 9.2. Percentage of Non-federal, acute care hospitals using CEHRT

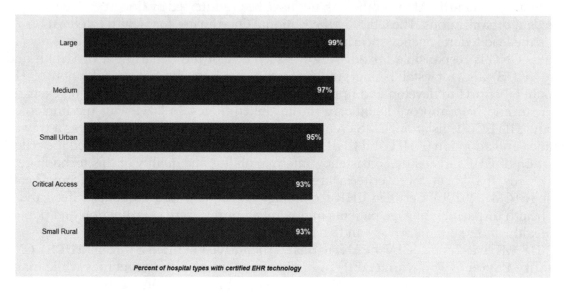

Large — 99%
Medium — 97%
Small Urban — 95%
Critical Access — 93%
Small Rural — 93%

Percent of hospital types with certified EHR technology

Source: ONC 2019a.

Of course, there are still obstacles to be overcome. Interoperability is still a sticking point. Standards for EHR systems and implementation lack specificity, resulting in variability as to how HIT stakeholders interpret and apply federal policies and regulations. Although HIT has improved patient safety in many areas, best practices have yet to be refined, publicized, and consistently implemented. HIT vendors and developers are hesitant to collaborate with competitors regarding data use agreements, hindering the exchange of health information. In addition to the lack of collaboration, health information blocking is also an issue. **Health information blocking** occurs when "persons or entities knowingly and unreasonably interfere with the exchange or use of electronic health information" (ONC 2016a). Blocking stems from healthcare providers or HIT vendors protecting their own proprietary and business interests above the interests of the patient and healthcare improvement. These efforts actively impede the progress sought by the concept of EHRs and health information exchange. For example, if Vendor A implements their health IT product in nonstandard way, that may substantially increase the complexity or burden of accessing, exchanging, or using electronic health information; or Vendor B implementing their health IT product in a way that may lead to fraud, waste, or abuse, or impede innovations and advancements in health information access, exchange, and use, including care delivery enabled by health IT (ONC 2016c). The ONC has established a complaint process whereby health information blocking efforts can be reported and investigated.

Certified EHR Technology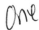

CEHRT is an absolute necessity to provide a nationwide infrastructure to promote interoperability for enhanced care coordination. It provides a baseline guarantee that the EHR product is compliant with interoperability standards and user-centered design (ONC 2019). CEHRT is intended to promote interoperability between all healthcare organizations, expand health data exchange and access, standardize all HI technologies regardless of practice, further demographic data capture, and provide sensitive data segmentation. In order to meet the base EHR definition as specified by the ONC and the 2015 edition of the health IT certification criteria, the EHR must have the following:

- Patient demographic and clinical health information capabilities such as: problem List, medication List, smoking status, medication allergy list;

- Capacity for clinical decision support (CDS);
- Capacity for physician order entry (CPOE);
- Capacity to query information relevant to health care quality such as Clinical Quality Measures (CQM); and
- Capacity to exchange electronic health information with, and integrate information from other sources such as Transitions of Care and Direct Project (Monica 2018; ONC 2019).

Certified EHR technology (CEHRT) has been evaluated by a member of the **Office of the National Coordinator–Authorized Certification Bodies (ONC-ACBs)** and verified that it meets the criteria set by the MU incentive programs, now referred to as the Promoting Interoperability Program. There were two programs, one for Medicare providers and the other for Medicaid providers. Providers had to choose one or the other, as participating in both programs was prohibited. The MU incentive EHR program created first a temporary certification organization, which was then replaced with permanent certification organizations. The testing of the EHR product is performed by Accredited Testing Laboratories (ATLs). Once the testing confirms that all standards have been met, the ONC-ACB awards the certification status. "A single organization can serve as both an ONC-ACB and an ATL, as long as a firewall is established between testing and certification activities" (ONC 2017a).

It is the responsibility of these organizations to evaluate EHR technologies to ensure that they perform specific functions and developed standards for structured data. The EHR certification program has evolved to encompass other HIT initiatives, interoperability, care quality improvement plans. HIT that is certified is subject to surveillance activities as a condition of certification. Surveillance of certified EHR products and vendors ensures the continued maintenance of the functionalities required by certification (ONC 2016b). The **National Voluntary Laboratory Accreditation Program (NVLAP)** maintains the Healthcare Information Technology Testing Laboratory Accreditation Program and accredits organizations that contract to perform HIT conformance testing in the ONC Health IT Certification Program (ONC 2017a).

As shown in Figure 9.3, the ONC oversees the Health IT Certification Program while delegating the specific function areas (testing, accreditation, and surveillance) and program operations to the designated and vetted agencies and entities. These vetted groups then accredit the testing organizations and certification bodies that evaluate specific products from HIT vendors. The **ONC–Approved Accreditor (ONC-AA)** is an entity designated by the ONC to accredit and oversee the certification bodies (ONC-ACBs). The ONC approves only one ONC-AA at a time, and approval status lasts for three years (ONC 2017a).

Organizations that wish to become accredited certification bodies must seek authorization from ONC-AA to participate in the ONC Health IT Certification Program. Once authorized, the responsibility for certifying EHR products is delegated to them, and they are called ONC-ACBs.

As shown in Figure 9.4, when developers and vendors seek ONC certification, they must contact an ATL to have their product tested. Only after the HIT product meets administrative requirements and passes all analyses and evaluations can the vendor apply to have its product certified. The vendors can then apply to an ONC-ACB to have their product certified (ONC 2017a).

An ONC-ACB certifies a vendor's HIT product has been successfully tested against the certification criteria by an ATL. The ONC-ACB submits the certifications of the HIT product for posting on the Certified Health IT Product List (CHPL) on the ONC's website. The CHPL provides the authoritative, comprehensive listing of Health IT Modules that have been tested and certified through the ONC Health IT Certification Program. The CHPL is updated, at minimum, once per week (ONC 2017a).

The ONC Certified Health IT Mark Certification and Design (Mark) is available to represent products that have been certified by an ONC-ACB under the ONC Health IT Certification Program and meet the 2015 Edition Standards and Certification Criteria. This means that a product was tested in accordance with the ONC-approved test method, and certified in accordance with the standards and certification criteria adopted by the HHS secretary and all other requirements of the ONC Health IT Certification Program.

Figure 9.3. ONC Health IT Certification Program schematic

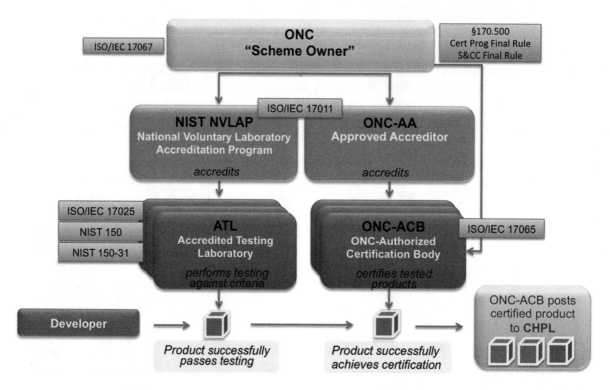

Source: ONC 2017a.

Figure 9.4. ONC certification process

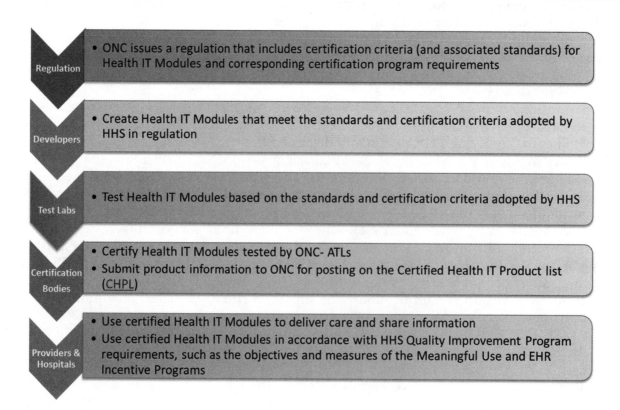

Source: ONC 2018b.

Once a vendor's product is certified, it does not end there. All certified products are subject to surveillance to make sure the product's capabilities are maintained by the vendor and that it is capable to perform its functions "in the real world" and not just in a testing laboratory. Surveillance is required and must be completed by ONC-ACBs. These surveillance activities can be randomized in reaction to a specific issue (ONC 2017a). Since 2017, the U. S. Department of Justice (DOJ) has actively enforced these requirements and has settled several fraud cases involving EHRs for more than $275 million. Various EHR companies falsely claimed they were in compliance with CEHRT criteria, misrepresented the functional status of their EHR, and manipulating their test-run software to appear to meet certification requirements when in reality, it did not (Reizen 2019).

Components of EHR

There are four main areas or systems within an EHR, and each system has specific components. Although there is variation between inpatient and outpatient EHR systems, Figure 9.5 shows the basic systems and components of an EHR.

Figure 9.5. Conceptual model of EHR

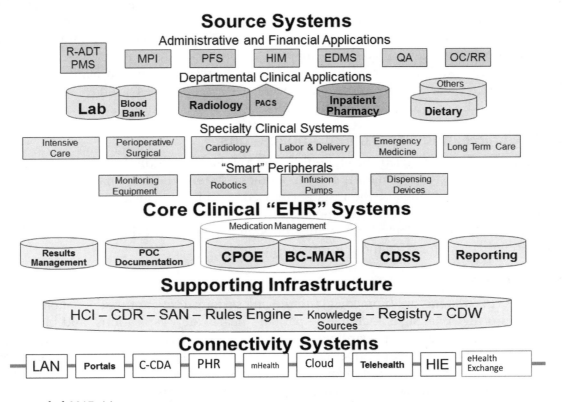

Source: Amatayakul 2017, 14.

The consolidation of these functions and systems allows health information to be used in ways that were impossible with the paper health record. The time and staff required to go through a paper health record to analyze data are much costlier compared to the readily available information contained within the EHR. For this reason, EHRs can be a significant source of information for identifying trends and ensuring that protocols are followed. For example, a healthcare organization can analyze data to determine that compliance practices are being followed, such as whether or not physicians performed a routine foot examination for patients with diabetes. A brief overview of each of these components follows.

Registration—Admission, Discharge, Transfer

The registration—admission, discharge, transfer (R-ADT) system collects patient demographic information such as name, address, and phone number. It also collects insurance information that will be used in billing and includes the master patient index. Refer to chapter 7 for details on the R-ADT system.

Patient Financial Services

The patient financial services (PFS) department receives the information collected by the R-ADT system. It then adds further information including charges for services provided and then creates the bill. It also has the capability to verify insurance coverage and copayments, determine the status of a claim, and manage prior authorizations (Amatayakul 2017, 17).

Order Communication and Results Retrieval

The order communication system notifies clinical departments, such as the laboratory, radiology, physical therapy, and dietary departments, of orders made by the physician. These orders are not typically entered by the physician, but rather by the nurse, unit secretary, or other authorized user (Amatayakul 2017, 18). When the orders are generally written down on paper and then transcribed into the order communication system, the healthcare organization does not receive the benefits of a **computerized provider order entry (CPOE)** system. The CPOE contains preprogrammed clinical decision support designed to assist the user through making an entry appropriately (Amatayakul 2017, 21). Once tests are performed, results of the diagnostic studies are compiled from their respective clinical information systems (that is, laboratory information system or radiology information system) and transferred into the EHR. The results are then available for viewing, which in turn speeds access to the information because the report does not have to be printed, filed in the health record, and transported to the healthcare provider before it is available for use.

Ancillary, Clinical, and Department Applications

Various clinical systems are used throughout the hospital and include the laboratory information system and the radiology information system. Clinical systems both manage the department as well as document the findings of the tests performed. Specialty clinical applications collect and manage information in specialty areas, such as the intensive care units, anesthesia, and labor and delivery. The information collected can include nursing notes, anesthesia records, delivery records, and more. Refer to chapter 8 for more information.

Patient Monitoring Systems

Patient monitoring systems are biomedical monitoring systems that capture data such as vital signs and fetal monitoring. Vital signs include the patient's heart rate, respirations, and blood pressure. Other smart systems collect electrocardiograms, electroencephalograms, and more advanced tests. The data captured by the smart peripherals are accessible through the EHR. This process can also be done outside of the healthcare organization. A patient's smart phone, watch, and/or other devices, has become very useful in tracking or evaluating heart rates, blood sugar levels, and other physiology markers on a regular basis so that healthcare providers can assess any changes that may occur.

Document Management System

The **document management system (DMS)** may utilize scanning to capture patient information from the paper health record. DMS also uses electronic document and content management systems that collect data from forms. Data may also be captured from an electronic source in another system or through voice recognition, e-mail, and e-fax systems. The DMS may utilize workflow technology to direct specific documents or patient health records to coders, risk management, analysts, and other users. Most DMS systems have the capability for indexing of forms. These information systems are referred to as electronic document/content management (ED/CM) systems and have methods to manage and retrieve some of the data on these forms (Amatayakul 2017, 17). For more information on DMS, refer to chapter 8.

Clinical Messaging and Provider-Patient Portals

Clinical messaging connects the medical staff and hospital by providing access to information systems such as order entry and results reporting and DMS. **Order entry and results reporting** is a software application in which healthcare professionals can enter patient care orders and then see the test results. Web-based technology often is utilized to access information in an internal system such as an intranet, or it can use the Internet. Clinical messaging is the function of electronically delivering data and automating the workflow around the management of clinical data. Clinical messages can use e-mail, portals, virtual private networks, and other means to provide the secure means of communication needed for patient information. These messages are shared in such a way as to protect the privacy of the patient (Amatayakul 2017, 19). Standards have been established to control clinical messaging. These standards are discussed later in this chapter.

The **patient–provider portal** is a secure method of communication between the healthcare provider and the patient, just the providers, or the provider and the payer. The patient–provider portal may include secure e-mail or remote access to test results and provide patient monitoring. Monitoring may include tracking pacemaker activity, blood sugar, and breathing sounds. Patients could also have access to patient education materials to help them manage their own care. This would be especially valuable for chronic conditions such as diabetes mellitus and chronic obstructive pulmonary disease (Amatayakul 2017, 15).

Results Management

Results management systems receive data from diagnostic tests and procedures. Laboratory test results, x-ray studies, and other scans are electronically reported to the originating provider. This data can be incorporated with other data such as medication administration and vital signs to get an accurate and timely view of how the patient is progressing with treatment (Amatayakul 2017, 14). The data can then be used to evaluate effectiveness in treating a patient. This ability makes the results management systems more sophisticated than results reporting systems (Amatayakul 2017, 14).

Point-of-Care Charting

Point-of-care (POC) charting, also called clinical documentation systems, may utilize many different systems to accommodate all of the different healthcare professionals who document in the health record (Amatayakul 2017, 20). There may be separate POC systems for physicians, nurses, physical therapists, respiratory therapists, and others. These POC systems may use bedside terminals, personal digital assistants (PDAs), and other wireless devices to enable the care provider to document in the health record as the information is obtained from the patient. These information systems generally allow entry of both structured and unstructured data. **Structured data** are generally found in checkboxes, drop-down boxes, and other data entry means whereby the user chooses from options already built into the information system. **Unstructured data**, also called narrative data, can be entered in a free text format by the user, usually by typing (Amatayakul 2017, 20). To ease the workload, these clinical documentation systems use handheld wireless devices, such as tablets or smartphones, so that nursing personnel can document at the patient's bedside. In some cases, laptops on movable carts are used, and are referred to as workstation on wheels or wireless on wheels (WOW) (Amatayakul 2017, 20).

Computerized Physician or Provider Order Entry System

As previously discussed, the computerized physician or provider order entry system (CPOE) is designed for orders to be entered by the healthcare providers. The use of a CPOE can lead to significant improvements in patient safety because of the reminders and alerts built into the system, improved legibility, reduced risk of data entry errors, and integrated clinical decisions support capabilities (Amatayakul 2017, 21). These alerts and reminders are provided to the physician or other healthcare provider as data are entered, thus identifying problems and key information at the point of capture rather than after review by nurses, pharmacists, or others. These alerts and reminders are controlled by clinical decision support built into the system, which is able to help prevent medication errors and improve the quality of care through its validation mechanisms (Amatayakul 2017, 21). Alerts may notify the physician of medication contraindications or that a prescription is about to expire. Reminders usually notify the physician of laboratory test results and preventive measures such scheduling for a mammogram. See Figure 9.6 for a sample CPOE screen.

Figure 9.6. Sample CPOE screen

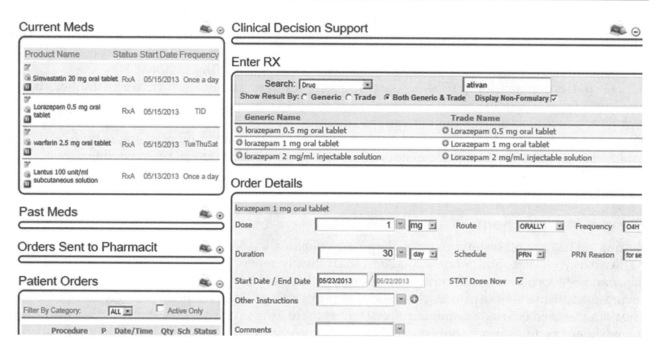

Source: CPOE developed by The Shams Group (n.d.). Reprinted with permission. The Shams Group (TSG), a privately held healthcare software and service provider, has served over 400 hospitals and healthcare systems worldwide.

Although alerts and reminders are useful, too many can become frustrating to the physician who is constantly interrupted during data entry to address the alerts and reminders (Amatayakul 2017, 21). CPOE can be used to avoid duplicate testing and ordering of medications not covered by the patient's insurance by reminding the physician a recent test or by telling the physician that the test is not covered or requires preapproval from the insurer.

Using CPOE can be time consuming for physicians; many are reluctant to adopt the information system or try to pass the responsibility of entering the orders to the nurses or other support staff. The benefits of CPOE are realized when the physicians are the users of the information system. Because of the importance of physician users and the decision support such as recommending alternative medications, catching inappropriate dosages, and other edits, the providers must be involved in developing it.

Electronic Medication Administration Record

The **electronic medication administration record (EMAR)**, also referred to a **barcode medication administration record (BC-MAR)** automates many of the medication administration processes in a healthcare organization. The level of sophistication varies by system and can be as simple as printing out a list of medications to be administered to the patient and documenting the medications given to the patient. It can be much more sophisticated by using barcodes or **radiofrequency identification devices (RFIDs)** to properly identify the patient. RFID is a microchip implanted in an item to allow tracking of that item (Sandefer 2020, 378). The EMAR can also provide alerts to assist in medication timing and provide the nurse with reference material on the medication itself (Amatayakul 2017, 22). Some EMARs can automate the entire medication administration process. This process includes identifying the drug to administer, identifying the patient, and documenting the administration of the medication or the exception. An example of an exception would be to record that medication was administered late. Some EMAR systems are designed to store commonly used medications in the nursing unit for dispensing through the use of kiosks. This capability is particularly important when addressing the eight rights of medication administration: the right patient, right medication, right time, right dose, right route, right position, right documentation, and the right of the patient to refuse medication.

Distinctions must be made between what has been prescribed or ordered and what has actually been taken by or administered to the patient. Specific prescribing information on the medication, such as dose, how it is given, and when it is given, is provided through the pharmacy information system (PIS) to the healthcare provider. The EMAR system documents the actual administration of the specific medication to the patient at the point of care, typically in real time.

Clinical Decision Support System

The **clinical decision support (CDS) system** is the process in which individual data elements are represented in the computer by a special code to be used in making comparisons, trending results, and supplying clinical reminders and alerts (AHIMA 2017, 45). The CDS system may be active, which means that it has alerts or reminders the user must address, or passive, which means the user may choose to utilize or ignore the alerts. Alerts may notify the care provider of patient allergies or contraindications for the medication or other treatment. It may notify the user that the drug being ordered is off-formulary (Amatayakul 2017, 23). The CDS system may also have the clinical practice guidelines advice installed and provide access to knowledge-based systems. Clinical guidelines advice provides recommendations to the physician on how to care for the patient given the patient's circumstances. Rules engines are used to control the reminders and alerts as well as the clinical practice and knowledge base (Amatayakul 2017, 23). Benchmarking compares internal data to external data. In a CDS system, benchmarking is used to standardize practice patterns and reduce the usage of high-cost drugs and other treatments.

Health Information Exchange

Health information exchange (HIE) is the exchange of health information electronically between providers and others with the same level of interoperability, such as laboratories and pharmacies. The organization signs a contract to share information between members of the health information organization (HIO). See chapter 11 for more information on HIE.

Population Health

The CDC refers to **population health** as "an interdisciplinary, customizable approach that allows health departments to connect practice to policy for change to happen locally. This approach utilizes non-traditional partnerships among different sectors of the community – public health, industry, academia, health care, local government entities, etc. – to achieve positive health outcomes" (CDC 2019b). It is slightly different from public health which works to protect and improve the health of communities through policy recommendations, health education and outreach, and research for disease detection and injury prevention. Public health works within its defined structure of local, decentralized health departments with a state-wide coordinating office. Population health has a broader scope in that it brings community organization (listed above) to collaborate to solve local issues (CDC 2019b).

The population health component in an EHR is designed to capture and report healthcare data that are used for public health purposes. It allows the healthcare provider to report infectious diseases, immunizations, cancer, and other reportable conditions to public health officials. This reporting is required at the local, state, and national levels and includes infectious diseases. A population health system also can connect with public health officials to receive alerts regarding health issues (Amatayakul 2017, 635). The traditional methods are cumbersome because of the manual processes and disparate information systems. The use of technology can speed up the reporting process, thus speeding up the management of disease outbreaks such as COVID-19.

HIT has a significant role in improving the health of not only a medical practice's population, but the population on the community level. The Affordable Care Act (ACA) and the Healthy People 2020 campaign set forth the following as goals to be achieved through the monitoring of population health:

- Attain high-quality, longer lives free of preventable diseases, injury, and disability and premature death
- Achieve health equity, eliminate health disparities, and improve health for all groups
- Create social and physical environments that promote good health for all
- Promote quality of life, healthy development, and healthy behaviors across all life stages (CDC 2019)

CHECK YOUR UNDERSTANDING 9.2

1. When Kelly, the EHR Coordinator for XYZ Hospital, does the EHR presentations to senior communities and assisted living facilities, she tries to promote more patient engagement by telling participants about how much more active they can be involved in their healthcare decisions and goals. The component of the EHR that she discusses frequently that allows patients to manage their own data is _____.

   a. Population health
   b. PHR
   c. Patient-provider portal
   d. Clinical decision support system

2. The Pediatric Clinic estimates that their physicians have saved five hours per day using their new EHR system to electronically send all of their orders for various services. Identify the component of the EHR allows physicians to direct the patient's care by sending orders for prescriptions, lab tests, or x-rays.

   a. Order communication and results reporting
   b. PHR
   c. CPOE *- Not Just drugs*
   d. Patient-provider portal

3. Since the 2004 Presidential Directive and the increased active direction and control of the ONC regarding the EHR implementation, identify the trend of adoption of EHRs in the United States

   a. All healthcare providers use an EHR throughout the United States.
   b. The United States adoption rate is rapidly decreasing.
   c. The United States is rapidly increasing the rate of adoption of EHRs. *b/c of incentive program*
   d. The United States adoption rate is gradually decreasing.

4. The Health People 2020 campaign is being used by Juanita, Operations Manager for Community Relations at XYZ Hospital. She is developing strategic goals for the hospital in working with community leaders to improve the health outcomes within the local population. Identify the strategic goal that would not be a goal of the hospital for the health of the general population.

CHECK YOUR UNDERSTANDING 9.2 (*Continued*)

  a. Health equity
  b. Prevent injuries
  c. Decrease physical environments that promote healthy behavior
  d. Promote healthy behaviors across all life stages

5. Christopher is Coordinator of the PIS at XYZ Hospital. In developing a quality improvement training session, he wants to emphasize methods to prevent medication errors. Identify the technology that supports the eight rights of medication administration for patients.

  a. CPOE
  b. EMAR *electronic admin*
  c. DMS
  d. PHR

Benefits of the EHR

The many benefits to the EHR, some of which are listed below, are economic, clinical, and administrative:

- The EHR offers easier access to clinical information. The EHR provides immediate access, which in turn speeds diagnosis and treatment to improve the quality of care provided.

- The EHR provides current information on tests, medications, allergies, and past diagnoses and treatments (among many more) required for decision making and disease management.

- As previously discussed, the use of tools such as reminders and alerts can remind a physician to schedule mammograms and colonoscopies and to avoid adverse drug events and allergies.

- The EHR can also enhance the documentation captured because the traditional paper health record is frequently illegible, incomplete, inaccurate, and redundant. These problems can be avoided with the use of required fields, uniform data entry practices, and trained personnel. Patient education is important for the continued improvement of a patient's condition. The EHR supports patient education materials such as discharge instructions and medication information can be personalized for the individual patient.

- The EHR allows healthcare providers to spend more time with patients because of the benefits in workflow and administrative tasks; for example, most documentation can occur at the bedside (Amatayakul 2017, 9).

- Test results can also be available immediately upon completion.

- The EHR supports various data analytics functions such as predictive modeling and application and contribution of evidence-based medicine to improve health outcomes (Lee-Eichenwald 2020, 381).

- It provides accurate, up-to-date, and complete information about patients at the point of care.

- It enables quick access to patient records for more coordinated, efficient care.

- It securely shares electronic information with patients and other clinicians.

- It helps providers more effectively diagnose patients, reduce medical errors, and provide safer care.

- It improves patient and provider interaction and communication, as well as health care convenience.

- It enables safer, more reliable prescribing.
- It helps promote legible, complete documentation and accurate, streamlined coding and billing.
- It enhances privacy and security of patient data.
- It helps providers improve productivity and work-life balance.
- It enables providers to improve efficiency and meet their business goals.
- It reduces costs through decreased paperwork, improved safety, reduced duplication of testing, and improved health. (ONC 2014)

Barriers to EHR Use

The EHR is a powerful tool that can revolutionize healthcare. The EHR provides a multitude of benefits, but there are many issues and barriers that must be addressed in order to encourage adoption and interoperability.

One of the primary barriers to EHR implementation is cost. Implementing an EHR is expensive, and many are hesitant to invest in one without a guarantee of a return on their investment. Accurate and flexible budget planning must be completed for a successful implementation. The healthcare organization must be sure to account for every cost in planning the budget. Costs will include items such as hardware, software, construction or reconstruction of space, training, and maintenance, to name a few. Additional technical staff may be required to address technical issues that arise, such as the system crashing or virus infection.

Other barriers include:

- Prohibitive cost of many EHR systems/limited access to capital and infrastructure
- Limited access to EHR vendor information and technical assistance
- Suitability of EHR products for practice and rural health care settings
- Difficulty connecting to or obtaining broadband service
- Limited health information technology (IT) workforce and training programs
- Difficulty in obtaining community buy-in
- Limited opportunities for collaboration with other health stakeholders
- Limited buy-in from practice/hospital/health center staff with multiple roles and busy schedules (ONC 2013a)

Signatures

Signatures are an important part of the EHR because the authentication of health record entries is a requirement of state licensing, accreditation, and other standards. The purpose of signatures, in both the paper and electronic environment, is to record the identity of the individual who performed the entry.

With electronic systems, digital signature management technology is a key authentication mechanism. To be in compliance with Joint Commission, Health Insurance Portability and Accountability Act (HIPAA), and the Affordable Care Act requirements, authentication means the corroboration that a person is who he claims to be. Digital signatures are the most secure way for a healthcare provider to acknowledge the order, progress note, discharge summary, or any other patient care–related document (Reynolds 2020, 127). The security capability of an EHR system to identify the individual who digitally signed the document is called signer authentication. Another security aspect of the digital signature management technology is to ensure that the document and the signature cannot be changed or altered, which is referred to as document authentication (Sandefer 2016, 350).

One of the benefits of the electronic signature is that it automatically stamps medical record entries with the date and time of the entry. It also records user identification so that the identity of the individual who created the entry into the system is automatically recorded. There are three levels of signatures found in the EHR. The **digitized signature** is a scanned image of an individual's actual signature. This method is unsecure because anyone who has access to the image can use the signature. The next level is the **electronic signature**, which requires at least a password but can use a two-factor authentication method (discussed in chapter 12). The **digital signature** is similar to the electronic signature except that it uses encryption to provide nonrepudiation to prove the authenticator's identity, used to secure a document, is authorized and regulated by certification authorities, and is verifiable, all of which makes it most secure (Trevor 2019).

most Secure

Copy and Paste Concerns

Copying is the process of moving information from an existing health record. Pasting is the process of entering the copied data into the current record. Using the copy and paste functions to enter data into the EHR saves time because the information does not have to be retyped, but the process is not without problems. The EHR is the legal health record for the healthcare organization and therefore must be managed in a way that protects the hospital from risk. The health record must contain quality information that can be used for patient care and other purposes.

Using the copy and paste functions without checks and balances can cause legal issues, quality of care issues, and other problems. For example, a user could copy information from one patient's health record and accidently paste it into another patient's record. This should not be condoned as it can easily enter data into a patient's health record that does not apply. Health record problems, such as those that follow, can result from improper use of the copy and paste functions:

- An entry can be nullified.
- An entire record can be suspect.
- Healthcare practitioners may not notice additional information.
- Healthcare practitioners may not notice missing information.
- The entry may misrepresent the case.
- Fraudulent claims for reimbursement may be made.
- The patient is harmed.
- There might be a sentinel event that must be reported. (Amatayakul 2017, 352)

There should be policies and procedures in place to specify when copy and paste functions can be used and when they cannot. Productivity is important, but the accuracy of the information is more important because of the impact that erroneous information can have on patient care and in the courtroom. Audit logs must be checked on a frequent and regular basis to determine the usage of the copy and paste function. An **audit log**, or audit trail, is an electronic footprint of the actions that occurred in a particular file in an information system or that were performed by a specific individual. It maps when a file was accessed, who accessed it, how long they were in the file, what was done to the file (including printing and saving), which terminal or device was used to access the file, and so forth. As a key security feature, it is permanently maintained within the information system. See chapter 12 for additional information regarding this security feature.

EHR Tools

The EHR utilizes a multitude of tools to assist in the usability of the EHR. The software controls screen layout, data entry, and data retrieval. The flexibility of the presentation layer is what allows the various healthcare providers to manipulate it. This flexibility allows users to control the screens to meet their needs. The EHR also makes it possible for users to graph information to identify trends over time. Other tools in the EHR are used to facilitate data retrieval, alerts, and data entry.

Data Retrieval

When developing the EHR, the healthcare organization should understand how the data are to be used to ensure that all data will be present and in the desired format for retrieval. Data retrieval should also take into account printing format. Because of privacy issues, the EHR should also allow for identifying information to be removed automatically. This process is called deidentification.

Graphical User Interface

Graphical user interface (GUI) technology is used to navigate through an information system. Tools such as icons, colors, buttons, menus, and other tools are used to help make the system user-friendly by being visually appealing and intuitive. For example, an icon containing an image of a printer would notify the user that clicking it will trigger printing the document.

Color and Icons

Color and icons can be used to assist in retrieval, ease of use, and functionality in the EHR. Icons are graphic indicators that can be used to alert the user to important information. The user can click on the icon to access data, such as text, audio, pictures, or video. The icon picture would indicate the data type. For example, a picture of an ear might be used to indicate audio. The picture should be self-explanatory so that the user understands what lies behind the icon. Color can be a useful tool but must be used judiciously as some people are color blind. The colors used and the amount used must be carefully chosen; otherwise, they can put a strain on the user's eyes.

Data Entry

Data entry is important to the EHR. Data entry can take a lot of time, and errors can cause mistakes that could be detrimental to the patient. Because of this, a lot of care should be taken to improve data quality and speed data entry. A full discussion of data quality is presented in chapter 2. Typing, voice recognition, transcription, and other means of data entry can be used to get data into the system. When entering data, unstructured and structured data—or a combination of these—may be used.

Unstructured Data

Unstructured data, also called narrative or free text data when referring to clinical care documentation, are usually entered using a keyboard, but other methods such as dictation may also be used. Unstructured data allow the data entered to be more specific and detailed for each patient than structured data. In these fields, the provider could enter a patient's history of present illness, level of compliance with medical regimen, or anything else not captured in the structured data. The user can use his or her own words to enter the data. Because of its unstructured nature, this data does not appear in a structured reports and cannot be interpreted by a an formation system (Brinda 2020). A disadvantage of unstructured data is that reporting is not as strong as with structured data entry for reporting purposes. Because unstructured data do not have a data model, it will be difficult for the system to identify and gather desired information provided in a report. Other examples of unstructured data also include images (x-rays and CT scans), audio (fetal heart rates and electrocardiograms), notes and scanned documents, and emails.

Structured Data

Drop-down lists, checkboxes, radio buttons, and other forms of controlled data entry are used in structured data entry. The choices must be clearly defined, comprehensive, and applicable. "Structured data enable standardized values to be supplied for specific variables, so the data can be used in clinical decision support systems and provide standardized meaning for reporting purposes" (Amatayakul 2017, 20). Once the user learns the structure, data entry is quick and easy. There is a learning curve in the beginning while users get familiar with the choices and the graphical user interface. For example, when entering a patient's gender, the options are male, female, and unknown; or if the data being entered were the number of dilation centimeters for an obstetrical patient, the choices would range from 0 to 10.

Structured data entry is frequently used for physician EHRs, with the menus developed specifically for the physician's medical or surgical specialty. Because it is easy for the user to overlook entry, defaults should not populate an entry but rather should be left blank, forcing the user to address the field. The EHR should be able to convert structured data into a narrative format. An example would be structured data of "no tobacco use" and "no alcohol use" converts to "Patient denies the use of tobacco and alcohol." One of the advantages of structured data is that it can be used for reporting purposes. Data can also be graphed, allowing for trending. An example of the use of graphing is the ability to trend blood sugar or blood pressure levels over time.

Template-Based Entry

Template-based entry can be a blending of both free text and structured data entry. The user is able to pick and choose data that are entered frequently, thus requiring the entry of data that change from patient to patient. Templates can be customized to meet the needs of the organization as data needs change by physician specialty, patient type (surgical, medical, newborn), disease, and other classifications of patients.

Natural Language Processing

Natural language processing (NLP) is the conversion of unstructured data into structured data through the use of computer algorithms or statistical methods (Sayles 2020, 82). This requires sophisticated computer software to separate the narrative into little packets. These packets can be stored for later analysis, and retrieval (Amatayakul 2017, 354). NLP is what allows individuals to interact with personal assistant apps such as "Siri", "Alexa", and "Google Assistant". NLP has the ability to mine and obtain dictated and transcribed structures or unstructured words or phrases and convert this data into CPT Current Procedural Terminology (CPT) or *International Classification of Diseases, 10th Revision* (ICD-10) codes for health record coding or patient bills (Lee-Eichenwald 2020, 359). Uses of NLP include dictation and computer-assisted coding. NLP is sophisticated enough to consider the different meanings of terms in order to correctly identify the word; one use of NLP is automated coding of diagnoses and procedures. NLP can analyze data entered and apply algorithms or statistical methods to the data to determine the correct code from either the *International Classification of Diseases, 10th Revision, Clinical Modification* (ICD-10-CM) or other coding systems. To be successful, automated coding must be able to understand the relationships between the terms. For example, the ICD-10-CM code for hypertensive heart disease is different from hypertension and heart disease; thus, algorithms must be able to understand these differences. NLP may also be utilized in clinical information systems and the EHR to convert narrative text into data that can be easily analyzed.

Legal Issues

There are a number of legal issues facing the EHR. Some of these issues are being addressed as laws and regulations catch up with technology. The EHR must be designed so that it is admissible in court as the legal health record. State laws vary as to what is and is not acceptable in a court of law regarding EHRs. Healthcare providers frequently receive subpoenas requesting the production of the health record. Data in the EHR will be used to meet the requirements contained in the subpoena. The documentation provided to the court must be in a usable and readable format, not just screen prints or other unformatted data. The subpoena may require the production of audit trails, decision support rules, clinical guidelines, and other information that was never an issue with the paper health record. A number of other legal issues that must be addressed are retention, storage, security, privacy, signatures, and data quality.

Unanticipated Issues in EHR Use

Several unanticipated consequences have arisen with the use of the EHR:

- Increased work for clinicians
- Unfavorable workflow changes
- Ongoing demands for system changes
- Conflicts between electronic and paper-based systems
- Unfavorable changes in communications
- Negative user emotions
- Generation of new kinds of errors
- Unexpected and unintended changes in institutional power structure
- Overdependence on technology (ONC 2017b)

Healthcare organizations must anticipate a variety of issues that will arise. Adequate planning, efficient decision-making, and early responses to problems can mitigate the negative effects of these unintended consequences. There must be acknowledgment of the trade-offs of implementing this new technology; indeed, this new way of thinking and performing medical care will be worthwhile in the end when increased patient safety and improved outcomes justify all of the angst that accompanied this massive undertaking (ONC 2017b).

Transition Period—Hybrid Record

The conversion to an EHR does not happen overnight. Throughout the information system and implementation life cycle, the healthcare organization will have to manage paper health records, microfilms, scanned images, and the EHR. Because the health information is fragmented, there may be some risk to the quality of patient care. The fragmentation comes from the information being on several different sources such as paper, microfilm, and the EHR. The healthcare organization must have a means of pulling all information together when it is needed.

In order to make paper health records available, healthcare organization have provided many different options. Some healthcare organizations backscan paper health records into the EHR, while others manually enter in basic information so that it is quickly available for patient care. Some even keep the paper health records as they are and maintain the same system and processes until the EHR is fully functional. The **hybrid record** is a combination of paper and electronic health records. Hospitals need policies and procedures to define the sources of the components of the patient's health information and to ensure easy and accurate access, use, and disclosure.

Some healthcare organizations print out documents from the electronic sources to compile the contents of the legal health record. This practice prevents the healthcare organization from realizing the benefits of the electronic system. Unnecessary printing is not only costly but also complicates operational issues in managing the hybrid health records; healthcare organizations frequently establish policies that discourage superfluous printing of documents.

Impact on Health Information Management

The EHR does not eliminate the health information management (HIM) department; however, the functions performed by the HIM department undergo significant changes and evolve to meet the current and future challenges that new technology brings. Issues facing the HIM department in a hybrid environment include authoring and printing issues, and access and disclosure issues.

As the EHR is implemented, some of the traditional HIM functions, such as assembly, are eliminated. Other functions, such as analysis, are significantly reduced as the information systems require authentication at the time of entry. Many functions such as coding are significantly changed. For example, computer-assisted coding technologies can be used to assign codes but coders are still needed to audit and monitor the codes assigned.

Transcription is a very labor-intensive process. The EHR decreases the dependence on transcription as providers more often perform data entry, including voice recognition, into the EHR, and the system can create discharge summaries and other documents automatically from data entered into the system.

Disclosure of health information traditionally has been a slow process because the paper health record had to be retrieved, copied or faxed, and then refiled. With the EHR, a few keystrokes will print or fax the document(s) needed to fulfill requests.

Health record processing varies widely by healthcare organization but generally includes assembly, analysis, and health record completion. The assembly process is eliminated completely with the implementation of the EHR because there is no need to organize paper documents. Dependent on healthcare organization's policy and quality levels, the analyst may or may not have to verify that all pages belong to the same patient, which will reduce the time needed for analysis. Finally, the information system will not allow an entry to be made without a signature, thus reducing the number of deficient health records.

In a hybrid health record environment, paper health records do not cease to exist immediately with the advent of the EHR but rather the paper health records disappear over time. The file room will ultimately be eliminated as the existing paper health records are destroyed according to the retention schedule or the health records are scanned into the EHR. For a discussion of disposal of electronic data, see chapter 12.

These changes do not signal the end of the HIM department or the HIM profession; rather, this is only the beginning. The knowledge and skill set of the HIM professional are needed to maintain and manage data quality, evaluate the system, evaluate standards, perform project management, and more. The HIM profession as we know it will change with some tasks being eliminated, others changed, and still others created. AHIMA has developed a plan to address these issues and move the profession forward. It is referred to as Health Information Management Reimagined (HIMR).

Public or population health surveillance reporting also uses ICD-9-CM and ICD-10-CM/PCS. Reporting and population health is one of the core aspects of an EHR and still required under the Promoting Interoperability Program (Green 2019). Public health professionals rely on these diagnostics and procedural coding schemes for their databases. For example, immunization data is necessary to help public health officials monitor, prevent, and manage various diseases. Immunization reporting from healthcare provider's EHR will support patient safety efforts and disease surveillance. This can also work in the reverse direction. Public health officials can use the EHR to notify local healthcare organizations of immunization forecasts, public health notices and alerts (ONC 2019b).

Using the ICD-10-CM/PCS codes for influenza and its immunizations, immunization and disease rates can be tracked and compared to previous years. This is particularly important when evaluating cyclical disease trends and patterns and the mapping between ICD-9-CM and ICD-10-CM/PCS will enable health professionals to see decades of trends (ONC 2019b). There have been several large influenza epidemics in the last several decades. With the COVID-19 pandemic continuing into the 2020-2021 influenza season, this data will be crucial in determining what impact COVID-19 will have on the rate of influenza in the US and globally, and to what extent does the rate of influenza have on the status and severity of COVID-19. Only by evaluating several decades of influenza data will healthcare professional truly know the extent to which each of these diseases has on the other and the world's population. Use cases are frequently used to create maps. The **use case** is part of the information system design process. It describes how the user will interact with the system and what the system will do. Use cases are tools that provide very detailed information for programmers to use when developing the system. The health information management (HIM) professional has this knowledge as well as an understanding of classification systems (Palkie 2016, 165). This makes the HIM professional a qualified candidate for this job.

A common mapping system is **General Equivalence Mappings (GEMs)**. GEMs were created by the Centers for Medicare and Medicaid Services (CMS). GEMs are used to convert ICD-9-CM codes to ICD-10-CM or ICD-10-PCS codes or the reverse. Because the two systems are not identical, the user would have to decide which code to select. For example, in ICD-9-CM, obstetrical codes record whether the condition was antepartum, postpartum, and so forth. ICD-10-CM obstetrical codes record trimester rather than antepartum and so forth. Because of this difference there is no exact match. If everything was an exact match there would not be a need for the new coding system. As a result of the differences GEMs were very important during the transition to ICD-10-CM and ICD-10-PCS and continue to be important for any medical research that must use historical coded data (prior to 2015). Table 9.1 shows an example of mapping between ICD-9-CM and ICD-10-CM.

Table 9.1. Example of mapping ICD-9-CM to ICD-10-CM

ICD-9-CM	Description	≈ =	ICD-10-CM	Description
742.0	Encephalocele	≈ =	Q01.9	Encephalocele
			Q01.0	Frontal encephalocele
			Q01.1	Nasofrontal encephalocele
			Q01.2	Occipital encephalocele
			Q01.8	Encephalocele of other sites

Some key terms used when mapping ICD-10-CM and ICD-10-PCS are:

- Source code: The origin of the map, or the data set from which one maps
- Target code: The destination map, or the data set in which one attempts to find equivalence or establish the code relationship
- Forward map: A map that translates an ICD-9 code, as source code, to ICD-10 as its target code
- Backward map: A map that links the two coding systems in the opposite direction, moving from ICD-10 to ICD-9
- 1-to-1, cluster, combination, and complex: The types of mapping relations between source and target codes that exist in both forward and reverse directions
  - Cluster map: This is an entry in a GEM where one code from the many target codes can become a map to the source code (OR)
  - Combination map: This is an entry where more than one code is required in the target code set to replicate the complete meaning of the source system (AND)
  - Complex map: This mapping represents multiple code combinations and alternatives that are required to translate a source to a target code (AND and OR) (De 2012)

CHECK YOUR UNDERSTANDING 9.3

1. The CFO of ENRG Orthopedic Clinic expresses concern about investing a considerable portion of the organization's budget to purchasing a new CEHRT. He's asking for a cost-benefit analysis, needs assessment, facility upgrades costs, and personnel training expenses. In this case, money and the initial cost investment is an example of a(n) _____ to the EHR.

   a. Barrier
   b. Benefit
   c. Component
   d. Asset

2. In response to the CFO above, the IT Director, discusses how the CEHRT will improve scheduling, patient data collection, faster billing and claims processing, and increasing patient volume seen by all practitioners. Identify the benefit of the EHR.

   a. Improved efficiency
   b. Costs
   c. Fear of technology
   d. Security concerns

3. When an EHR reminds a physician to schedule preventive medicine techniques such as mammograms and colonoscopies for all her patients that may have an impact within the surrounding community, this is an example of the _____ functions and reportings in a EHR.

   a. Population health
   b. Results reporting
   c. BC-MAR
   d. CPOE

4. Zachary is the new EHR Coordinator. He's written all the training material for employees about the EHR. During the initial training, he stresses an important concept that different systems must be able to communicate and exchange information without corrupting the data. The ability of different information systems and software applications to communicate and exchange data is referred to as _____.

   a. Interoperability
   b. Certification
   c. NLP
   d. Meaningful Use

5. As ABC Hospital transitions to their new EHR system, the HIM Department's management team is developing policies to address procedures for working with and protecting both the electronic and paper versions of the medical records. Identify the term that the management team is using to describe the combination of the paper and electronic medical record.

   a. Mash-up
   b. Hybrid
   c. Cross mix
   d. Fusion

(Continued)

6. Marion, the Coding Supervisor, was talking with her coders about discussing the similarities between cholecystitis and cholelithiasis. Edward asked his iPhone, "Siri, why are cholecystitis and cholelithiasis different?" Identify the software that converts unstructured data into structured data to help assist in automated coding functions and other processes in the EHR.

   a. SQL
   b. C++
   c. HTML
   d. NLP

Real-World Case 9.1

Many new assisted living and memory care complexes are being constructed in north Florida due to a significant increase in the population of individuals over age 50. Local medical societies and HCO administrators are actively working with these companies to establish relationships for continuing care services. As director of HIM at a local hospital, Larry Green has been asked to develop a slide presentation on the EHR and patient portals to members of these assisted living complexes and active senior citizens' educational centers.

Since the audience has somewhat limited medical terminology and technology knowledge, he is tailoring the presentation to meet their needs. Within the presentation, Larry stresses the importance of the EHR and the benefits it provides to patients, such as increased communication between providers, enhanced continuity of care, and improved patient safety.

He gives a brief overview and examples of the basic functions such as e-prescribing, CPOE, results management, and public health reporting. Larry also gives a demonstration of the patient portal for his hospital. He shows the audience how they can access their patient information, follow-up on lab test results, monitor their blood pressure or glucose levels, ask questions about prescriptions, request or change appointments, schedule educational or health-monitoring sessions, and address their insurance and account issues.

Larry is aware that confidentiality is a topic of concern. Therefore, he addresses interoperability and secure transmission of data between HCOs and providers in his presentation. He also incorporates the HIPAA confidentiality and security information audience members receive when visiting their physicians. Larry concludes his presentation with a discussion of frequently asked questions, and then he allows a significant amount of time to address any other questions the audience may have.

Real-World Case 9.2

A local internal medicine and cardiology practice has recently implemented their new EHR system from Company A. Some relatively minor building renovations were required, and additional hardware was installed. Extensive training sessions and onsite support staff spent several months meeting with all users. Superusers and managers were identified and given additional training.

During the testing phases, there were several glitches that needed to be addressed. Because of the practice's long-standing relationship with a local hospital, they had to electronically communicate seamlessly to coordinate ongoing patient care throughout the healthcare continuum. The EHR from Company B is used by the hospital. Technology and software issues had to be addressed to ensure interoperability so that complete patient information was transmitted securely. The application of the HL7 messaging standards were evaluated for each system, and then the firewall and encryption software were adapted to meet data integrity and secure transmission requirements per the required standards. The patient portal for the physician practice had to be coordinated with the hospital's EHR so that patients were able to see information generated from their hospital admission. The cardiologists and internal medicine physicians were incorporating this information into their outpatient treatment plan. These issues have been addressed and care coordination has become more efficient thanks in part to the new electronic processes incorporated into both EHR systems.

REVIEW QUESTIONS

1. The ability of the EHR system to identify the person who signed the document electronically is called:

    a. Signer authentication
    b. Document authentication
    c. Password authentication
    d. Biometric authentication

2. The publication, _____, highlighted the large number of medical mistakes that kill tens of thousands of patients every year.

    a. The *Federal Register*
    b. *To Err is Human*
    c. The Affordable Care Act
    d. *Crossing the Quality Chasm*

3. The acronym, _____, is used to describe the hardware, software, and other integrated technologies used in the creation of electronic patient health information.

    a. HIPAA
    b. HIM
    c. HIT
    d. ACA

4. Identify the example that can be used to justify a policy against using the copy/paste function.

    a. Improves the quality of care
    b. Decrease the chances of fraudulent claims
    c. Provides more detailed documentation
    d. Documentation cannot be used for quality improvement purposes

5. Identify the concept that is considered an electronic footprint of what has occurred within a file.

    a. Audit log
    b. Digital signature
    c. Template-based entry
    d. Unstructured data

6. Dr. Wesson is looking for a new EHR system for her practice. Since you are the HIM Director, she asks you what is the most important thing an EHR system should have. You tell her EHRs must prove they have been tested to perform up to national standards. Identify the term that is used to describe health information technologies that have been tested and certified to perform up to national standards.

(Continued)

REVIEW QUESTIONS (*Continued*)

   a. CEHRT
   b. CERT
   c. CPOE
   d. ONC

7. The Physical Therapy Director wants to know how all the patient information is put into the EHR. You explain that the information systems of radiology, lab, R-ADT demographic information, and billing each feed their material electronically into the EHR. The phrase, _____, is used to describe the foundation systems that collect administrative and clinical data that make up the EHR.

   a. Source systems
   b. Connectivity systems
   c. Specialty clinical systems
   d. Smart peripherals

8. The acronym, _____, is used to describe the activities and charting that happen at the patient's bedside or while the patient is actively receiving care.

   a. POC
   b. CPOE
   c. CDS
   d. BC-MAR

9. All of the following are barriers to EHR adoption except

   a. Cost
   b. Limited HIT workforce
   c. Suitability of products to meet practice needs
   d. Ability to prescribe medication safely

10. The Nursing Director wants her staff to be consistent when discussing patient information either within the paper medical record or the EHR. She's heard various terms bantered about on the nursing floors and it seems to be causing confusion. You inform her that the combination of paper and electronic health records is called: _____

   a. Hybrid
   b. Half and half
   c. Mixed
   d. Interoperable

11. The Lab Manager was talking to the Radiology Director who directed her to see you about her concerns of transmitting so much lab information to other providers outside the hospital. These files can be very large given that most patients have several sets of labwork done on them each day. Identify the standards used for the exchange of laboratory data.

   a. NDC
   b. NCPDP
   c. RIM
   d. LOINC

12. The cardiologist group wants to add some terms and abbreviations that have been developed in their clinic. Their IT coordinator comes to you and asks to put these into the EHR system. You inform him that to happen these must be recognized and meet standard requirements of the most widely recognized nomenclature in healthcare which is:

    a. ICD-10
    b. ICD-9
    c. SNOMED-CT
    d. ANSI

13. A new procedure is implemented during patient check-out from the clinic. Patients are given a brochure that has a temporary username and password in order for them to access their health information online from their respective doctor. They are informed they can also see their bill, check lab results, and schedule appointments. Technicians tell the patients that the name of this process is referred to as the:

    a. Patient-provider portal
    b. EMR
    c. CCR
    d. EHR

14. There have been consistent issues with the R-ADT system regarding the identification of the primary and secondary insurance carriers for patients being admitted. Identify processes that would help the HIM and Registration managers determine who, when, and where these mistakes were constantly happening.

    a. Interoperability standards
    b. Source systems
    c. Audit logs
    d. Patient-provider portal

15. The Jackson Orthopedic Clinic has a high percentage of Medicare patients. The QPP gives monetary rewards to healthcare providers who show improved value and patient outcomes. Identify the area that the clinic should prioritize their review efforts since this section has the highest weight of 45%.

    a. Quality of care
    b. Promoting interoperability
    c. Improvement activities
    d. Cost

16. Fredericka, the CIO of XYZ Hospital, has brought together the directors of HIM and IT and the hospital's' attorney. The goal for this team is to update policies and procedures for information security and disclosures of health information in the new EHR system scheduled to go live in six months. Identify the level of interoperability used.

    a. Level 1
    b. Level 2
    c. Level 3
    d. Level 4

(*Continued*)

REVIEW QUESTIONS (*Continued*)

Abbreviations/Acronyms Matching

1. NLP
2. EMR
3. CEHRT
4. EMAR
5. ONC
6. CCR
7. HL7
8. POC
9. RFID
10. GUI

A. a standard and complete set of patient information during an encounter for service sent to the next provider to ensure optimal continued care

B. any patient care or discussions that happen at the bedside or during the services being provided to the patient

C. the use of graphic displays on computer screens, such as icons, colors, and buttons, to increase the ease of use

D. the federal agency in charge of all things associated with the implementation and functioning of the EHR by US healthcare providers

E. an electronic method, usually by a computer chip of tracking an object

F. the evaluation of an EHR system against specific established criteria to ensure its proper functioning by a healthcare provider

G. computer software that changes voice or dictation into electronic format to be input into the EHR system

H. a safety mechanism to track the drugs given to patients to make sure it is the proper drug, in the correct amount, given the right way, and has no contraindications

I. this is the computerized version of the actual paper health record containing all patient information

J. a standards organization that establishes criteria and protocols for the sharing of patient information

References

Abdelhak, M. and M. A. Hanken. 2016. *Health information: Management of a Strategic Resource*, 5th ed. St. Louis, MO: Elsevier.

Amatayakul, M. K. 2017. *Health IT and EHRs: Principles and Practice*, 6th ed. Chicago: AHIMA.

Brinda, d. 2020. Data Management. *Health Information Management Technology, An Applied Approach*, 6th ed. Chicago: AHIMA.

Centers for Disease Control and Prevention. 2019. Healthy People 2020. Accessed 9/25/2020. https://www.cdc.gov/nchs/healthy_people/hp2020.htm

Centers for Disease Control and Prevention. 2019b. What is Population Health? Accessed 9/28/2020. https://www.cdc.gov/pophealthtraining/whatis.html

Centers for Medicare and Medicaid Services (CMS). 2018. Historical National Health Expenditure Data. https://www.cms.gov/Research-Statistics-Data-and-Systems/Statistics-Trends-and-Reports/NationalHealthExpendData/NationalHealthAccountsHistorical.html.

Centers of Medicare and Medicaid. 2020a. Merit-based incentive payment system (MIPS) 2020 MIPS Quick Start Guide. Accessed 7/19/2020. https://qpp.cms.gov/mips/overview

Centers of Medicare and Medicaid. 2020b. Promoting Interoperability Programs. Accessed 9/25/2020. https://www.cms.gov/Regulations-and-Guidance/Legislation/EHRIncentivePrograms/index?redirect=/EHRIncentivePrograms

De, S. 2012. 8 steps to success in ICD-10-CM/PCS mapping: Best practices to establish precise mapping between old and new ICD code sets. *Journal of AHIMA* 83(6):44–49. http://bok .ahima.org/doc?oid=106975#.WpHQFqinFRY

Green, J. 2019. What are the core functions of EHR? https://www.ehrinpractice.com/ehr-core -functions.html

Health Level 7 (HL7). 2018. About HL7. Accessed 1/22/2018. http://www.hl7.org/about/index .cfm?ref=common.

Health Level 7 (HL7). 2019. FHIR Overview. Accessed 9/25/2020. http://hl7.org/fhir/overview .html

Healthcare Information and Management Systems Society. 2020. Interoperability in Healthcare. Accessed 9/25/2020. https://www.himss.org/resources/interoperability-healthcare

Institute of Medicine (IOM). 2003. Key Capabilities of an Electronic Health Record System. https://www.nap.edu/catalog/10781/key-capabilities-of-an-electronic-health-record-system -letter-report.

Lee-Eichenwald, S. 2020. Health Information Technologies. Chapter 12 in *Health Information Management: Concepts, Principles, and Practice, 6th ed.* Edited by P. Oachs and L. Watters. Chicago: AHIMA.

Mayo Clinic. 2020. Personal health records and patient portals. Accessed 7/20/2020. https:// www.mayoclinic.org/healthy-lifestyle/consumer-health/in-depth/personal-health-record/art -20047273

Myrick KL, Ogburn DF, Ward BW. Table. Percentage of office-based physicians using any electronic health record (EHR)/electronic medical record (EMR) system and physicians that have a certified EHR/EMR system, by U.S. state: National Electronic Health Records Survey, 2017. National Center for Health Statistics. January 2019.

National Academy of Medicine (NAM). 2000. *To Err Is Human: Building a Safer Health System.* The National Academies Press. https://www.nap.edu/read/9728/chapter/1

Office of the National Coordinator for Health Information Technology (ONC). 2019a. Health IT Dashboard, Quick Stats. Accessed 7/7/2020. https://dashboard.healthit.gov/quickstats /quickstats.php

Office of the National Coordinator for Health Information Technology (ONC). 2019b. Improving Public and Population Health Outcomes. Accessed 9/27/2020. https://www .healthit.gov/faq/how-can-electronic-health-records-improve-public-and-population-health -outcomes#:~:text=Electronic%20health%20records%20(%20EHR%20s,public%20 health%20reporting%20and%20surveillance

Office of the National Coordinator for Health Information Technology (ONC). 2019c. Health IT Playbook: Certified Health IT. Accessed 10/25/2020. https://www.healthit.gov/playbook /certified-health-it/

Office of the National Coordinator for Health Information Technology (ONC). 2018a. https:// www.healthit.gov/providers-professionals/medical-practice-efficiencies-cost-savings.

Office of the National Coordinator for Health Information Technology (ONC). 2018b. https:// www.healthit.gov/policy-researchers-implementers/about-onc-health-it-certification -program

Office of the National Coordinator for Health Information Technology (ONC). 2018c. Individuals' use of online medical records and technology for health needs; ONC Data Brief, No. 40, April 2018. https://www.healthit.gov/sites/default/files/page/2018-03/HINTS-2017-Consumer-Data -Brief-3.21.18.pdf

Office of the National Coordinator for Health Information Technology (ONC). 2017a. About the ONC Health IT Certification Program. https://www.healthit.gov/policy-researchers -implementers/permanent-certification-program-faqs#a1.

Office of the National Coordinator for Health Information Technology (ONC). 2017b. Introduction to Unintended Consequences. https://www.healthit.gov/unintended-consequences/content /module-i-introduction-unintended-consequences.html.

Office of the National Coordinator for Health Information Technology (ONC). 2017c. Standards to Promote Health Information Exchange. https://www.healthit.gov/providers-professionals /health-it-curriculum-resources-educators.

Office of the National Coordinator for Health Information Technology (ONC). 2017d. Basic Health Data Standards. https://www.healthit.gov/providers-professionals/health-it -curriculum-resources-educators.

Office of the National Coordinator for Health Information Technology (ONC). 2016a. 2015 Report to Congress on Health IT Adoption, Use, and Exchange. http://bok.ahima.org /PdfView?oid=301962.

Office of the National Coordinator for Health Information Technology (ONC). 2016b. Health IT Certification Program Overview. https://www.healthit.gov/sites/default/files /PUBLICHealthITCertificationProgramOverview.pdf

Office of the National Coordinator for Health Information Technology (ONC). 2016c. Information blocking. Accessed 7/21/2020. https://www.healthit.gov/topic/information-blocking

Office of the National Coordinator for Health Information Technology (ONC). 2014. Advantages of Electronic Health Records. https://www.healthit.gov/providers-professionals/faqs/what -are-advantages-electronic-health-records.

Office of the National Coordinator for Health Information Technology (ONC). 2013. Implementing Consolidated-Clinical Document Architecture (C-CDA) for Meaningful Use Stage 2. https://www.healthit.gov/sites/default/files/c-cda_and_meaningfulusecertification .pdf.

Monica, K. 2018. What Is the ONC Health IT Certification Program? Accessed 10/25/2020. https://ehrintelligence.com/features/what-is-the-onc-health-it-certification-program

Palkie, B. 2013. Clinical Classifications and Terminologies. Chapter 15 in *Health Information Management: Concepts, Principles, and Practice*, 4th ed. Edited by K. LaTour, S. Eichenwald Maki, and P. Oachs. Chicago: AHIMA.

Palkie, B. 2020. Other Healthcare Terminologies, Vocabularies, and Classification Systems. Chapter 5 in *Health Information Management: Concepts, Principles, and Practice*, 6th ed. Edited by P. Oachs and A. Watters. Chicago: AHIMA.

Reizen, M. and Thompson, K. 2019. Multiple DOJ Settlements Relating to Electronic Health Records Systems—What Does This Mean for Health Care Entities Today? Accessed 9/25/2020. https://www.foley.com/-/media/files/insights/publications/2019/06/ahla_rapsheet_may2019 _reizen_thompson.pdf

Reynolds, R. and Morey, A. 2020. Health record content and documentation. Chapter 4 in *Health Information Management: Concepts, Principles, and Practice, 6th ed*. Edited by P. Oachs and L. Watters. Chicago: AHIMA.

Sayles, N. B. 2020. Health Information Functions, Purpose, and Users. Chapter 3 in *Health Information Management Technology: An Applied Approach, 6th ed*. Edited by N. B. Sayles and L. L. Gordon. Chicago: AHIMA Press.

The Shams Group. n.d. CPOE Portal. Accessed February 12, 2018. http://shamsgroup.com /healthcare-solutions/clinical-innovation/cpoe-portal/.

Trevor, M. 2019. Difference Between Digital Signature and Electronic Signature. Accessed 9/25/2020. http://www.differencebetween.net/technology/difference-between-digital-signature -and-electronic-signature/.

Consumer Informatics

Learning Objectives

- Explain consumer informatics.
- Describe the importance of health literacy to the state of health.
- Describe the role of consumer informatics in the elimination of health disparities.
- Differentiate between the patient portal and a personal health record.
- Clarify telehealth's impact on the delivery of healthcare.

Key Terms

Blue Button
Consumer
Consumer engagement
Consumer health applications
Consumer informatics

E-patients
Health disparities
Health literacy
Jargon
Patient portal

Population health
Public health
Shared data record
Social media

A **consumer** is a patient, client, resident, or other recipient of healthcare services. Therefore, **consumer informatics**, also known as consumer health informatics, is "the field devoted to informatics from multiple consumer or patient views" (AMIA 2017). More and more consumers are using technology to keep in touch with their healthcare providers and to access health information. Consumer informatics includes health literacy, consumer health applications, patient portals, personal health record (PHR), health information literature, and other consumer applications. An important concept within consumer informatics is population health. The CDC refers to **population health** as "an opportunity for health care systems, agencies and organizations to work together in order to improve the health outcomes of the communities they serve" (CDC 2019). It is different from public health. **Public health** "works to protect and improve the health of communities through policy recommendations, health education and outreach, and research for disease detection and injury prevention" (CDC 2019). The reporting of population health metrics, such as immunizations and colon cancer screenings, is a key function of EHRs. Consumers also contribute to population health by the increased engagement in their healthcare. Consumer informatics can help patients become more knowledgeable about what questions to ask and what processes need to be done to help increase their chances of a positive health outcome. This can be achieved by health information on a particular condition being provided through the patient portal, providing regular reminders about immunizations and various health screenings, and/or exercise and nutrition plans to meet weight goals. One aspect of this engagement is the use of patient portals, which will be discussed later in this chapter.

Along this line are three significant events occurring in the 2010's would drastically influence the delivery of healthcare:

- The socio-political Black Lives Matter (BLM) movement starting 2013
- The medical and health crisis of the corona virus (COVID-19) pandemic starting in late 2019
- The hospital price transparency rule passed in 2019 (implementation date of 2021)

These issues brought attention to one important obstacle in healthcare –health disparities. Healthy People 2020 defines **health disparities** as "a particular type of health difference that is closely linked with social, economic, and/or environmental disadvantage. Health disparities adversely affect groups of people who have systematically experienced greater obstacles to health based on their racial or ethnic group; religion; socioeconomic status; gender; age; mental health; cognitive, sensory, or physical disability; sexual orientation or gender identity; geographic location; or other characteristics historically linked to discrimination or exclusion." Just because an individual identifies as different from the "norm" of the surrounding population, doesn't mean there should be a systematized negative health outcome associated with it.

The Black Lives Matter movement and COVID-19 has shown a spotlight on the extent of health disparities in the US. There is a disproportionate effect of the pandemic on populations of color and lower socioeconomics, which has provided the additional motivation to thoroughly evaluate the delivery of health services and patient outcomes. Initial data indicate in most states 1.) African Americans have significantly higher death rates than whites given their proportion within the population; and 2.) Hispanic/Latinos suffer from significantly higher incidence rates of COVID-19 given their proportion in the population (Godoy and Wood 2020). Having complete, accurate, comprehensive quality data is imperative to precisely identify all trends within healthcare. However, data reporting and collection has been unreliable and erratic during the pandemic due to lack of consistent case definitions, reporting guidelines, shortage of public health professionals performing testing, tracking and tracing, lack of COVID-19 testing capabilities, and so forth. Hopefully as time progresses, the use of EHRs will fill in some of the information gaps that exist. EHRs will also be used to investigate, research, and amend missing data in order to provide a clearer picture of the impact this pandemic will have on society. An individual's socio-economic status has long played a negative role in the delivery of services; the less money and insurance you have, the less likely you are to seek healthcare services in a timely manner. Since the US does not have a national healthcare system or universal healthcare coverage at this time, prices for healthcare services vary wildly depending on geographic location, insurance coverage (or lack thereof), and inconsistent access to healthcare services. This applies to both inpatient and outpatient services. Starting 2021, hospitals will be required to publish online standard charges for all services and items, publicize shoppable services to allow consumers to compare prices between providers, health insurance and plans must publish negotiated rates for in-network providers and allowed payments for out-of-network providers, and daily monetary penalties will be applied for non-compliance (Ellison 2019). Due to the emphasis on the need for data quality, the knowledge, skills, and role of HIM professionals will be essential to better prepare for future pandemics and health challenges. The use of quality data leads to more informed decisions, better planning, and comprehensive after-action analyses. Provided that decisions and protocols are made with quality data and scientific evidence and not on political interference, mitigation efforts can be more successful.

Health Literacy

Health literacy, more recently referred to as personal health literacy, is the degree to which individuals have the capacity to obtain, process, and understand basic health information and services needed to make appropriate health decisions (HRSA 2019). Patients need to be able to understand consent forms, discharge instructions, how and when to make appointments, be able to determine when they need to seek treatment or referrals, and where to go to get healthcare services. According to the Institute of Medicine (n.d.a), 90 million adult Americans have limited health literacy. Low personal health literacy rates contribute to the high levels of health disparities among certain populations since low literacy rates are more commonly found in older adults, minority populations, individuals with lower socioeconomic status, and medically underserved people (HRSA 2019). Knowing and understanding that preventive health screenings, such as colonoscopies and mammograms, help to identify and treat diseases in their early phases, can lead to improved outcomes for the patients. In Health People 2030, the definition of health literacy not only includes the personal aspect mentioned above, but also **organizational health literacy**. Organizational health literacy "is the degree to which organizations equitably enable individuals to find, understand, and use information and services to inform health-related decisions and actions for themselves and others" (HHS 2020). There is now more emphasis on the responsibility of healthcare providers to adopt health literacy and help people use the information, not just understand it. This compels healthcare organizations to have a more public health perspective regarding their services since helping more individuals make well-informed decisions impacts the health outcomes of a target audience or population.

Even patients with advanced education frequently do not understand their health information and the healthcare delivery system, which are complex even for healthcare professionals. The Department of Health and Human Services (HHS) is working to solve this problem by developing a comprehensive action plan based on two overarching principles: 1.) All people have the right to health information that helps them make informed decisions, and 2.) Health services should be delivered in ways that are easy to understand and that improve health, longevity, and quality of life (HRSA 2019). The National Action Plan to Improve Health Literacy has established seven goals to improve health literacy:

- Develop and disseminate health and safety information that is accurate, accessible, and actionable
- Promote changes in the health care system that improve health information, communication, informed decision-making, and access to health services
- Incorporate accurate, standards-based, and developmentally appropriate health and science information and curricula in child care and education through the university level
- Support and expand local efforts to provide adult education, English language instruction, and culturally and linguistically appropriate health information services in the community
- Build partnerships, develop guidance, and change policies
- Increase basic research and the development, implementation, and evaluation of practices and interventions to improve health literacy
- Increase the dissemination and use of evidence-based health literacy practices and interventions (HRSA 2019)

Health literacy is not necessarily about a patient's reading ability or education level, but about understanding the terms and concepts related to their healthcare (HRSA 2019). Anything that affects the patient's ability to make decisions related to his healthcare, including understanding insurance coverage and billing or his rights as a patient, is related to health literacy.

A number of factors contribute to an individual's health literacy:

- Communication skills of the patient and the healthcare professional providing the information
- Level of educational knowledge of healthcare

- Culture-based experiences with or knowledge of healthcare
- Demands on the healthcare organization (HHS 2010, 5)

Other health literacy factors include:

- Age greater than 65
- Nonwhite ethnicity
- Recent immigrant
- Poverty level or below
- English is second language (HHS 2010, 8)

Patients for whom English is a second language may struggle with everyday communications, much less the complex language of medicine. However, communication goes far beyond the words or language used by the patient and the physician, extending to the ability of the patient to understand implications beyond the fundamental meaning. Aspects of culture, beliefs, and customs derived from the patient's ethnicity, religion, and interpersonal values all influence how health information is received (AHRQ 2015). The American Sociological Association defines culture as "the languages, customs, beliefs, rules, arts, knowledge, and collective identities and memories developed by members of all social groups that make their social environments meaningful" (ASA 2020). These factors influence patients' beliefs and the way that they communicate, as well as how they understand and react to health information (National Library of Medicine n.d.b).

Health literacy is important for a number of reasons, including the patient's:

- Ability to find the way through the healthcare delivery system
- Knowing what information to share with the healthcare provider
- Ability to care for himself
- Ability to understand risk (HHS 2010, 3)

The patient's struggle to find the way through the healthcare delivery system is shown in many ways including having trouble completing forms, understanding the healthcare claim, knowing who to call, and knowing what questions to ask. The inability to understand health information and remember instructions is even more difficult when the patient is not feeling well (HHS 2010, 5). See Figure 10.1 for a graphic display of how to improve health literacy within a community.

Upwards of 80% of people research a diagnosis, medication, or symptoms on the Internet and it is the top choice as to where to get medical information (Weaver 2019, Cohen 2017). The search engine Google reports that queries for health information occur at more than 70,000 per minute which is more than one billion per day (Drees 2019). Some websites provide quality information on diseases, procedures, and other healthcare issues. Others provide erroneous, outdated information. Consumers do not always know how to determine the difference. Basing healthcare decisions on erroneous or outdated health information can have a negative impact on the patient. For example, a patient may decide not to take the physician's advice based on the outdated information.

However, not everyone has an equal opportunity to research the Internet for their health questions. An issue that must be addressed is the "digital divide." This "refers to the growing gap between the underprivileged members of society, especially the poor, rural, elderly, and handicapped portion of the population who do not have access to computers or the Internet; and the wealthy, middle-class, and young Americans living in urban and suburban areas who have access" (Steele 2019). This divide within any population is influenced by the level of education of its citizens, the broadband infrastructure in the geographic area, and people's computer literacy knowledge. In developing countries, the digital divide is influenced by gender since the vast majority of women do not have cell phones or any type of computer, nor have access to the Internet (Steele 2019). In the US, this became readily apparent when many communities had to shutter K-12 schools due to the corona virus pandemic. Schools located in the higher socioeconomic zip codes had students who

Figure 10.1. Approaches to improve health literacy

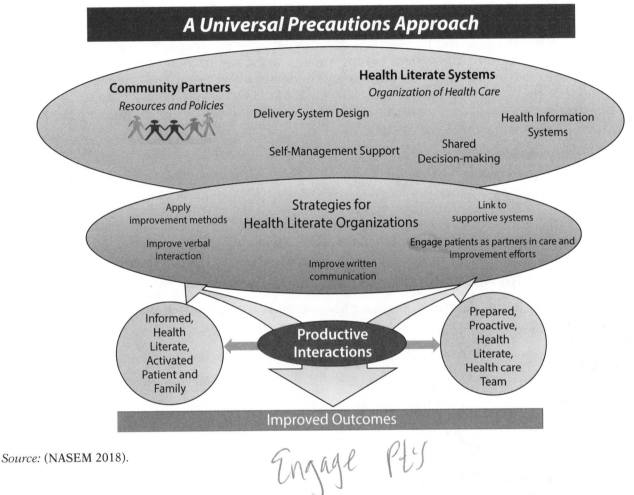

Source: (NASEM 2018).

Engage Pts

were much more prepared to attend school online than the poorer neighborhoods. A recent study found that 40% of the students in the lowest socioeconomic areas accessed online learning once a week or less but that more than 80% of more affluent students were using online learning every day for at least 2 hours per day. A third of low-income families reported that the child did not have access to a device or had to share with a sibling and more than 10% said their schools did not have any online learning material (Kamenetz 2020).

The healthcare provider may believe that he/she is explaining the patient's condition in simple terms when, in fact, advanced medical terminology and jargon are being used. **Jargon** is specialized terminology used by a specific group; in this case healthcare professionals. For example, in health information management (HIM) terms such as MS-DRGs, health information exchange, and notice of privacy practices are familiar to providers and HIM professionals, but patients do not necessarily understand them if they have heard of them at all. Problems with understanding healthcare jargon makes it difficult for patients to make informed decisions about their healthcare or for them to understand the decisions that they make. This can lead to negative outcomes. For example, a patient may agree to have her "tubes tied" and not realize that it means she cannot have any more babies. Medicaid requires patients undergoing surgical sterilization to sign a document stating that the patient realizes he or she cannot have a baby. This form came about because patients did not realize the significance of the procedure.

There are tools, such as pictures, and strategies, such as Teach Back and Ask Me 3, available to healthcare providers in order to help improve patient's understanding of their health.

There is an old adage that says a picture is worth a thousand words. Pictures, graphs, and other visual aids can present health information in a way that is easy to understand. These pictures should not be the only method of communication but rather reinforce the verbal communications (CDC 2019a).

The Teach Back communication strategy involves using simple language to explain the patient's condition and then asking the patient to repeat the information in their own words. This enables the healthcare provider to ensure that the patient understands her condition, her plan of care, and the provider's directions (Always Use Teach-Back n.d).

The Ask Me 3 initiative is a method promoted to patients to help them get the information that they need. It consists of three questions:

- What is my problem?
- What should I do?
- Why do I need to do this?

These three questions are designed to bring patients into their own care process, alongside providers, to achieve improved communication (IHI 2018).

Consumer Health Applications

Consumer health applications are healthcare-based applications designed for use by the patient or provider on smart phones, tablets, and other computers. Patients use consumer health applications to:

- Access health information
- Promote a healthy lifestyle
- Track calories and other information
- Manage their conditions
- Access the PHR

The healthcare provider uses it to:

- Access patient information
- Communicate with patients and other healthcare professionals
- Monitor patients
- Provide telemedicine (Athenahealth 2017)

Telehealth

Telehealth is defined as "the use of electronic information and telecommunication technologies to support and promote long-distance clinical health care, patient and professional health-related education, public health and health administration. Technologies include videoconferencing, the Internet, store-and-forward imaging, streaming media, and terrestrial and wireless communications. It is used in dentistry, counseling, both physical and occupational therapy, disease management, patient information, and more (Center for Connected Health Policy 2018, Kadlec 2017). AHIMA has defined telemedicine as "telecommunications systems that link healthcare organizations and patients from diverse geographic locations and transmit text, data, and images for (clinical) consultation and treatment" (Kadlec 2017).

In addition to being more convenient for patients, telehealth has led to better outcomes, reduced cost of care, and higher patient satisfaction. As a result, the number of patients using telehealth is rapidly increasing. (AHA 2019). See Figure 10.2 to see how much the use of telehealth has increased over the last decade.

Figure 10.2. Increased growth of telehealth usage in hospitals since 2010

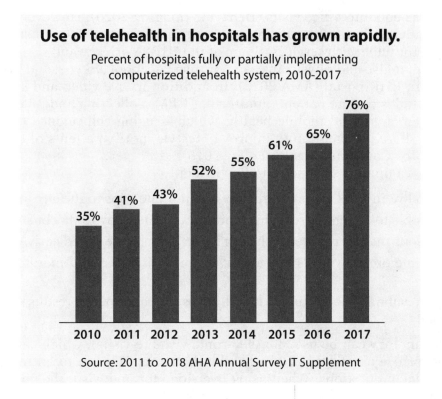

Use of telehealth in hospitals has grown rapidly.

Percent of hospitals fully or partially implementing computerized telehealth system, 2010-2017

Source: 2011 to 2018 AHA Annual Survey IT Supplement

Source: AHA 2019.

Several factors are contributing to this increase:

- Patients are more engaged in their healthcare.
- Affordable Care Act provided incentives to healthcare facilities to implement various telehealth models.
- Some states are mandating that insurers pay for telehealth services.
- Employers are offering telehealth to employees as part of their benefit program. (AHA 2019)
- The Veteran's Administration offers these services to veterans. (Blackburn 2020)

Despite its many benefits, telehealth has its disadvantages:

- Lack of funds to start telehealth program.
- Decreased face-to-face interaction.
- Issues with patient's technology.
- Reimbursement for e-visits. (AHA 2019)

The costs of creating a telehealth program include more than the hardware. It also includes planning, training, new technologies, and staff to manage the technologies. Because the patient and healthcare provider are not actually face to face, efforts must be taken to create a personalized, interactive environment in which the patient is engaged so that the experience does not feel impersonal. Although many Americans have computers or other technology and access to the Internet, their computers often do not have the security measures and speed required for the best experience. This can result in issues such as low-quality video. In spite of the fact that telehealth is a significant trend, many insurers have been slow to cover it (Anderson et al. 2017, 13–14). State legislation regarding reimbursement for telehealth has been an issue. Various levels of telehealth legislation and reimbursement were approved in 42 states. However, less than 20 of the states had full payment parity legislation, meaning reimbursement was equal to office visits (Behavior Imaging 2020). However, since the start of the COVID-19 pandemic in the US, this has put extra pressure on many insurance companies to now reimburse for telehealth services. Some of the HIPAA privacy and security requirements have eased somewhat also and physicians can now use Facebook, Skype, and Zoom and not just their organization's EHR portal (AMA 2020). In addition to live video and store-and-forward, telehealth also includes remote patient monitoring (RPM) collecting and reviewing health data patients submit remotely) and mobile health, which is using cell phones, tablets, and other mobile devices to share information to improve lifestyle, notify patients of disease outbreaks, and more (Center for Connected Health Policy 2018).

Telehealth offers a number of benefits to the patient:

- Patients who live in rural areas can reduce or eliminate trips to the city to see specialists.
- Patients are able to be monitored while going about their day-to-day business.
- Hospitalizations may be reduced as health issues may be identified early.
- Amount of time out of work is less as travel time is reduced and monitoring is performed remotely.
- Patients can submit blood sugar, blood pressure, and pulse results to the healthcare professional.

Telehealth technology can be used for electronic visits (e-visits), which can take the form of real-time videos, or use a patient portal whereby the patient logs in to an information system and asks the physician questions. When using live video for an e-visit, the patient and provider communicate synchronously (both online at the same time). Synchronous communication requires an appointment, but an appointment is not necessary to communicate with a provider through asynchronous (not online at the same time) methods, such as store-and-forward. The store-and-forward method includes videos that have been prerecorded, pictures, e-mail, and more.

Due to the COVID-19 pandemic, the use of telehealth has skyrocketed with estimates ranging anywhere from 50 to 175 times more than before the pandemic (Zarefsky 2020). The American Medical Association has been instrumental in expanding the use of telehealth and providing greater flexibility. It is also helping ease some of the restrictions that originally hindered its application by working with the Centers for Medicare and Medicaid and other entities to assist in the delivery of healthcare services during this time. They have provided information to states to address the urgent need for telehealth regarding patient populations eligible for telehealth, coverage and reimbursement policies, providers and practitioners eligible to provide telehealth, technology requirements and pediatric considerations. Payment for telehealth visits are now the same as regular office visits, even if it is not for COVID-19 (AMA 2020). The Office of Civil Rights will also not impose penalties to providers for noncompliance of HIPAA regulations relating to telehealth services during the pandemic (Davis, 2020).

Patients are also using telehealth to take daily ownership of their healthcare by using wearable devices, such as fitness trackers or their smart phones and watches, to monitor a number of aspects of their health including exercise, blood sugar, and vital signs. These wearable devices can notify the patient when there is a problem. For example, the technology could notify the patient of a spike or drop in blood sugar. This notification could be through a text or a message on the device or smart phone. When a problem is identified, the patient or the technology can contact the physician (Majumder and Deen 2019). One prediction is that there will be 213 billion wearable devices, including watches, wristbands, clothing, and eyewear, sold by 2020 (Marbury 2017). For additional information on technical aspects of telehealth, refer to chapter 8.

Consumer Informatics Applications

One of the benefits of consumer informatics is that these technologies encourage consumer engagement. **Consumer engagement** is "a diverse set of activities that can include interacting with healthcare providers, seeking health information, maintaining a PHR, and playing an active role in making decisions in regard to personal healthcare" (Aschettino et al. 2016a, 7). Research shows that for consumer informatics to have a positive impact on patient's health, three factors are key: individual tailoring of the interaction based on the characteristics of the patient; personalization, which is customizing the program specifically for the patient; and behavior feedback, which provides messages to the patient about how well he is doing and where he is in the program (AHRQ 2009, 97).

In order to encourage patient engagement, the **Blue Button** campaign was established by The Office of the National Coordinator for Health IT (ONC). It is a consumer-motivated method to improve healthcare by having the patient or caretaker actively involved in decisions and planning by having direct access to personal health information. Many healthcare providers, health plans, pharmacies, laboratories, and other healthcare businesses are now offering this service. The Blue Button logo signifies that consumers can electronically access their health information in a secure and easy manner. See Figure 10.3 showing the Blue Button logo. Many studies have shown that the more actively involved patients are in their healthcare, the healthier they are likely to be (ONC 2016). "Individuals who are equipped, enabled, empowered and engaged in their health and health care decisions" are called **e-patients** (Society for Participatory Medicine 2017).

Figure 10.3. Logo for the Blue Button campaign

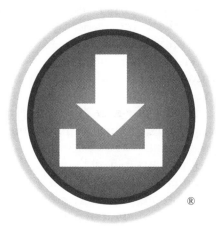

https://www.healthit.gov/topic/health-it-initiatives/blue-button

Source: ONC 2019.

The benefits of consumer engagement include reduced costs, increased communication between physicians and patients through the use of technology, improved patient satisfaction, and population health.

Three key consumer informatics applications are patient portals, PHR, and social media. Patients using these consumer informatics applications, described in the following sections, provide additional information about their health habits, care, and outcomes.

Patient Portals

A **patient portal** is an information system established and maintained by the healthcare organization that allows patients to log in to obtain their health information, register for appointments, and perform other functions such as using secure e-mail, downloading forms, updating demographics, scheduling appointments, and requesting a prescription refill. The information contained in the patient portal is a subset of the patient's electronic health record (EHR). Patients can access their health information through the patient portal at all times. Information available in the portal varies but can include lab results, summary of hospitalization, medications, radiographic reports, and much more. Patients must log in, typically with a username and password to protect the patient's privacy. The benefits of using patient portals include:

- Strengthening communication between the healthcare provider and the patient
- Providing patients with healthcare information
- Providing resources to the patient between patient visits
- Promoting patient engagement (Aschettino et al. 2016b)
- Reducing the amount of time that healthcare staff spend answering the phone, processing requests for information, and related activities (Kadlec et al. 2015)

Unfortunately, little if any training in the portal is provided to patients, and many patients are unable to understand the information available to them because of health literacy issues (Grebner and Mikaelian 2015). The healthcare provider can supply training for patients that addresses how to log in and navigate the site, privacy concerns, and health literacy.

There are two types of patient portals: standalone and system integrated. Standalone portals do not have all of the features of a system integrated portal and are typically used by smaller healthcare providers. System integrated portals are typically a function of the EHR and are, therefore, a fully functioning system (Aschettino et al. 2016b). The portal itself is owned by the healthcare provider or some other agent, such as a vendor or insurance company, who controls the portal, but the information is owned by the patient.

Some of the trends in patient portals include personalization, mobile devices, wearable technology, and communication. Personalization allows the healthcare provider to dispense educational material and other resources specific to the patient's condition. Mobile devices are used by the patient to enter data, such as blood sugar levels, into the portal for review by the physician. Data captured by wearable technology, such as fitness trackers and other monitoring devices, can be uploaded and reviewed by the physician. The patient portal supports two-way communication, which allows the patient to work with physicians between patient visits, request appointments, and receive reminders (Aschettino et al. 2016b). These reminders can be for appointments, need for follow-up, and more.

Even with the majority of EHRs having patient portals, studies indicate they are underutilized by patients. While almost 60 percent of patients review their health information through the portal, only 20 percent use the information in order to make decisions. Those that did use the information were more likely to see improvement in their care with more efficient medication refills and new treatment methods being employed (Health 2016). Even though patient portals are quite prevalent, most patients do not use them because they are not aware that under HIPAA, they have the right to review their health information. The ONC have produced a three-video series on teaching patients about their privacy rights and usage of their health information. Of course, interoperability still remains an issue. Whether the patient does not have access because of their level of health literacy, personal device or connectivity issues, or has multiple providers using multiple platforms, this roadblock still remains. However, many IT companies are working together to resolve these issues and the ONC quality program rewards providers for increasing interoperability of their systems for patients (Health 2016).

Personal Health Record

The personal health record (PHR) is an electronic or paper health record maintained and updated by an individual for himself or herself; it is a tool that individuals can use to collect, track, and share past and current information about their health or the health of someone in their care. The PHR contains health information that comes from both the physician and the patient, but the PHR is controlled by the patient. It is estimated that 75 percent of adults will be using PHRs by 2020 (Landi 2016). Personal health records are commonly being tied to patient portals of their healthcare provider's EHR. While 90 percent or insured patients have providers with patient portals and have established accounts, only approximately one-third had actually used it in the previous year (Crist 2019).

The PHR is important because it links health information from all of the patient's care providers into one central location, which will help to improve the overall quality of the care provided. The PHR has no uniform format and is independent of any specific provider's EHR or patient portal and therefore not constrained by those requirements. The patient's health information from a provider can be downloaded to the PHR. A **shared data record** is a popular and effective model for a PHR. The shared data record is maintained by the patient and provider, health plan, or employer. The PHR may be managed by a healthcare provider, vendor, employer, or other (Amatayakul, 2016, 305).

Several items should be included in the PHR:

- Personal identification, including name and birth date
- People to contact in case of emergency
- Doctor's names and phone numbers
- Allergies, including drug allergies
- Medications, including dosages
- List and dates of illnesses and surgeries
- Chronic health problems, such as high blood pressure
- Living will or advance directives
- Family history
- Immunization history
- Home blood pressure readings
- Exercise and dietary habits
- Health goals, such as stopping smoking or losing weight (Mayo Clinic 2020)

Much of the information in the PHR is the same as in the patient portal. The distinction between the two is that PHR is created and controlled by the patient whereas the patient portal is created and controlled by the healthcare organization (Aschettino et al. 2016b). A PHR that is part of an EHR is called a patient portal (Mayo Clinic 2020). There are currently four common formats of PHRs: paper, personal computer, Internet, and portable devices such as smart phones and tablets. Obtaining copies of health records and organizing them into a folder or a three-ring binder is one way to start a PHR. However, because there is only one source, accessibility is limited. The health information can also be scanned documents on a USB drive or other portable device. Although much more portable than a folder or three-ring binder, the physical nature of the USB format still limits accessibility. A personal computer-based product uses the patient's computer for storage of information that can be printed or copied to a portable device to take to the care provider. The Internet PHR provides access at anytime from anywhere. Internet PHRs can be obtained by the patient in several ways. One way is for the patient to purchase a PHR service from a vendor who stores the data and provides basic services to the user. In this case, the patient must collect health records from his or her physicians and other providers and enter the information into the PHR. The patient's healthcare provider or insurer may provide the service automatically, populating it with clinical information and claims data.

Internet-based PHRs may be tethered or untethered. Tethered PHRs are connected to the EHR and allow patients to access information contained within the EHR. Untethered PHRs are not connected to the EHR. One of the benefits to tethered PHRs is that patients can identify any errors and therefore request a correction to the EHR (Lester et al. 2016). The PHR allows the patient to share information from other healthcare providers, exercise regimen, medications, dietary supplements, and other information that the patient wants the healthcare provider to know. The patient controls who has access to this information and what information it contains.

The PHR is not without its challenges. Studies have identified a number of challenges to the patient's adoption or continued use of the PHR include:

- Age: older people typically use less technology
- Race/ethnicity: non-whites less likely to adopt/use PHR
- Socioeconomic status (SES): higher levels of SES had higher rates of adoption
- Level of education
- Internet access
- Text/numeracy literacy
- Personal health literacy
- Health/chronic disease status: those who were healthy more likely to use the PHR
- Disability: disabilities may affect ability to use PHR even with adaptive equipment
- Usability or user-friendliness status of PHR
- Lack of information regarding availability of PHR
- Privacy and confidentiality concerns
- Lack of motivation to use PHR (Showell 2017)

Figure 10.4 addresses some issues related to the PHR. The use of the PHR has created roles for health information management professionals. For a discussion of these roles, refer to figure 10.5.

Social Media

Social media are online tools that allow people to communicate. Healthcare organizations use social media to advertise services, promote wellness, provide health education, provide support forums, and provide other communications to their patients and the general public (Backman et al. 2011). It does not utilize any patient-specific information and none of the postings are included in the legal health record. The benefits of using social media in healthcare include:

- Building a sense of community for patients with chronic diseases
- Patients are better informed and can track their health
- Patients can search for clinical trials that they might quality for
- Building awareness of conditions (Glaser 2016)

Figure 10.4. Challenges the PHR presents

1. **Who owns the data?** The consumer, employer, insurance carrier, or provider? Can you take the data with you when you switch doctors or stop paying the subscription fee?
2. **Who can access that data?** Will the information be sold to or shared with a third party? If personal health information is stored on an employer's database, will employers have access to it?
3. **How does the PHR get populated** with the patient's health information? Data must be accurate and traceable so that physicians know information is the right information about the right patient.
4. **Is there adequate technology** in place to keep personal health information secure in an Internet-based PHR?
5. **Are there adequate laws and regulations** that protect privacy and security of health information in a PHR or EHR format? For example, independent, third-party PHR websites are not subject to HIPAA regulations. Some states are filling the gap, but others do not.
6. **How can information from an EHR populate the PHR** securely and conveniently—and at the same time meet privacy and security guidelines?

Source: AHIMA 2008, 3–4.

Figure 10.5.   Roles of health information management in PHR

Design and testing of PHRs. HIM professionals can be active advocates in designing PHR tools that are sensitive to underserved populations. Well-designed forms can overcome health literacy deficits. They should be designed to capture accurate information and be understandable to both the patients and providers. Testing of resources in development should include minority populations so their concerns are identified.

Distribution of PHRs to consumers. Cultural differences can be a barrier to PHR adoption. HIM professionals can address various groups using lay terminology to tout the benefits of PHRs and train consumers to become effective users.

Training providers and consumers. Having active, informed patients is often a paradigm shift for both providers and consumers. HIM professionals can facilitate information exchange between providers and patients, who often use differing language to describe medical conditions. They can also assist consumers, especially the elderly, in overcoming the digital divide.

Protecting confidentiality. HIM professionals can communicate safeguards to protect privacy for various PHR formats. Many consumers do not trust electronic systems to protect their privacy. HIM professionals are experts on privacy regulations and procedures for both the paper and the electronic world.

Source: Garvin et al. 2009.

Patient information cannot be exchanged via social media due to privacy laws, but healthcare facilities may use social media to share emergency room wait times, list new services, gain information about patient satisfaction, and more (Glaser 2016). The healthcare organization's policies and procedures should address:

- Who can access social media websites from within the healthcare organization
- Improper usage of social media
- Penalties for improper use of social media
- Responsibility of employees to report improper use
- Ensuring that employees know that statements on their personal social media accounts can impact the healthcare organization (Backman et al. 2011)

Patients can use social media to text, blog, and post status updates to share information about their condition with their family and friends, access support groups for their particular disease, and raise money for medical research.

Real-World Case 10.1

During the COVID-19 pandemic, a disproportionate number of persons of color were affected by the diseases. A concerted effort was made in Southville to address the needs of these populations. The state health department, local community health clinic, and the nursing, allied and public health, and pharmacy programs of a historically black college university (HBCU), combined forces to offer a comprehensive screening and testing process. A walk-in/drive-in testing station was set up at the football stadium of the university, staffed by public health nurses, and student interns/volunteers. After registration, patients were given contact information and patient portal access the community clinic's EHR system. Additional educational material was posted to the patient portal. Testing kits were processed by the public health laboratory. After a stated period of time, patients were told to access the patient portal to get their results. If treatment was warranted, patients would be instructed how to proceed, either through the community clinic, public health department, or personal physician. If the patients had an established relationship with a physician, test results were also referred to their practice. Local churches provided additional educational sessions manned by public health personnel. The local public libraries also participated in the educational sessions and by providing computer and Internet access for patients who did not have this capability at home.

Real-World Case 10.2

Due to the COVID-19 pandemic, the Southtown Medical Group (SMG) has increased the services and support functions of their patient portal to better serve their needs of their patients. SMG now have dedicated clinical staff manning the information system from 6:00 am to 11:00 pm. They are able to communicate through email, Skype, Facetime, and regular landline phone. Patient communication is triaged, much like they would have been if the patients had come to the Emergency Department. Most of the communications are addressed by nurse practitioners (NP) and physician assistants (PA). This has not only increased the volume of business due to the calls/telehealth visits, but also better streamlined the process of determining what services the patients need and/or what specialist they need to see. The physicians, in turn, are also happy because they are able to spend more quality time with patients who actually do need to see the doctors in person.

The NPs and PAs had specialized training regarding the documentation of services provided through the telehealth services, but also to identify the appropriate CPT codes and modifiers needed for accurate billing. If the patient was not able to satisfy their needs by using the established protocols already on the patient portal, they can immediately be funnelled into the que to speak to an NP or PA directly. Patients have been very pleased with these new services since many of them are concerned about going out of their home in the midst of the pandemic.

REVIEW QUESTIONS

1. Connie has met with her new primary care physician and nurse practitioner (NP). The NP has explained in detail to her the patient portal for the practice. Since Connie has some unusual conditions, the NP has shown her how to find more information on her conditions. The NP called it "consumer informatics". An example of consumer informatics includes

   a. Health information literature
   b. EHR
   c. Telehealth
   d. Health record

2. New patients at ABC Clinic are given an orientation to the clinic's services. The health literacy orientation includes contact information and pictures of the providers as well as material on specific medical conditions. The material includes websites, articles, and diagrams to help patients and their caregiver/family better understand their conditions. Health literacy is important because patients need to be able to: _____

   a. Understand risk
   b. Use patient portal
   c. Utilize telehealth technologies
   d. Use social media

3. The ABC Clinic is a member of the Blue Button campaign. It wants to help improve the health of the community it serves by better educating its patients. The staff is trained as to how to increase the number of e-patients it has. An e-patient is one who:

   a. Is engaged in her healthcare
   b. Is using telehealth technologies
   c. Has not signed up to use patient portal
   d. Uses social media

REVIEW QUESTIONS (*Continued*)

4. You are discussing material that can be posted to the hospital's website and its Facebook page by the Public Relations Department for ABC Hospital. Identify what they can post to their social media.

   a. Support groups
   b. Sharing clinical information with physician
   c. Obtaining clinical information from physician
   d. Wearable technology

5. The XYZ Clinic is consulting with the hospital about social media. It is working with the CIO to strengthen its policies and procedures. The clinic's social media policies should address:

   a. Improper usage of social media by the staff regarding clinic business and communications
   b. How patients can use social media
   c. How employees can use social media at home
   d. Use of wearable technology

6. An excellent way to increase patient engagement is to have patients keep their own PHR. Not only will they have access to their lab results for themselves, but also to track exercise and dietary information. PHRs allow patients to: _____

   a. Add other personal health-tracking information
   b. Experience e-visits
   c. Request prescription refill
   d. Schedule appointments

7. The ABC Clinic wants to make sure patients are more prepared for medical procedures by getting them involved in patient education. One of the patient education sessions involves a tour of an operating room suite and they encourage the patients to be involved and ask questions. Benefits of this type of patient engagement include: _____

   a. Focus on the individual
   b. Improved patient satisfaction
   c. Telehealth
   d. Social media

8. Deborah really likes the ability to go online and schedule her appoints with her internal medicine doctor. She just has to go the clinic's website and click into the patient scheduler and choose the day and time available that best meets her needs. She doesn't need to wait and talk to a staff member unless something unusually is going on. The information system that is controlled by the healthcare organization that allows patients to register is known as: _____

   a. PHR
   b. Wearable device
   c. Social media
   d. Patient portal

9. To better the rural community it serves, XYZ Hospital has instituted a remote patient monitoring system for patients with pacemakers. Patients use a smart phone app to download

(*Continued*)

the information collected by the pacemaker that is then sent to their physicians on a more frequent basis than a regularly scheduled doctor's appointment. Because the data is collected more frequently, the doctor's can identify cardiac issues before they become a real problem requiring the patient to be admitted. Benefits to telehealth include: _____

   a. Access to patient information
   b. Reducing hospitalization
   c. Providing information to healthcare providers
   d. Population health

10. Critique this statement: Consumer health applications are used solely by patients.
   a. This is a true statement.
   b. This is a false statement as it is also used by insurers and healthcare providers.
   c. This is a false statement as it is also used by healthcare providers.
   d. This is a false statement as it is only used by physicians.

11. Identify the accurate statement about health literacy.

   a. Health literacy is all about the patient's reading level.
   b. Health literacy is not impacted by the patient's culture.
   c. Health literacy includes understanding discharge instructions.
   d. Health literacy applies to healthcare professionals only.

12. Dr. Tate told his patient James that he was going to "perform a CABG due to James's CAD before he had an AMI". Of course, James had no idea what Dr. Tate said or meant by that statement. The terms or phrases used for specialized terminology by a specific group is called _____.

   a. Jargon
   b. Culture
   c. Telehealth
   d. Portal

13. Sarah needs to schedule an appointment for her yearly physical exam. Her physician's office has a very interactive EHR. Identify the aspect of the EHR she should use to request an appointment.

   a. Health record
   b. PHR
   c. Telehealth
   d. Patient portal

14. Kyle wants to ensure his physician knows about the dietary supplements he is taking for his irritable bowel syndrome. Identify where Kyle should record this.

   a. Health record
   b. PHR
   c. Telehealth
   d. Patient portal

15. ABC Hospital is working with the surrounding physician offices and health clubs to encourage more physical conditioning activities within the community. They have provided incentives

to patient who join health clubs, lose weight, or decrease their cholesterol levels. This type of program is an example of:

a. Population health
b. Public health
c. Health disparities
d. Health literacy

16. A local university is now the site for COVID-19 testing. After meeting with the state health department and local hospital officials, they have devised a plan for the notification of positive test results. This plan includes notifying the patient, followed by contact with health professionals regarding treatment, tracing anyone the patient came in contact with, and follow-up care. This process is an example of:

a. Population health
b. Public health
c. Health disparities
d. Health literacy

17. Black women die at a higher rate from breast cancer than white women even though white women get breast cancer more frequently. Because the patient outcomes are unequal based on population statistics, this is an example of:

a. Population health
b. Public health
c. Health disparities
d. Health literacy

18. The health data collection process during the COVID-19 pandemic has been inconsistent when collected by state agencies. At a future point in time, hospitals, clinics, physician offices, and other healthcare providers will be submitting additional information about any COVID-19 cases they may have treated during this time. Identify the professionals who would be best suited to conduct and manage this data collection process to ensure the quality, accuracy, and completeness of the data.

a. HIM
b. Nursing
c. Public health
d. Physician assistants

19. Identify the federal agency responsible for developing an action plan to improve health literacy.

a. HHS
b. AHIMA
c. HRSA
d. AMA

References

Adamson, S. C. and J. W. Bachman. 2010. Pilot Study of Providing Online Care in a Primary Care Setting. Mayo Clinic Proceedings. https://www.ncbi.nlm.nih.gov/pmc/articles/PMC2912730/.

Agency for Healthcare Research and Quality (AHRQ). 2009. Impact of Consumer Health Informatics Applications. https://www.ahrq.gov/downloads/pub/evidence/pdf/chiapp/impactchia.pdf.

Agency for Healthcare Research and Quality (AHRQ). 2015. Health Literacy Universal Precautions Toolkit, 2nd Edition Consider Culture, Customs, and Beliefs: Tool #10. Accessed 7/11/2020. https://www.ahrq.gov/health-literacy/quality-resources/tools/literacy-toolkit/healthlittoolkit2-tool10.html

Always Use Teach-Back. n.d. Welcome to the Always Use Teach-back Training Toolkit. Accessed February 11, 2018. http://www.teachbacktraining.org/.

Amatayakul, M. 2020 Health Information Technologies. Chapter 11 in *Health Information Management Technology: An Applied Approach*, 6th ed. Edited by N. B. Sayles and L. L. Gordon.

American Health Information Management Association. 2008. The Power of the PHR. *AHIMA Advantage* 12(3). http://bok.ahima.org/PdfView?oid=79608.

American Hospital Association. 2019. Fact Sheet: Telehealth. Accessed 7/8/2020. https://www.aha.org/system/files/2019-02/fact-sheet-telehealth-2-4-19.pdf

American Medical Association. 2020. CARES Act: AMA COVID-19 pandemic telehealth fact sheet. Accessed 7/8/2020. https://www.ama-assn.org/delivering-care/public-health/cares-act-ama-covid-19-pandemic-telehealth-fact-sheet

American Medical Informatics Association (AMIA). 2017. Consumer Health Informatics. https://www.amia.org/applications-informatics/consumer-health-informatics.

American Sociological Association (ASA). 2020. Culture. Accessed 7/11/2020. https://www.asanet.org/topics/culture

Anderson, R., B. Beckett, K. Fahy, E. Gordon, A. Gray, S. Kropp, S. LePage, E. Liette, F. McNicholas, B. Phillips, K. Pulda, and L. Renn. 2017. Telemedicine Toolkit. https://healthsectorcouncil.org/wp-content/uploads/2018/08/AHIMA-Telemedicine-Toolkit.pdf

Aschettino, L., K. M. Baldwin, L. Bouma, B. Burton, D. Collier, M. Davis, M. Dolan, K. Fahy, C. Gardner, E. Gorton, L. Grebner, M. Hennings, L. Kadlec, A. Kirby, N. LaFianzo, M. Nelson., P. Reinger, and A. R. Smith. 2016a. Consumer Engagement Toolkit. http://bok.ahima.org/PdfView?oid=301404.

Aschettino, L., L. Bouma, B. Burton, M. Davis, C. Gardner, E. Gorton, L. Grebner, M. Hennings, N. LaFianza, K. Baldwin, M. Nelson, P. Reisinger, A. Rose, and A. Smith. 2016b. Patient Portal Tool Kit. http://bok.ahima.org/PdfView?oid=301419.

Athenahealth. 2017. What is mobile health technology?. https://www.athenahealth.com/knowledge-hub/healthcare-technology/what-is-mobile-health-technology/healthcare

Backman, C., S. Dolack, D. Dunyak, L. J., Lutz, A. Tegen, and D. Warner. 2011. Social Media + Healthcare. *Journal of AHIMA* 82(3), 20–25.

Behavior Imaging. N. a. 2020. Telehealth Reimbursement Progress by State. Accessed 9/27/2020. https://behaviorimaging.com/2020/03/05/telehealth-reimbursement-progress-by-state/

Center for Connected Health Policy. 2018. What is Telehealth? https://www.cchpca.org/about/about-telehealth

Centers for Disease Control and Prevention (CDC). 2019a. Health Literacy: Visual Communication Resources. https://www.cdc.gov/healthliteracy/developmaterials/visual-communication.html

Centers for Disease Control and Prevention (CDC). 2019. What is population health? Accessed 7/12/2020. https://www.cdc.gov/pophealthtraining/whatis.html

Cohen, J. 2017. 72% of consumers use the internet to find healthcare info: 6 survey findings. Accessed 7/12/2020. https://www.beckershospitalreview.com/healthcare-information-technology/72-of-consumers-use-the-internet-to-find-healthcare-info-6-survey-findings.html

Crist, C. 2019. Most U.S. patients not using online medical portals. https://www.reuters.com/article/us-health-disparities-patient-portals/most-u-s-patients-not-using-online-medical-portals-idUSKCN1OX1HO

Department of Health and Human Services (HHS) Office of Disease Prevention and Health Promotion. 2020. https://health.gov/our-work/healthy-people-2030/about-healthy-people-2030/health-literacy-healthy-people

Davis, J. 2020. OCR Lifts HIPAA Penalties for Telehealth Use During COVID-19. Accessed 7/8/2020. https://healthitsecurity.com/news/ocr-lifts-hipaa-penalties-for-telehealth-use-during-covid-19

Department of Health and Human Services (HHS). 2020. National Action Plan to Improve Health Literacy. Accessed 7/8/2020. https://health.gov/our-work/health-literacy/national-action-plan-improve-health-literacy

Department of Health Resources and Services Administration (HRSA). 2015. Telehealth Programs. https://www.hrsa.gov/rural-health/telehealth/index.html.

Drees, J. 2019. Google receives more than 1 billion health questions every day. Accessed 7/12/2020. https://www.beckershospitalreview.com/healthcare-information-technology/google-receives-more-than-1-billion-health-questions-every-day.html

Ellison, A. 2019. CMS finalizes hospital price transparency rule: 6 things to know. Accessed 9/26/2020. https://www.beckershospitalreview.com/finance/cms-finalizes-hospital-price-transparency-rule-6-things-to-know.html

Garvin, J. H., B. Odom-Wesley. W. J. Rudman, and R. S. Stewart. 2009. Healthcare Disparities and the Role of Personal Health Records. http://bok.ahima.org/doc?oid=91677#.WoCi9-Ry5jo.

Godoy, M. and Wood, D. 2020. What Do Coronavirus Racial Disparities Look Like State By State? Accessed 7/7/2020. https://www.npr.org/sections/health-shots/2020/05/30/865413079/what-do-coronavirus-racial-disparities-look-like-state-by-state

Graham, S. and J. Brookey. 2008. Do Patient's Understand? *The Permanente Journal* 12(3). https://www.ncbi.nlm.nih.gov/pmc/articles/PMC3037129/.

Grebner, L. A. and R. Mikaelian. 2015. Best practices in mhealth for consumer engagement. *Journal of AHIMA* 86(9), 42–44.

Health Resources and Services Administration (HRSA). 2019. Health Literacy. Accessed 7/9/2020. https://www.hrsa.gov/about/organization/bureaus/ohe/health-literacy/index.html#:~:text=Health%20literacy%20is%20the%20degree,Older%20adults

Healthy People 2020. 2020. Disparities. Accessed 7/12/2020. https://www.healthypeople.gov/2020/about/foundation-health-measures/Disparities

Health, S. 2016. Top 3 Challenges Limiting Patient Access to Health Data. Accessed 7/22/2020. https://patientengagementhit.com/news/top-3-challenges-limiting-patient-access-to-health-data

Hicks, R., J. Talbert, W. W. Thombury, N. R. Perin, and A. J. Goodin. 2015. Online medical care: the current state of "eVisits" in acute primary care delivery. *Telemedicine and e-Health*. https://www.ncbi.nlm.nih.gov/pubmed/25474083.

Institute for Healthcare Improvement (IHI). 2018. Ask Me 3: Good Questions for Your Good Health. http://www.ihi.org/resources/Pages/Tools/Ask-Me-3-Good-Questions-for-Your-Good-Health.aspx

Kadlec, Lesley; Buttner, Patty. "HIM's Role in Telemedicine and Telehealth Technology". *Journal of AHIMA* 88, no. 11 (November 2017): 48–49.

Kadlec, L., A. D. Rose, and D. Warner. 2015. HIM engaging the patient portals. *Journal of AHIMA* 86(1).

Kamanetz, A. 2020. Survey Shows Big Remote Learning Gaps For Low-Income And Special Needs Children. https://www.npr.org/sections/coronavirus-live-updates/2020/05/27/862705225/survey-shows-big-remote-learning-gaps-for-low-income-and-special-needs-children

Kohn, D. (2012). AHIMA Advance: The Impact of Social Media on the Integrity of Patient Record Information. http://www.mobihealthnews.com/news/ahima-advance-impact-social-media-integrity-patient-record-information.

Landi, H. 2016. Study: 75% of Adults Will Use Personal Health Records by 2020, Exceeding MU Targets. https://www.hcinnovationgroup.com/policy-value-based-care/news/13026586/study-75-of-adults-will-use-personal-health-records-by-2020-exceeding-mu-targets

Lester, M., S. Boateng, J. Studeny, and A. Coustasse. 2016. Personal health records: Beneficial or burdensome for patients and healthcare providers? *Perspectives in Health Information Management.* 13(Spring):1h.

Majumder, S., & Deen, M. J. 2019. Smartphone Sensors for Health Monitoring and Diagnosis. Sensors (Basel, Switzerland), 19(9), 2164. https://doi.org/10.3390/s19092164

Marbury, D. 2017. Top 10 Healthcare Wearables. https://www.managedhealthcareexecutive.com/view/ten-healthcare-wearables-health-execs-should-watch

Mayo Clinic. 2020. Personal health records and patient portals. Accessed 7/8/2020. https://www.mayoclinic.org/healthy-lifestyle/consumer-health/in-depth/personal-health-record/art-20047273

National Academies of Sciences, Engineering, and Medicine (NASEM). 2018. *Building the case for health literacy: Proceedings of a workshop.* Washington, DC: The National Academies Press. doi: https://doi.org/10.17226/25068.

National Library of Medicine. n.d.a. Clear Communication. Accessed February 10. 2018. https://www.nih.gov/institutes-nih/nih-office-director/office-communications-public-liaison/clear-communication/.

National Library of Medicine. n.d.b. Health Literacy. Accessed February 7, 2018. https://nnlm.gov/professional-development/topics/health-literacy.

Nielsen-Bohlman, L., A.M. Panzer, and D. A. Kindig. 2004. *Health Literacy: A Prescription to End Confusion.* Washington, D.C: National Academies Press. https://www.ncbi.nlm.nih.gov/books/NBK216032/.

Office of the National Coordinator of Health Information Technology (ONC). 2016. About Blue Button. https://www.healthit.gov/patients-families/blue-button/about-blue-button.

Sandefer, R. 2020. Consumer Health Informatics. Chapter 14 in *Health Information Management: Concepts, Principles and Practice*, 6th ed. Edited by Oachs and Watters.

Showell C. 2017. Barriers to the use of personal health records by patients: a structured review. PeerJ, 5, e3268. https://doi.org/10.7717/peerj.3268

Society for Participatory Medicine. 2017. About Us. https://participatorymedicine.org/epatients/about-e-patientsnet.

Steele, C. 2019. What is the digital divide? Accessed 7/12/2020. http://www.digitaldividecouncil.com/what-is-the-digital-divide/

Ventola C. 2014. Social media and health care professionals: benefits, risks, and best practices. Pharmacy & Therapeutics, 39(7), 491–520. Accessed 11/1/2020. https://www.ncbi.nlm.nih.gov/pmc/articles/PMC4103576/#:~:text=HCPs%20can%20use%20social%20media,health%20information%20to%20the%20community.

Weaver, J. 2019. NBC News More people search for health online. Accessed 7/11/2020. http://www.nbcnews.com/id/3077086/t/more-people-search-health-online/#.Xwoj-ChKg2w

Wolf, M. S., L. M. Curtis, K. Waite, S. C. Bailey, L. A. Hedlund, T. C. Davis, W. H. Shrank, R. M. Parker, and A. J. J. Wood. 2011. Helping patients simplify and safely use complex prescription regimens. *Archives of Internal Medicine* 171(4): 300–305. https://jamanetwork.com/journals/jamainternalmedicine/fullarticle/226687.

Zarefsky, M. 2020. Five huge ways the pandemic has changed telemedicine. https://www.ama-assn.org/practice-management/digital/5-huge-ways-pandemic-has-changed-telemedicine?gclid=Cj0KCQjwzbv7BRDIARIsAM-A6-2BIm81f21ehn6xsYL5rOHZWcpyda6EBbwjdZZE4q4V72X66E0he9AaAlPOEALw_wcB

Health Information Exchange

Learning Objectives

- Illustrate why the health information exchange (HIE) is a positive step for healthcare.
- Describe the role and function of the health information organization (HIO) in the HIE efforts.
- Explain the concept of interoperability and its importance in healthcare.
- Compare and contrast the benefits and barriers of HIE.
- Compare and contrast the models and methods of HIE.
- Explain the requirements of Meaningful Use and its role in the Merit-based Incentive Payment System.

Key Terms

American Recovery and
    Reinvestment Act (ARRA)
Bring your own device
    (BYOD)
Consent management
Consolidated (centralized)
    model
Consumer-mediated exchange
Directed exchange
eHealth Exchange
Federated (decentralized)
    model
Health information exchange
    (HIE)
Health information
    organization (HIO)

Health Information
    Technology for Economic
    and Clinical Health
    (HITECH) Act
Hybrid model
Identity management
Identity matching
Infrastructure
Interoperability
Local health information
    organization
    (LHIO)
Meaningful Use (MU)
Medicare Access and
    CHIP Reauthorization
    Act (MACRA)

Merit-based Incentive
    Payment System
    (MIPS)
Nationwide health
    information network
    (NwHIN)
Opt-in or opt-out consent
Population health reporting
Query-based exchange
Record locator service
    (RLS)
Regional health
    information organization
    (RHIO)
Value-based healthcare
Vetting

One of the major ideas in the early 2000's, when discussions and plans about electronic health records became serious, was the vision that an individual's health information, regardless of where the information originated, would be quickly, easily, securely, and reliably delivered electronically to any legitimate healthcare provider at any point along the continuum of care anywhere in the country.

The federal government encouraged state-wide **health information exchange (HIE)** to support the **nationwide health information network (NwHIN)**, now referred to as **eHealth Exchange**. According to the ONC, the NwHIN

> "is broadly defined as the set of standards, specifications and policies that enable the secure exchange of health information over the Internet. This program provides a foundation for the exchange of health information across diverse entities, within communities and across the country, helping to achieve the goals of the HITECH Act. The Nationwide Health Information Network Exchange is the first community that implemented these standards, specifications and policies in production (ONC n.d.).

The term **infrastructure** is defined as the foundation and resources (such as personnel, equipment, policies and procedures, and buildings) necessary for an organization or system to function. The eHealth Exchange can be thought of as the required infrastructure in order for HIE to succeed. HIE is defined as the formal agreed-upon process for the seamless exchange of health information electronically between providers and others with the same level of interoperability, according to nationally recognized standards. According to the Office of the National Coordinator for Health Information Technology (ONC), "health information exchange (HIE) allows doctors, nurses, pharmacists, other health care providers and patients to appropriately access and securely share a patient's vital medical information electronically—improving the speed, quality, safety and cost of patient care" (ONC 2019a).

HIE is a revolutionary and evolutionary step in the delivery of healthcare services. It is no longer sufficient to gather information and store it in health records (paper or electronic) or in secondary databases such as tumor registries and consider it a static resource. This data and information must become dynamic to be transformed into knowledge and wisdom not only to make better decisions for individualized patient care but also to make an impact on the health of the population, both regionally and nationwide. HIE requires collaboration between healthcare providers, patients, government and public health agencies, health information technology (HIT) companies, professional associations, and payers. These parties must work jointly and cooperatively in order to achieve individual, organizational, and national goals of improving health status, efficient coordination of services, financial viability, and producing valid and reliable healthcare research.

The **eHealth Exchange** is a group of "federal agencies and non-federal organizations that came together under a common mission and purpose to improve patient care, streamline disability benefit claims, and improve public health reporting through secure, trusted, and interoperable health information exchange" (Lee-Eichenwald 2020, 392). Currently, it is now the largest query-based, health information exchange network in the US, operating in all 50 states, supports more than 120 million patients, 75% of all US hospitals, and 50% of all of the nation's HIEs. Organizations taking part in the eHealth Exchange "mutually to agree to support a common set of standards and specifications that enable the establishment of a secure, trusted, and interoperable connection among all participating Exchange organizations for the standardized flow of information". Although it initially found its footing with the guidance of the ONC under the title Nationwide Health Information Network (NHIN), eHealth Exchange is now an independent enterprise for secure health information transmission, but it does not store any data (eHealth Exchange 2019).

HIE requires a shift in mindset for healthcare professionals, from treating individuals within a specific practice or healthcare organization to understand how healthcare organizations impact the health of the entire community in which they practice. HIE can improve patient outcomes by reducing medical errors and increasing the efficiency of care by decreasing unnecessary tests and services because the health information is readily available for all providers. These steps, in turn, support healthy, productive citizens. HIE encourages patients to become active participants in their healthcare and well-being by offering information and education about health conditions, managing chronic diseases, working with diet and exercise tracking apps, and decreasing completion of repetitive paperwork needed by providers. HIE works to bolster community health by coordinating with public health officials by identifying disease trends, implementation of immunization programs, and developing health education programs for at-risk populations (ONC2019b). These new cultural norms must permeate through every personnel layer and work process in the healthcare organization. The traditional silos of information or territories exclusive to one aspect of care must be broken down to allow free exchange of information and ideas and foster better coordination of healthcare services for the duration of a patient's life. **Value-based healthcare** is an evolving concept focused on three areas: better care for the individual, better health for the community, and lower cost of healthcare through improvement of services and delivery methods (CMS 2017). HIE is a way to bridge the gaps in the disjointed healthcare system of the United States. Figure 11.1 shows the connectivity that can be achieved by the use of HIE.

Figure 11.1. Health information connectivity with the HIE

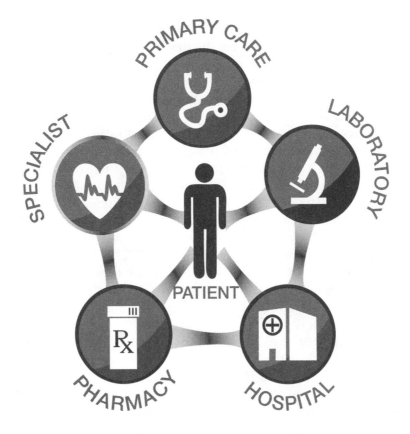

Source: ONC 2019a.

Interoperability and Health Information Exchange

The exchange of health information between entities is possible only if interoperability is in place. **Interoperability** is the ability of different information technology systems and software applications to communicate; to exchange data accurately, effectively, and consistently; and to use the information that has been exchanged. E-prescribing, in which pharmacies receive electronic prescriptions from hospitals, physician practices, and health departments, is an example of interoperability. It is likely that each of these healthcare organizations has a different electronic health record (EHR) or information system. Nonetheless, the pharmacy must be able to securely receive a verified prescription from a licensed provider and accurately provide the correct medication and dosage for the specified patient, this is termed e-prescribe. Another example is a primary care provider (PCP) referring one of her patients to a specialty provider, such as an oncologist or cardiologist. The PCP would electronically send, over a secure network, all pertinent medical and health information of the patient to the specialist for the specialist to have all the background health information to develop a tailored and comprehensive care plan. Again, each of these practitioners would have different EHRs, but these systems must be able to communicate effectively to benefit the patient.

Interoperability must be both an internal and external application and can be difficult to achieve. To achieve interoperability internally, software across an health care organization's departments must communicate and exchange information with each other. Many health care organizations have several information systems to coordinate internally, such as laboratory, radiology, and pharmacy, and some could be years older (and, therefore, potentially obsolete) compared to others. For example, coordinating and converting a radiology information system that is five years old with a newly implemented EHR will be a challenge for the healthcare organization, the EHR vendor, and the old radiology software vendor, who must work together to make sure all old information on the original system can be accessed and used. Other challenges of coordinating with older information systems include a change in workflow because the newer information system may have automated functions that were manual in the older information system, software programming most likely would be different, and reporting functions and formats would change. The healthcare organization may be using the phased-in approach to implement the EHR, and the new radiology administrative information system may be two years out. Converting or updating these older information systems can put a financial strain on even the most efficiently run facilities.

If the healthcare organization is part of a large corporation of healthcare providers, each satellite facility must be able to exchange information with the others easily. Because most healthcare organizations are independent, this is where external interoperability gets very problematic. For example, ABCD Medical Center is a Level-1 trauma facility that treats the most severely injured patients from a very large geographic region. Once the patient has recovered sufficiently from the initial injury, they may still require hospitalization or treatment. ABCD Medical Center would then transfer the patient to the XYZ Rehabilitation Center closer to the patient's home. The health record and documentation of their trauma care at ABCD will be essential in order to continue subsequent treatment without interruption at XYZ. Since most healthcare organizations have different EHR systems, the ability to exchange health information must be smooth, complete, timely, and efficient.

As mentioned in chapter 9, health information blocking has created a challenge to interoperability by impeding the flow of data between healthcare organizations or providers, which may be detrimental to the patient. Healthcare organizations that are owned by corporations typically have similar systems, but this is not necessarily the case with independent providers. In order to address issues with either internal or external interoperability, ensuring that the following four types of interoperability are evaluated and tested, will facilitate a successful exchange of health information:

- **Technical:** Based on the hardware and equipment connectivity used in the exchange, this type of interoperability allows any computer or device to exchange data with another computer or device without corrupting the data or creating errors.

- **Syntactic:** Message format standards identify how the data should be formatted or structured to allow the exchange. Interface software (programming where one application or entity is told how the other application or entity formats its data so that the receiving entity can appropriately convert the data it receives for processing) must be employed for compatibility to enable the exchange. These interoperability standards are not specific to healthcare, as they are applied to any electronic transmission between two entities.

- **Semantic:** This process involves the use of standardized terminologies (such as SNOMED-CT which is covered in chapter 9) to provide clarity, consistency, and appropriate meaning in HIE. This area of HIE is still undergoing development.

- **Process:** The most difficult of all the types of interoperability, process refers to the "degree to which the integrity of workflow can be maintained between systems and includes maintaining and conveying information such as user roles, data protection, and system service quality between systems" (Amatayakul 2017, 398). An example of this would be the patient authorization for disclosure of health information, which varies by state. healthcare organizations requesting protected health information (PHI) (any individually identifiable health information of the patient) across state lines or with other healthcare organizations that have less reputable security and access standards impede the exchange of data (Amatayakul, 2017, 398–399).

The **Office of the National Coordinator for Health Information Technology (ONC)** is the principal federal entity charged with the coordination of nationwide efforts to implement and use the most advanced HIT and the electronic exchange of health information and, in so doing, establishing interoperability among all health information systems (ONC 2017a). The ONC was established in 2004 as a result of an executive order by President George W. Bush and is a permanent agency within the Department of Health and Human Services (HHS). The ONC was the first federal agency empowered to coordinate and modernize the use of HIT and infrastructure to seamlessly and securely transmit electronic health data to improve patient care and administrative functions. It has grown to include branches that address standards and technology, ethics and compliance, care transformation, quality and safety, planning, evaluation, and analysis (ONC 2017a). This allows for improved strategic planning and communication to address concerns from healthcare providers and organizations, patients, HIT industry leaders, other stakeholders to effectively confront the challenges of this massive overhaul of the US healthcare system.

In 2009, the **American Recovery and Reinvestment Act (ARRA)** was enacted to stimulate the US economy during a recession. A significant portion of ARRA was dedicated to expanding the use of HIT to improve the business efficiency and effectiveness of healthcare organizations while increasing patient safety and positive health outcomes. This part of the ARRA legislation is the **Health Information Technology for Economic and Clinical Health (HITECH) Act** which dedicated more than $19 billion to developing HIT, implementing workforce education and training, certifying EHR products, establishing standards and vocabularies, and driving electronic security and privacy regulations into the 21st century (Miller 2020, 56).

The HITECH Act was the foundational legislation for the development, adoption, promotion, and use of electronic and computerized applications to create an interoperable health information exchange system. The HITECH Act added new regulations and requirements toughening enforcement and increasing penalties for security breaches and privacy violations. Fortifying privacy and security standards in HIE helped foster more connectivity and communications and therefore interoperability between information systems. It also mandated the establishment and strengthening of transmission standards and protocols to help establish interoperability among US health information systems. The HITECH Act emphasizes use of real-time health information on current and emerging technology at the time health services are administered to help providers make better decisions for the benefit of the patient and society (Lee-Eichenwald 2020, 356).

In 2014, the ONC published *Connecting Health and Care for the Nation: A 10-Year Vision to Achieve an Interoperable Health IT Infrastructure*, which lays out the goals and objectives for the improvement of HIT interoperability. An infographic road map, shown in figure 11.2, was developed to visualize a path to achieving this goal.

Figure 11.2. Shared nationwide interoperability roadmap

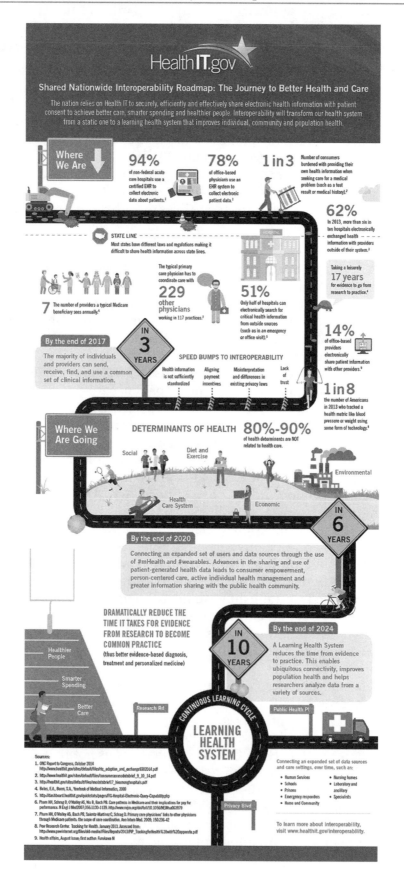

Source: ONC 2014b.

CHECK YOUR UNDERSTANDING 11.1

1. Identify the legislation that provided the economic stimulus money to help the US out of a recession and provided specific funding for the advancement of HIT.

   a. HIPAA
   b. HITECH
   c. ADA
   d. ARRA

2. Dr. Michaels orders an antibiotic for her patient, Millie, who has been diagnosed with a UTI. The nurse verified which pharmacy Millie uses when she did the initial assessment for the appointment. Millie can now leave the doctor's office and the antibiotic will be ready for pick up on her way home. This process of a physician ordering medication to a specified licensed pharmacy is termed:

   a. E-prescribe
   b. E-drugs
   c. E-meds
   d. EMAR

3. Dr. Willis is a pediatric cardiologist in Atlanta, GA. He has a former colleague, Dr. James, now located in Tallahassee, FL. Dr. James wants a consult regarding heart surgery for his seven-year-old patient. Scans, x-rays, and all diagnostic notes are sent electronically to Dr. Willis. They have several video meetings to discuss the case. Identify the concept that describes the ability for healthcare providers and their associates, regardless of location, to swap healthcare data seamlessly and meeting all interoperability and national standards to provide patient-centered care.

   a. RHIO
   b. HIE
   c. NHIN
   d. ONC

4. Simone, the EHR Coordinator, is performing part of the annual review of HIE efficiency. Since there are several new providers in town, she wants to verify the integrity of all authorized health information that is sent and received to various healthcare organizations through the HIE. Identify the principle that Simone is testing that describes the unified and smooth exchange of information among various healthcare providers and information systems and software applications.

   a. Privacy
   b. Confidentiality
   c. Infrastructure
   d. Interoperability

5. Peter, the IT Director, has nicknamed the hospital's EHR system after the president who initiated the push for health information to be completely computerized. President _____ (and hence the nickname) is responsible for the establishment of the ONC and laying the foundation for HIE.

(Continued)

CHECK YOUR UNDERSTANDING 11.1 (*Continued*)

a. Barack Obama
b. Bill Clinton
c. George W. Bush
d. Donald Trump

6. Viola, the HIM Director, is discussing new hardware her department needs in order to accommodate the increased volume of electronic requests for health information. Identify the type of interoperability that Viola is addressing that deals with the functions of actual computers and other hardware used during HIE?

a. Process
b. Technical
c. Semantic
d. Syntactic

History of Health Information Exchange

The HIE concept has evolved over the last several decades from a myriad of attempts at transmitting data from one healthcare organization to another. However, without oversight and coordination from one designated governing body, previous attempts were piecemeal at best. Over these decades there have also been technological advances that could hardly have been imagined at the inception of the HIE.

HIE is typically conducted through an intermediary called an healthcare organization. A **health information organization** is typically a public–private partnership organization that oversees, governs, and facilitates the transmission of health data between different types of healthcare organizations that have various EHR systems, according to nationally recognized standards. Many HIOs started as a **local health information organization (LHIO)** or **regional health information organization (RHIO)**. The Health Information Management Systems Society (HIMSS) defines RHIO as "a group of organizations with a business stake in improving the quality, safety and efficiency of healthcare delivery that comes together to exchange information for these purposes. The terms RHIO and Health Information Exchange, or 'HIE', are often used interchangeably" (HIMSS 2018). An LHIO is a small-scale version of an RHIO. LHIOs and RHIOs are groups of healthcare organizations in specific geographic areas that share electronic health information according to accepted standards. HIOs help the healthcare organizations and providers by delivering the services of patient identification functionality, identity management and security services, and data exchange management (Amatayakul 2017, 418). Inconsistent federal oversight and financial support, particularly prior to mid-2000s, has limited tracking of HIOs in the United States, making it difficult to determine exact numbers. Public–private partnerships with state governments have facilitated the stability of HIOs and contributed to the development of the eHealth Exchange, a network of healthcare organizations and associated businesses that can exchange health information securely, privately, and efficiently through established transmission protocols (Amatayakul 2017, 422).

Benefits and Barriers to Health Information Exchange

In 2000, the Institute of Medicine (IOM), later renamed National Academy of Medicine, identified a conservative estimate of 98,000 people who die annually due to the lack of quality in healthcare, including incorrect medications; untimely or incomplete tests results; lack of timely access to health information that could influence healthcare decision making, and lack of continuity of care in all realms of medicine and healthcare (IOM 2000). In addition to the deaths, lack of quality in healthcare can also result in wrong-limb amputations, medication errors and poisonings, hospital-acquired infections, and faulty communication leading to delayed or incorrect treatment and follow-up. The IOM's data led to a call for action to reduce the number of quality-related deaths and improve health and safety of patients by implementing HIT and HIE. The authors of the IOM study hypothesized that better and more timely information and the use of technology for monitoring patient care and safety can contribute to the decrease in the number of medical mistakes. A more recent study by Johns Hopkins University, confirming the IOM study, estimates that more than a quarter of a million deaths in the US can be attributed to medical mistakes (Cha 2016).

Implementing and using current HIT and HIE has many benefits for healthcare organizations, providers, patients, and society:

- Ability to improve quality of care by increasing the amount of patient-specific data available and decreasing the time it takes to make treatment decisions
- Reduction of healthcare costs by eliminating the repetition of diagnostic tests, unnecessary paperwork, and unnecessary diagnostic testing
- Use of clinical decision support software by healthcare providers to assist with more comprehensive and effective care
- Increased public health monitoring and reporting for immunizations, health screenings, communicable and infectious diseases such as influenza, Zika virus, or COVID-19 outbreaks, and other major health events
- Reporting and monitoring of population health trends such as a decrease in diabetic complications due to patient education and notification
- Increased use of mobile technology such as cell phones, tablets, laptops that can communicate anywhere and anytime; the new phrase is **bring your own device (BYOD)**, which refers to healthcare practitioners using their personal smartphones or other devices rather than devices provided by the healthcare organization. While acceptable, the personal device must meet specific encryption and other security protocols to protect PHI as required by the healthcare organization.
- Increased and improved effectiveness and efficiency of healthcare treatments and business operations
- Improved connection between evidence-based health research and actual medical practice
- Provides basic level of interoperability among EHRs (Biedermann and Dolezel 2016, 112, 499; Bowe and Williamson 2020, 381; ONC 2017b)

Because patients are the priority, their involvement, treatment, and successful outcomes must be evaluated to determine best practices to improve patient care. HIT and HIE benefits for the patients include:

- Patient safety—reduce unnecessary treatment and testing, decrease medication errors, more coordinated healthcare, longitudinal documentation of healthcare among all providers
- Automatic appointment and health reminders such as follow-up instructions, patient education information, and medication prescriptions sent directly to patient's pharmacy

- Saving patient's time throughout continuum of care by decreasing time spent on completing paperwork and briefing providers on health history allowing more time spent on interactive discussions regarding decisions about their health status and treatment with providers
- Equity of treatment and services with improved health outcomes leading to a reduction of health disparities
- Emergency and urgent care personnel can quickly determine the patient's medications, allergies, and other significant medical history to aid in diagnosing current episode of care
- More engaged patient education and patient involvement in the decisions that affect their health (Biedermann and Dolezel 2016, 506; Amatayakul 2016, 305; ONC 2017b)

Patient health affects more than just that individual, extending into his or her network of communities into society at large. Benefits to society include:

- Equity of treatment and services with improved health outcomes leading to a reduction of health disparities
- Decreased response time for disaster response—many population/public health issues have links to homeland security such as newly emerging diseases such as Ebola and bioterrorism attacks
- Public health surveillance of outbreaks, epidemics, or pandemics of large-scale food-borne illnesses, epidemics/pandemics of mutated influenza, Zika virus, and COVID-19 spread
- Alerts can be sent to appropriate government and health officials to speed response and mitigation efforts. This is particularly helpful when outbreaks or epidemics cross state lines (Amatayakul 2017, 9; Biedermann and Dolezel 2016, 498)

However, along with the good comes the bad. Implementing computerization for a large portion of the healthcare industry creates many changes and problems. Barriers to implementing Health IT are numerous and include:

- Financial issues of supporting the HIOs and HIE and increased cost of hardware and software, trained professionals, and infrastructure
- Lack of complete operational and interoperability standards and vocabularies and inadequate computer interfaces across all vendors and organizations
- Healthcare information ownership between patients and providers
- Patient identification and matching capabilities and protocols along the entire continuum of care
- Competition and proprietary issues between healthcare organizations
- Many rural hospitals lack financial stability and strength to provide new hardware, software, up-to-date IT personnel, and regional geographic infrastructure for reliable transmission of data (Biedermann and Dolezel 2016 268; ONC 2015a)

The ONC has developed an infographic (shown in figure 11.3) on how HIT can improve the state of healthcare in the United States.

Figure 11.3. Infographic on HIT impact

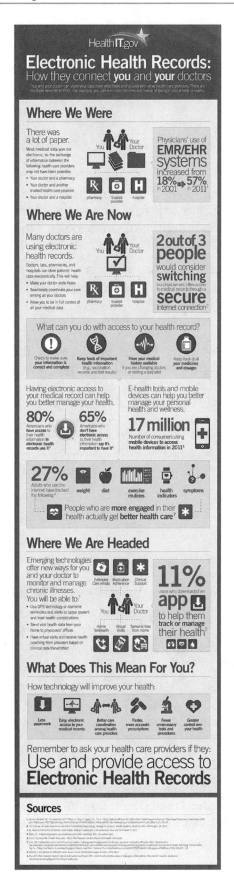

Source: ONC 2016.

CHECK YOUR UNDERSTANDING 11.2

1. The hospitals within a seven-county area in Montana have agreed to set up an information exchange for their area according to national standards to share electronic health data to meet the needs of their constituents that is referred to as a:

   a. RHIO
   b. healthcare organization
   c. HIO
   d. NHIN

2. Because Southtown has a much larger percentage of African-Americans and Latinos due to several large universities in the city, ABC University Medical Center wants to compare patient outcomes in all the various subpopulations to see if there are any differences. Identify the societal benefit of an HIE.

   a. Ability to schedule appointments with healthcare provider
   b. Equality of treatments and decreasing health disparities
   c. Cost of implementation of HIT
   d. Reducing unnecessary tests and treatments

3. ABC University Medical Center wants to review all deaths that have occurred in the facility for the past two decades. The chief residents for all the services want to evaluate how much other causes of death contribute to the hospitals death rate. They are interested in doing a follow-up to recent research from Johns Hopkins University. This study supports the original Institute of Medicine/National Academy of Medicine report identifying the leading cause of death that could be decreased or prevented with the implementation of health information technology. This leading cause of death is

   a. Medical mistakes
   b. Physician shortage
   c. Nursing shortage
   d. Opioid overdoses

4. Dr. Martinez has joined the Medical Staff at Southtown Hospital. At his previous healthcare organization in a large urban area with a high tourism rate, he treated many patients who were from out of town. Getting their health information was relatively easy since his previous healthcare organization was a member of the largest HIE in the country. He stated that _____ is a nationwide project with federal and non-federal agencies providing the data stewardship for most US hospitals in all 50 states initially starting as the NHIN.

   a. eHealth Exchange
   b. HIPAA
   c. BYOD
   d. NHIN

5. Dr. Davis is always the first physician to get the latest iPhone model. He doesn't like using the older smart phone models the hospital provides. He requests the privacy and security policies and procedures be updated so that he can continue to use his personal smart phone to conduct his business with the hospital. Healthcare providers using their

CHECK YOUR UNDERSTANDING 11.2 (*Continued*)

personal smart phones and other devices and the increase in mobile technology is referred to as:

a. eHealth Exchange
b. HIPAA
c. BYOD
d. NHIN

Meaningful Use

Meaningful Use (MU) was a regulation that was issued by the Centers for Medicare and Medicaid (CMS) on July 28, 2010, outlining an incentive program for eligible professionals (EPs), eligible hospitals, and critical access hospitals (CAHs) participating in Medicare and Medicaid programs that adopt and successfully demonstrate meaningful use of certified EHR technology (CEHRT) (ONC2019c). The EHR product in question must meet HIT and HIE criteria and standards for functionality and interoperability in order to be certified by the ONC or its designee. healthcare organizations using a CEHRT can then applied and qualified for the MU incentive program (Amatayakul 2017, 6).

ARRA and the HITECH Act specified three components for MU, all requiring the use of CEHRT:

- Must be used in a meaningful way such as e-prescribing (eRx) and computerized provider order entry (CPOE).
- The exchange of health information must be used to improve quality of health care.
- EHR must be used to submit clinical quality measures (CQMs) and other specified measures identified by the ONC and HHS (CMS 2020).

Since 2004, when HIT became a major focus of healthcare delivery, most recent health legislation has addressed many of the negative issues that have been identified in the US healthcare system such as patient safety, healthcare outcomes, and health disparities. In order to tackle these negative issues, specific guidelines, standards, and levels of treatment and patient care must be followed. Using CQMs is one of the ways to evaluate the delivery of care and patient outcomes. CQMs are criteria and tools to measure or quantify healthcare processes, outcomes, patient perceptions, and organizational structure and systems that relate to one or more of the quality goals for healthcare: effective, safe, efficient, patient-centered, equitable, and timely. The CQMs were specifically designed to use HIT effectively to combat the negative issues (CMS 2020).

MU emphasized **population health reporting**, the aggregate data on immunizations, communicable diseases, and other health events and CQMs that healthcare entities, providers, and public health agencies are required to report and is a standard function in EHRs. Population health, or public health, focuses on preventing, diagnosing, and treating an entire group of people rather than one person at a time. Figure 11.4 shows how the EHR and HIE used by acute care facilities is providing real-time reporting of diseases such as influenza to public health officials. Electronic reporting improves the timeliness and accuracy of health data to identify outbreaks and health trends (ONC 2017b). Using HIE, healthcare providers electronically submit reportable lab results, provide electronic syndromic surveillance data (health data which is used by community and public health officials to plan, respond, evaluate to a disease and its spread throughout the population), and submit electronic data to immunization registries to public health agencies.

Research on the state of health outcome disparities between genders, race, and socioeconomic status that exist within the United States has helped to identify priority populations where much

Figure 11.4. Public health syndromic surveillance

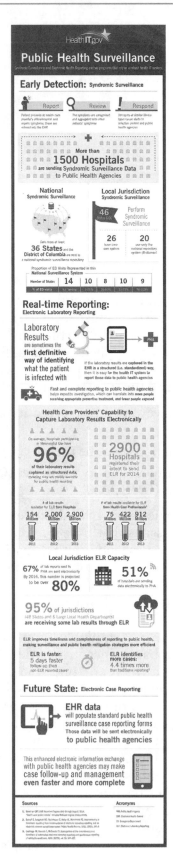

Source: ONC 2015b.

of the work needs to be implemented to alleviate and eventually eliminate these inequities. Data collection of health outcomes and treatment patterns is used to identify specific disparities, and the subsequent epidemiological information is used to support evidence-based action plans for HIT and EHR adoption to improve healthcare delivery and help reduce health disparities. A health disparity occurs when there are unequal differences in health access, status, or outcome based upon factors such as gender, race, socioeconomic status, sexual identity/orientation, disability, and geography. After this phase, language barriers and health literacy can be addressed, and more effective and efficient communication can be employed to help educate specific populations about their health status. Refer to chapter 10 for additional information on health literacy. Healthcare coordination as well as planning and implementing identified services to best meet the needs of underserved populations can help to decrease the occurrence of health disparities. CMS has given priority to research and development of action plans that address health disparities in the following populations:

- Racial and ethnic minorities
- Immigrants (and those with limited English proficiencies)
- Individuals with low health literacy
- Socioeconomically disadvantaged
- Disabled and those with special needs
- Older adults
- Rural residents
- Children and adolescents
- Lesbian, gay, bisexual, and transgender (LGBT) people (CMS 2020)

Meaningful use has now morphed into the **Merit-based Incentive Payment System (MIPS)** due to the implementation of the **Medicare Access and CHIP Reauthorization Act (MACRA)** (ONC 2019c). The MACRA legislation rewarded providers for providing higher quality of care, consolidated MU into MIPS (see Figure 11.5), and repealed flawed physician payment formulas (AAFP 2019). MU has been renamed "Promoting Interoperability" to continue the emphasis on the use of CEHRT to improve the patient's access to their health information, the exchange of information between providers, and the systematic collection, analysis, and interpretation of healthcare data (CMS 2020b).

Figure 11.5. Components of MIPS

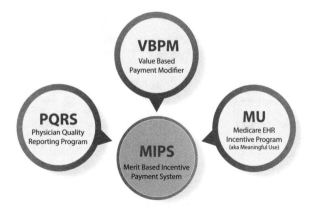

Source: ONC 2019c.

While the MU program was the incentive to get more providers to adopt HIT and EHRs, MIPS takes it further by ensuring the use of technology delivers actual positive changes to healthcare processes and patient outcomes. See Figure 11.5 showing the components of MIPS. MIPS is the current attempt to streamline the reporting and evaluation of quality care. MIPS goals are the following:

- Improve quality, safety, efficiency, and reduce health disparities
- Engage patients and family
- Improve care coordination, and population and public health
- Maintain privacy and security of patient health information

Models of Health Information Exchange Architecture

HIE architecture refers to the configuration, structure, and relationships of hardware (the machinery of the computers including input and output devices and storage devices) in an information system. There are three types of HIE architecture that are most commonly used in the United States. Each will be discussed in detail in the following pages. See Figure 11.6 for a diagrammatic comparison of the three types of HIE models.

Figure 11.6. Diagram of the three types of HIE models in the US

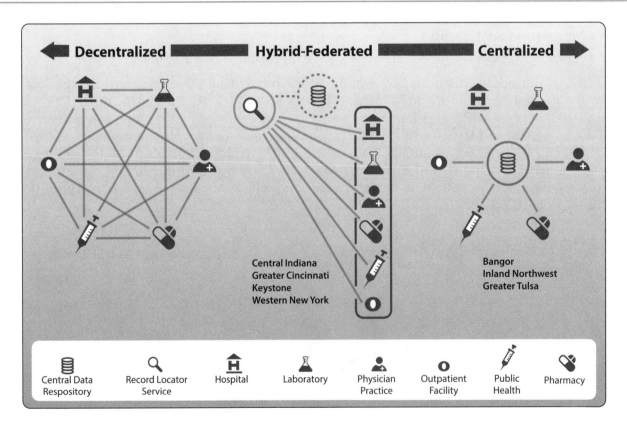

Source: McCarthy, 2014.

Consolidated or Centralized Model

The **consolidated (centralized) model** of HIE was typical of the early years of HIEs. Many independent healthcare organizations connected with the HIE and aggregate data was stored and shared within a central repository managed by the HIE (Amatayakul 2017, 417). This centralized data has a master patient index or a **record locator service (RLS)** (Biedermann and Dolezal

2016, 304). A RLS indicates where the patient's information is detected within the participating healthcare organizations based on patient identity information and record data type. With robust access and security controls (see chapter 12 for more information), each healthcare organization can access the appropriate information. However, because the US healthcare system is highly competitive and proprietary, healthcare organizations were concerned about competitors having access to their data. Advantages to the consolidated model include consistency of the data availability and rapid response to requests. Duplication of data, data that is not completely up-to-date, and costs for supporting software are some of the disadvantages to this model (Lee-Eichenwald 2020, 388).

Federated or Decentralized Model

The **federated (decentralized) model** of HIE occurs where there is no centralized database of patient information. The federated model is more common than the consolidated model because it works much like the Internet (Lee-Eichenwald 2020, 388). With the advent of cloud computing, the federated model may become the more common HIE model (Hochman, Garber, and Robinson 2019).

Each healthcare organization is responsible for maintaining its own patients' health records and is required to have the appropriate access and transmission safeguards operational. Each healthcare organization is also responsible for vetting user access. **Vetting** is the process of critically appraising the abilities of an organization or person to determine if they meet the stated criteria. For example, an healthcare organization establishes criteria for authorized access to the healthcare organization's health information. The healthcare organization uses the criteria to determine which external entities have authorized access the healthcare organization's health information. The external entities are vetted for their authority and security mechanisms to access the health information.

The federated model has several key benefits, including the lack of data ownership. Because each healthcare organization maintains its own data, the available data are always current, and this HIE has the capability to integrate with many EHR systems, providing redundancy, or the use of additional or back-up systems. This is particularly important in the case of disasters when an healthcare organization could be damaged or completely shut down. Disadvantages include data availability problems due to technical issues of a specific healthcare organization, and data may not always be available or complete because the patient may have data distributed across many of the healthcare organizations involved (Lee-Eichenwald 2020, 390).

Hybrid Model

The **hybrid model** combines the advantages of centralized and decentralized models. It has an RLS, and some data are stored in a central repository while the remainder stays with the other healthcare organizations within the HIE. The hybrid model also has a patient portal to itself, and not to a specific healthcare organization (Lee-Eichenwald 2020, 388).

However, after more than a decade, a true national HIE has yet to be achieved. Less than half of office-based physicians can exchange health information outside of their practice and less than a third are able to have this information easily incorporated into their EHR. In the spring of 2019, CMS and the ONC issued new guidelines that would require that all providers and insurers serving Medicare patients make their data electronically accessible by 2020. These new rules include:

- Financial penalties for non-compliance to new HIE regulations by 2020
- Would require emergency department and hospitals to notify primary care providers and other pertinent practitioners of admission, transfer, and discharge
- Require the use of HL7's technical standards Fast Healthcare Interoperability Resource (FHIR) to guarantee timely and accurate transmission of health information in a standardized format
- Additional penalties for healthcare organizations, plans, or providers that create impediments to HIE functions (Hochman, Garber, and Robinson 2019)

There are still challenges to this concept and these specific rules. The obstacles include who would govern the national HIE, what is the funding source, patient matching, and privacy concerns. The next decade will see the HIE experience growth, setbacks, and change.

Methods of Health Information Exchange

There are three methods in which health information is exchanged between appropriate healthcare entities or providers: directed exchange, query-based exchange, and consumer-mediated exchange.

Directed Exchange

Directed exchange is frequently referred to as a "push exchange" because it pushes authorized and secure information from one healthcare organization to another. For example, if a patient is being transferred from one hospital to another, the patient's health information would be "pushed" to the receiving hospital in order to provide the background health information to help the transition to continued care. As part of the stage 1 Meaningful MU requirements for EHRs, the Direct Project was initiated in 2010. The Direct Project is important for the secure messaging and transmission of laboratory results, summary care records, referrals, public health reporting, and conveying quality measures. Direct Project is a standards-based exchange platform to provide a secure, straightforward, scalable method to transmit encrypted information to collaborating providers. Direct messaging exchange acts like regular e-mail but with the added Health Insurance Portability and Accountability Act (HIPAA) security mechanisms for protection of both senders and recipients with Direct addresses. Any messages sent from a Direct e-mail address are encrypted, and can only be opened when received by another Direct e-mail address. If a nurse at ABC Hospital used her employee e-mail address to send a patient's health information to an emergency department physician at XYZ Hospital, it would fail because it was not sent through a Direct address (ONC 2014c).

DirectTrust, which oversees the Direct Project, "is a federally recognized, non-profit policy and governance body that makes it possible for Direct exchange to operate smoothly and reliably, giving Direct users much needed confidence in their exchange partners' privacy and security practices" (DirectTrust 2020). It is a collaboration of 124 HIT companies and healthcare providers to further the interoperable HIE and is federally recognized by the ONC. DirectTrust currently has more than 251,000 healthcare organizations, more than 2.4 million electronic addresses of DirectTrust participants, with more than 1.7 billion cumulative Direct messages as of 2020. For additional information on EHRs, refer to chapter 9. For additional information on PHRs, refer to chapters 9 and 10.

Query-Based Exchange

Query-based exchange is a find-and-seek request for information that is sent through the HIO to find any available health information on a specified individual. It is the opposite of the "push exchange," so it is thought of as a "pull exchange." This type of exchange is typically used in urgent and emergency care to seek information that would be relevant for the encounter at hand. For example, a Medicare patient is brought to the Emergency Department of a local hospital. The Emergency physician requests the patients' most recent EKG and bloodwork results from her cardiologist. The cardiologist's EHR is queried and it sends the EKG and labwork to the Emergency Department in response. The Emergency Physician is then able to compare the last EKG and bloodwork with the ones being done currently in order to make an informed decision about the patient's treatment. In order to use a query-based exchange, an interface is required within the HIO. The HIO broadcasts the request for information through the eHealth Exchange. It uses the internal tools of its patient registry, identification matching, and other programs to locate the appropriate health information. This method requires higher security, audit logging, and additional protection protocols because of its wider scope of exchange (Amatayakul 2017, 425).

Consumer-Mediated Exchange

Consumer-mediated exchange is a type of HIE that is controlled by patients who want to control the use and access of their health information. According to the ONC, "consumer-mediated exchange provides patients with access to their health information, allowing them to manage their health care online in a similar fashion to how they might manage their finances through online banking. When in control of their own health information, patients can actively participate in their care coordination by:

- Providing other providers with their health information
- Identifying and correcting wrong or missing health information
- Identifying and correcting incorrect billing information
- Tracking and monitoring their own health" (ONC2019a).

While some HIT professionals feel that consumer mediated exchanges would improve health information privacy and cooperation among healthcare organizations, others feel that the complexity and volume of data would overwhelm consumers, who would not be able to effectively and efficiently manage and control their information (Pak 2017).

Patients may have the ability to incorporate their PHR because, as discussed in chapter 10, consumer engagement and getting patients more involved in their healthcare and well-being is a component of MU requirements. Although not administered by a federal entity, consumer-mediated exchange is encouraged through the Blue Button campaign and commercial EHR enterprises (Amatayakul 2017, 425).

CHECK YOUR UNDERSTANDING 11.3

1. Dr. Patrick needs to order an antibiotic for her patient, Timothy, who has been diagnosed with strep throat. The term _____, is used to describe the process where Dr. Patrick will electronically order this antibiotic for Timothy and that Timothy can pick it up at a specified drugstore.

   a. E-meds
   b. E-drugs
   c. Compu-drugs
   d. E-prescribe

2. Several years ago, the pediatric clinic needed to upgrade their old EHR system. It did not have the functioning capability necessary to keep up with federal requirements. Due to the very high cost of new EHR systems, they enrolled into the new incentive program from CMS to help with the costs. Identify the regulations that required healthcare providers who participate in the incentive program to utilize computer-based patient health records effectively to improve patient outcomes.

   a. CEHRT
   b. MU
   c. HIPAA
   d. CQM

3. The first requirement that the physicians at the pediatric clinic decide the new EHR system must have is confirmation that the system will meet all federal requirements for privacy,

(Continued)

security, reporting, and quality monitoring functions. The requirement that vendors prove that their EHR products meet specific and optimal standards is termed _____.

a. CEHRT
b. MU
c. HIPAA
d. CQM

4. Dr. Brown wants to know the percentage of patients in the ABC Family Practice who received the flu shot last year after they were sent reminders through the patient portal. With the COVID-19 pandemic on-going, he is anticipating a higher number of flu cases in the upcoming winter season and wants to increase the number of reminders. He knows that flu shots help decrease the number of patients who need to be hospitalized and is a key measurement of population health. Identify the name of the criteria that healthcare providers must meet to show that they are efficiently using the EHR to show a positive impact on patient care.

a. CEHRT
b. MU
c. HIPAA
d. CQM

5. MU is not just to improve the health of one patient but to have an impact on a large portion of patients in a particular geographic area or diagnosis classification. One of the goals of the pediatric clinic is to increase the number of children who receive the MMR vaccine to decrease the number and size of measles outbreaks in their region. The way this is monitored is called _____.

a. Population health reporting
b. Vetting
c. Record locator service
d. Query-based exchange

6. Joe Smith is being treated at the Emergency Department at ABC Hospital. He can't remember the names of all of his doctors and the other hospitals he's been to for treatment. ABC Hospital initiates a "find and seek" request to all of the regional healthcare organizations to find as much information as they can on Mr. Smith. The "find and seek" method of HIE performed through an HIO is referred to as:

a. Population health reporting
b. Vetting
c. Record locator service
d. Query-based exchange

Patient Identification

Making sure that the correct patient is identified within the HIE is one of the major issues. In large or densely populated geographic areas, there could be hundreds of individuals with common names, such as John Smith. Many methods have been used to address this issue, from smart cards with magnetic strips or chips with identifying information, to advanced computer algorithms, to biometrics using fingerprints, facial recognition, or retinal scans. No one method has been found to be completely correct in its matching capabilities. To make matters worse, all this additional technology is expensive, meaning that many healthcare organizations cannot afford to implement these methods (Brinda and Watters 2020, 344).

Identity matching (also known as patient matching) is the process in which the HIO identifies the right person within the database to exchange information between healthcare organizations. The process examines "different demographic elements from different health information technology (health IT) systems to determine if they refer to the same patient. From an interoperability perspective, the ability to complete patient matching efficiently, accurately, and at scale has long been identified as a key element of the nation's health IT infrastructure. Patient matching is almost universally needed to enable the interoperability of health data for all kinds of purposes. Patient matching also requires careful consideration with respect to its effect on patient safety and administrative costs" (ONC 2017c).

Owing to privacy concerns, Congress had banned the Department of Health and Human Services (HHS) from trying to develop and implement a national unique patient identifier (Dimick 2016). However, because of the progression of EHR systems and the issues with patient identification and matching, a national unique patient identifier is being more aggressively addressed. Patient ID Now is a large coalition of a wide variety of healthcare organizations, including AHIMA and the Health Information Management Systems Society (HIMSS), who are working on methods allowing the HHS to work with private-sector healthcare organizations to develop a nationwide patient identification strategy (Patient ID Now 2020). In the meantime, HIOs must establish other methods for identity matching. The sophistication of the algorithms depends upon the type and amount of data needed to solve the query:

> Basic algorithms that compare selected data elements, such as name, date of birth, and gender, are the simplest technique for matching records. Intermediate algorithms use more advanced techniques to compare and match records by assigning subjective weights to demographic elements for use in a scoring system to determine the probability of matching patient records. Advanced algorithms contain the most sophisticated set of tools for matching records and rely on mathematical theory and statistical models to determine the likelihood of a match (Lusk et al. 2018)

Identity management is different from identity matching. **Identity management** ensures "that [the] individual who has been identified is who they say they are, that they have the authority to do what they want to do, and that their actions are tracked" (Amatayakul 2017, 419). Traditionally, identity management was performed as a part of patient registration or in health information management when the paper health record or master patient index were reconciled (AHIMA Work Group 2014). Individual healthcare organizations develop processes for identity management that are best suited to their needs. For example, at the time of registration, most healthcare organization's require the patient to provide a driver's license or state-issued identity card, his insurance card, and employment identification card as proof of employment (if applicable). These methods enforce identity management procedures within the healthcare organization and compel the patient to prove that he is who he says he is.

Because of the HIPAA, patients have the right to refuse to participate in the HIE and to limit who can view their information. A component of identity management within HIE is **consent management**. Consent management has nothing to do with the consent for treatment but rather the patient consents or approves the HIO to transmit health information between two or more authorized entities. According to the ONC, electronic consent management is

> a system, process, or set of policies that enables patients to choose what health information they are willing to permit their healthcare providers to access and share. Consent management allows patients to affirm their participation in electronic health initiatives such as patient portals, personal health records (PHR), and health information exchange (HIE) (ONC2018a).

Figure 11.7 shows key components for the implementation on an electronic consent management process.

Figure 11.7. Implementing meaningful consent

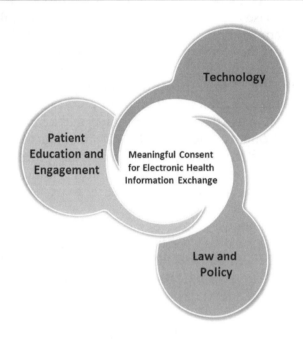

1. **Patient Education and Engagement**—including educating patients about their consent options, who may release their information and how, and the significance of the consent choice.
2. **Technology**—using technology to capture and maintain patient consent decisions, identify which sensitive portions of patient information are restricted from access, and communicate these restrictions electronically with others.
3. **Law and Policy**—ensuring alignment with federal and state law and other legal and policy requirements pertaining to consent, individual choice, and confidentiality.

Source: ONC2018a.

The process of obtaining approval or consent to transmit health information has two components. The first is to obtain consent from an authorized healthcare organization or provider to electronically request or transmit any patient's health information to or from other authorized healthcare entities. This part of the consent process is performed when healthcare providers enlist to be authorized users of an HIO. The second component involves the patient consenting to have the health information accessed and released. This is typically done the first time a patient is registered to receive healthcare services at the particular healthcare organization and then confirmed during any subsequent encounters or admissions. This may be a complete consent allowing all information to be accessed by authorized users. There can also be constraints on the type of accessed data and by whom it may be released or accessed (Amatayakul 2017, 419).

Opt-in or opt-out consent sets the default for health information of patients to be included in the HIO automatically (opt-in), but the patient can choose not to be included (opt-out) completely. Opt-in consent means that the patient must specifically agree to have the personal health information accessible for the HIE (Biedermann and Dolezel 2016, 306). A variation of this consent is the opt-in with restrictions, in which the default is "no patient health information," which is automatically made available and the patient must define what information is to be sent, who it is sent to, and for what purpose the information may be used. "Each HIE must determine how patients and consumers will consent or not consent to have their data and information transmitted by or included in HIE operations" (Biedermann and Dolezel 2016, 306).

The opt-out consent means that the patient data can automatically be exchanged within the HIO by default (Amatayakul 2017, 419). A variation on this consent is the *opt-out with exceptions* model that sets the default for health information for patients to be included, but the patient can opt-out completely or allow only select data to be included (Biedermann and Dolezel 2016, 306).

The AHIMA Work Group has recommended specific data elements that help the healthcare organizations and providers with patient identification issues. Some of the primary data elements include legal name (first, middle, last, maiden), date of birth (DOB), gender, race, mother's maiden name, and primary phone number. Examples of the secondary data elements are birth place, marital status, social security number, driver's license number, e-mail address, and some type of biometric. A biometric is a physical characteristic of the patient or users (such as fingerprints, voiceprints, retinal scans, iris traits) that systems store and use to authenticate identity of the patient or before allowing the user access to a system (AHIMA Work Group 2014). Patient identification integrity has always been a crucial principle of HIM. It is even more crucial now with HIE. Integrity refers to the ability of data to maintain its structure and attributes, including protection against modification or corruption during transmission, storage, or at rest. Maintenance of patient identification and data integrity are key aspects of data quality management and security.

Health Information Exchange Privacy Concerns

All health information is private, but mental health diagnoses, drug and alcohol treatment, and sexually transmitted disease identification are considered to be particularly sensitive. The healthcare organization must determine what additional privacy and security protections are in place because some HIEs may not be able to adequately protect that sensitive information (Brinda and Watters 2016, 331).

Other best practices addressing privacy issues with the HIE include:

- Workforce education programs are robust and timely, including the right of the patient to request restrictions: All employees involved in any patient data or information transaction, access to ePHI, PHI, or HIE operations must receive regular and documented training regarding HIPAA and healthcare organization rules, regulations, policies, and procedures.

- Up-to-date breach notifications policies and procedures for all HIPAA-covered entities: As recent news of data breaches and identity-theft events have shown, the public's trust has decreased regarding the ability of an organization to safeguard their information.

- All mobile devices have effective and strong encryption protection.

- Application of breach sanctions are as written in policy and procedures: Depending on the level of breach, sanctions must have commensurate severity of consequences and be established prior to the event following HIPAA guidelines.

- Business associate agreements are analyzed, evaluated, and updated on a regular basis: The rules are continually expanded and updated and the healthcare organization must make certain it follows suit.

- Current risk analysis is implemented and revised on a regular basis: Follow-up with business associates, covered entities and any others must be verified by the healthcare organization to be in compliance.

- Request for restrictions on disclosure of health information by patients is implemented and on the Notice of Privacy Practices: The enhanced privacy rule requires the healthcare organization to have a method to note that the information has been restricted. (Downing 2014).

CHECK YOUR UNDERSTANDING 11.4

1. XYZ Hospital is located in a large urban city. There are many people in the region who have the same name and birthdates. During registration, additional demographic information is collected to try and distinguish between these individuals. The process whereby the HIO has identified the correct person within a healthcare provider's database in order to send it to the requesting provider is termed _____.

   a. Identity matching
   b. Consolidated HIE
   c. Consent management
   d. Federated HIE

2. The five-state HIO, All-Info, is working with all of its members to update procedures for HIE. All-Info is streamlining the process where patients give their permission for health information will be automatically exchanged with other authorized providers when necessary within the HIO. The protocols for approving that the HIO can exchange health information between two or more authorized healthcare providers is called _____.

   a. Identity matching
   b. CDA
   c. Consent management
   d. ePHI

3. In order to increase the reliability of its patient identification and matching process at registration, the hospital now scans the patient's hand. Identify the name of the method of patient identification that uses a physical characteristic of the patient, such as a fingerprint.

   a. CQM
   b. Biometric
   c. PHR
   d. RLS

4. Because Spencer had his identity stolen several years ago, he wants to make sure his health information is extra protected. If he does not want his ePHI exchanged with other healthcare organizations, which is acceptable and allowable under HIPAA, the process he would participate in is referred to as:

   a. Opt-in consent
   b. Opt-out consent
   c. Privacy
   d. Confidentiality

5. Mary knows that she will be receiving treatment for her cancer from a number of healthcare providers in the region. To make it easier for all of them to get any of her health information, she agrees that her information will be available at any point during her treatment. When a patient gives consent for her personal information to accessible in the HIE, it is referred to as:

   a. Opt-in consent
   b. Opt-out consent
   c. Privacy
   d. Confidentiality

Real-World Case 11.1

Florida's Agency for Health Care Administration (AHCA) oversees the health information exchange activities within the state. On a quarterly basis, it publishes a dashboard of metrics regarding HIE activities. It has been promoting the adoption of e-prescribing since 2007. Part of the dashboard includes e-prescribing adoption and use trending data. It also shows a comparison to the national adoption and trending status. Florida has seen a steady increase in the rate of e-prescriptions since 2007. In 2017, the rate reached almost 75 percent relative to all prescriptions that could have been e-prescribed.

Based on some modifications and clarification to existing federal and state regulations, Florida providers can e-prescribe controlled substances (EPCS) through EHR systems that are certified for that purpose, meaning they must not only have a certified EHR system, it must also be certified to EPCS. Pharmacies must also have certified systems to receive EPCS orders. AHCA has been collecting data on e-prescriptions of controlled substances since 2015. Since this is relatively new process, rates are low but expected to increase. As of 2017, 7.4 percent of active e-prescribers have been enabled to EPCS. The rate that pharmacies are enabled to receive EPCS is almost 87 percent.

Real-World Case 11.2

In a small university town, two hospitals are trying to negotiate how to improve the health information exchange between themselves and the many physicians and other healthcare practitioners in the community. Each hospital has different EHR s, most of the physicians/providers have different EHR systems, with only some of them coordinating with one of the hospitals. The Chamber of Commerce, city and county government leaders, and the major employers have developed a task force to investigate the best HIO and processes to help improve the health of the population, streamline the continuum of care, and help reduce costs for not only the patients, but also for the medical community. The major employers also want an improvement in the efficiency of services being offered to keep insurance costs under control. The Chamber of Commerce has shown that the population is shifting to more retirees locating to the area because of the many amenities it offers. A timeline of 18 months has been established to complete this evaluation and to make recommendations for a public-private partnership to address these issues.

REVIEW QUESTIONS

1. The university medical center, the other private hospitals and the state agree to contract with an HIO to safely transmit patient health information between them. The type of management for this HIO is:

   a. ONC
   b. State agencies
   c. Private EHR vendors
   d. Public-private partnerships

2. The five-state HIO, All-Info, has grown significantly in the last three years. Several local and state health information exchange companies have banded together to offer services to more healthcare organizations and improve transmission capabilities. Once these companies got together, they renamed the company as All-Info. Identify the type of organization that was a precursor to today's HIO?

(Continued)

    a. HIM
    b. RHIO
    c. HIE
    d. ePHI

3. The HIM department is involved in data and information collection, storage, quality, protection. EIS and CDS manipulate data and information to make decisions and strategic planning. Identify the fourth stage in the following sequence of events: data, information, knowledge, and: _____

    a. Behavior change
    b. Wisdom
    c. Attitude
    d. Intelligence

4. The IT Department at ABC Hospital wants to make sure that the new demographic information and medical terms that the medical staff wants to add to their EHR is formatted correctly. This will prevent glitches or other problems with transmitting this information to other healthcare organizations that may need it at some point. Identify the type of interoperability that refers to how the data should be formatted and structured so that seamless exchange can take place.

    a. Technical
    b. Syntactic
    c. Semantic
    d. Process

5. One of the assignments that is given to new HIT students is to report on the organizational structure of the federal agency that is responsible for the coordination and implementation of EHR technology for the exchange of ePHI. Identify the federal agency that is responsible for the coordination and implementation of EHR technology for the exchange of ePHI.

    a. ONC
    b. NHIN
    c. Congress
    d. Department of Defense

6. In order to implement a meaningful consent process at an healthcare organization, consumers would need to be informed of the available possibilities and decisions, its importance in continued treatment, the process of releasing their health information and to whom, and what it means for them. This falls under which of the three key components of a meaningful consent program?

    a. Patient education and engagement
    b. Technology
    c. Law and policy
    d. Identity management

7. Dr. Tanaka is lead researcher for a COVID-19 treatment study involving six university hospitals in four states. Each research team will be evaluating the various treatment methods used for the patients. The study requires that researchers have access to any health information on all COVID-19 patients at the six hospitals. Dr. Tanaka wants to ensure that the research

REVIEW QUESTIONS (*Continued*)

teams will be able to access the necessary patient information. Identify the term that is used to describe the interconnected organizations that have the capability of sending and receiving confidential patient information anywhere in the country.

a. eHealth Exchange
b. LHIO
c. ePHI
d. EHR

8. One of the goals of the Women's Clinic is to increase the number of patients who receive mammograms and colon cancer screenings. They are working with the local health department to offer these services. Statistics indicate that the county population has a higher rate of breast and colon cancer than the rest of the state. Population health can also be known as: _____

a. Epidemiology
b. Biostatistics
c. Public health
d. ePHI

9. Dr. Ambrose wants to participate in an HIE but doesn't want the clinic's information in one large shared database and wants it to work like the Internet. The _____ HIE model does not have a centralized database of patient information, is more common, and works much like the Internet.

a. Consolidated
b. Federated
c. Hybrid
d. Direct exchange

10. To reduce patient fraud, the hospital wants to have policies and procedures that ensures that the person is who he says he is, has the authority to do what he needs to, and that his actions are tracked. Identify the process that ensures that the person is who they say they are, have the authority to do what they need to, and that their actions are tracked.

a. Identity matching
b. Identity management
c. Consent management
d. CDA

Abbreviations/Acronyms Matching

1. HIE   A. federal legislation that invests specifically in healthcare and health information technology

2. HIO   B. a group of businesses that all have a stake in the wellbeing of the community and its providers that band together to exchange information to achieve those goals

3. RLS   C. a precursor to the HIO in a specific geographic area

(*Continued*)

4. BYOD   D.   the basic infrastructure requirements for patient information to be transmitted to any other valid healthcare provider for the continuation of health services anywhere in the US

5. ARRA   E.   the incentive program for healthcare providers to adopt EHRs and HIT

6. RHIO   F.   the secure transmission of health data between two or more providers

7. NHIN   G.   the middle-man between healthcare providers that runs the exchange of health information between them

8. HITECH   H.   the concept that healthcare providers will use their personal cell phones and smart devices when conducting the business of healthcare

9. MU   I.   federal legislation used to stimulate the US economy and invest in the country's infrastructure

10. LHIO   J.   software that finds health information on a specific patient in a participating healthcare organization after a query is initiated

References

AHIMA Work Group. 2014. Managing the integrity of patient identity in health information exchange (2014 update). *Journal of AHIMA* 85(5): expanded web version. http://bok.ahima.org/doc?oid=300436#.WojcLainFRY.

Amatayakul, M. K. 2017. *Health IT and EHRs: Principles and Practice*, 6th ed. Chicago: AHIMA.

American Academy of Family Physicians (AAFP). 2019. Frequently Asked Questions: Medicare Access and CHIP Reauthorization Act of 2015 (MACRA). https://www.aafp.org/practice-management/payment/medicare-payment/macra-101/faq.html

Biedermann, S. and D. Dolezel. 2016. *Introduction to Healthcare Informatics*, 2nd ed. Chicago: AHIMA.

Bowe, H. and Williamson, L. 2020. Healthcare Information. Chapter 12 in *Health Information Management Technology: An Applied Approach*, 6th ed. Edited by N. B. Sayles and L. L. Gordon. Chicago: AHIMA.

Brinda, D. and A. Watters. 2020. Data Privacy, Confidentiality, and Security. Chapter 11 in *Health Information Management: Concepts, Principles, and Practice*, 6th ed. Edited by P. Oachs and A. Watters. Chicago: AHIMA.

Centers for Medicare and Medicaid (CMS). 2017. Value-based programs. https://www.cms.gov/Medicare/Quality-Initiatives-Patient-Assessment-Instruments/Value-Based-Programs/Value-Based-Programs.html.

Centers for Medicare and Medicaid (CMS). 2020. Clinical Quality Measures. https://www.cms.gov/Regulations-and-Guidance/Legislation/EHRIncentivePrograms/ClinicalQualityMeasures.html.

Centers for Medicare and Medicaid (CMS). 2020b. MIPS quick start guide. Accessed 9/29/2020. file:///C:/Users/FAMU/Downloads/2020%20MIPS%20Quick%20Start%20Guide%20(1).pdf

Cha, E. A. 2016. "Researchers: Medical Errors Now Third Leading Cause of Death in United States." *Washington Post*, May 3, 2016. https://www.washingtonpost.com/news/to-your-health/wp/2016/05/03/researchers-medical-errors-now-third-leading-cause-of-death-in-united-states/?utm_term=.64637f3a8bed.

Dimick, C. 2016. Petition calls for unique patient identifier solution. *Journal of AHIMA* 87(3) https://journal.ahima.org/petition-calls-for-unique-patient-identifier-solution/

DirectTrust. 2020. What is DirectTrust?: DirectTrust overview. https://www.directtrust.org/what -we-do Downing, K. 2014. "Seven select questions to ask your privacy officer (or yourself)" *Journal of AHIMA* 85(4): 42–44.

eHealth Exchange. 2019. What is eHealth Exchange? https://ehealthexchange.org/

HIMSS. 2018. Privacy & Security for RHIOs/HIEs. http://www.himss.org/privacy-security -rhioshies-0.

HL7. 2017. HL7/ASTM Implementation Guide for CDA® R2 Continuity of Care Document (CCD®) Release 1. https://www.hl7.org/implement/standards/product_brief.cfm?product _id=6.

Hochman, M., Garber, J., Robinson, E. 2019. Health Information Exchange after 10 years: Time for a more assertive, national approach. https://www.healthaffairs.org/do/10.1377 /hblog20190807.475758/full/

Institute of Medicine (IOM). 2000. *To Err Is Human: Building a Safer Health System*. https:// www.ncbi.nlm.nih.gov/books/NBK225179/.

Lee-Eichenwald, S. 2020. Health Information Technologies. Chapter 12 in *Health Information Management: Concepts, Principles, and Practice* 6th ed. Edited by P. Oachs and A. Watters. Chicago: AHIMA.

Lusk, K. N. Noreen, G. Okafor, K. Peterson, and E. Pupo. 2018 (Winter). Patient matching in health information exchanges. *Perspectives in Health Information Management.* http:// perspectives.ahima.org/patient-matching-in-health-information-exchanges/.

McCarthy, D. B., Propp, K., Cohen, A., Sabharwal, R., Schachter, A. A., & Rein, A. L. 2014. Learning from health information exchange technical architecture and implementation in seven beacon communities. EGEMS (Washington, DC), 2(1), 1060. https://doi.org/10.13063/2327 -9214.1060 Accessed 9/29/2020. https://www.ncbi.nlm.nih.gov/pmc/articles/PMC4371446/

Miller, K. 2020. Healthcare Delivery Systems. Chapter 2 in *Health Information Management Technology: An Applied Approach*, 6th ed. Edited by N. B. Sayles and L. L. Gordon. Chicago: AHIMA.

Office of the National Coordinator for Health Information Technology (ONC). N.d. Nationwide Health Information Network Exchange. Accessed 7/13/2020. https://www.healthit.gov/sites /default/files/factsheets/nationwide-health-information-network-exchange.pdf

Office of the National Coordinator for Health Information Technology (ONC). 2019a. Health Information Exchange (HIE). https://www.healthit.gov/topic/health-it-and-health -information-exchange-basics/health-information-exchange.

Office of the National Coordinator for Health Information Technology (ONC). 2019b. Why Is Health Information Exchange Important? https://www.healthit.gov/faq/why-health -information-exchange-important

Office of the National Coordinator for Health Information Technology (ONC). 2019c. Meaningful Use. https://www.healthit.gov/topic/meaningful-use-and-macra/meaningful-use.

Office of the National Coordinator for Health Information Technology (ONC). 2018a. Patient Consent for eHIE. https://www.healthit.gov/topic/meaningful-consent-overview.

Office of the National Coordinator for Health Information Technology (ONC). 2018b. Standards Collaboration. https://www.healthit.gov/topic/interoperability/standards-collaboration.

Office of the National Coordinator for Health Information Technology (ONC). 2017a. About ONC. https://www.healthit.gov/newsroom/about-onc.

Office of the National Coordinator for Health Information Technology (ONC). 2017b. Population /Public Health. https://www.healthit.gov/playbook/population-public-health/.

Office of the National Coordinator for Health Information Technology (ONC). 2017c. Demystifying Patient Matching Algorithms. https://www.healthit.gov/buzz-blog/interoperability /demystifying-patient-matching-algorithms/.

Office of the National Coordinator for Health Information Technology (ONC). 2016. Electronic Health Records Infographic. 2016. https://www.healthit.gov/infographic/electronic-health -records-infographic.

Office of the National Coordinator for Health Information Technology (ONC). 2015a. Key Barriers to Health IT Adoption. https://dashboard.healthit.gov/report-to-congress/2015-update-adoption-health-information-technology-full-text.php.

Office of the National Coordinator for Health Information Technology (ONC). 2015b. Public Health Surveillance. https://www.healthit.gov/sites/default/files/onc_public_health_surveillance_infographic-11042014.pdf.

Office of the National Coordinator for Health Information Technology (ONC). 2014b. Connecting Health and Care for the Nation: A Shared Nationwide Interoperability Roadmap. https://www.healthit.gov/sites/default/files/hie-interoperability/nationwide-interoperability-roadmap-final-version-1.0.pdf.

Office of the National Coordinator for Health Information Technology (ONC). 2014c. Direct Basics: Q&A for Providers. https://www.healthit.gov/sites/default/files/directbasicsforprovidersqa_05092014.pdf.

Office of the National Coordinator for Health Information Technology (ONC). 2018a. Patient Consent for eHIE. https://www.healthit.gov/topic/meaningful-consent-overview.

Office of the National Coordinator for Health Information Technology (ONC). 2018b. Standards Collaboration. https://www.healthit.gov/topic/interoperability/standards-collaboration.

Pak, H. 2017. Consumer Mediated Exchange. https://www.ehidc.org/sites/default/files/resources/files/Consumer%20Mediated%20Exchange-Pak.pdf.

Patient ID Now. 2020. What is Patient ID. Accessed 9/29/2020. https://patientidnow.org/about/

Sequoia Project. 2020. About the Sequoia Project. https://sequoiaproject.org/about-us/

Chapter 12

Security

Learning Objectives

- Educate staff on security issues.
- Discuss federal security regulation.
- Recommend security measures.
- Develop policies and procedures on security practices.
- Control access to protected health information.
- Conduct audit for security violation.

Key Terms

Access controls
Addressable standards
Administrative safeguards
Administrative simplification
Audit controls
Audit reduction tools
Audit trails
Baiting
Biomedical device
Biometric identifiers
Bots
Bring your own device (BYOD)
Business associate agreement (BAA)
Business associates
Completely automated public turning test to tell computers and humans apart (CAPTCHA)

Certified in Healthcare Privacy and Security (CHPS)
Certified Information Security Manager (CISM)
Certified Information Systems Security Professional (CISSP)
Code set
Context-based authentication
Contingency plan
Covered entity (CE)
Data at rest
Data in motion
Data in use
Data loss prevention (DLP)
Data recovery
Degaussing
Denial of service
Designated standard maintenance organizations (DSMOs)

Electronic protected health information (e-PHI)
Emergency access procedure
Emergency mode operation plan
Encryption
Firewalls
Forensics
Healthcare clearinghouse
Health Insurance Portability and Accountability Act of 1996 (HIPAA)
Health plan
Information access management
Information system activity review
Integrity
Intrusion detection system (IDS)

Intrusion protection system (IPS)

Malicious software

Mitigation

Network security

One-factor authentication

Organization access controls

Passwords

Penetration testing

Phishing

Physical safeguards

Pretexting

Privacy Rule

Protected health information (PHI)

Ransomware

Redundancy

Remote wipe

Required standards

Risk analysis

Risk management

Role-based authentication

Security

Security awareness training

Security event

Security incident

Security management plan

Security official

Security Rule

Single sign-on (SSO) system

Social engineering

Spoliation

Spyware

Technical safeguard

Termination process

Threats

Token

Transaction and Code Sets rule

Transmission security

Trigger

Trojan

Two-factor authentication

User-based authentication

Username

Virtual private network

Virus

Vulnerabilities

Workforce clearance procedure

Worm

The security of health information has always been a priority of health information management (HIM) professionals, but it was raised to a new level of importance with the implementation of information systems that document and retain health record information as well as other data that can identify the patient.

Data can be classified in a number of ways. One way is to classify data according to data type—clinical, administrative, financial, and so on. Data can also be classified into categories according to the level of security required. Different terms might be used, but one example is PHI, sensitive, and public. Who has access and how the information is used will be controlled by the classification allocated to it (UAB 2020).

Data must be protected in its three states: data at rest, data in motion, and data in use. Data at rest is when the data is stored on an electronic media such on a computer's hard drive. Data in motion is data that is moving from point A to point B such as being shared between a hospital and an insurer. Data in use is when the data is being accessed for review, updates, or other purposes.

With the paper record, access was limited to the health record itself. With the electronic health record (EHR) and other information systems, access is available from anywhere, including outside the healthcare organization.

Historically, security regulations were enacted at the state level, which led to a patchwork of very different laws across the country with no consistency among them. There were, and are, accreditation standards and the Medicare Conditions of Participation that address security, but these standards applied solely to accredited healthcare organizations and healthcare organizations that treated Medicare patients, respectively. Accreditation standards generally include broad security requirements that vary by accrediting organization. Because of security concerns of healthcare professionals and patients alike, federal laws were enacted. This chapter will address the Health Insurance Portability and Accountability Act of 1996 (HIPAA) including the revisions from the Health Information Technology for Economic and Clinical Health and security concepts such as security threats and safeguards.

Introduction to Health Information Portability and Accountability Act of 1996

The **Health Insurance Portability and Accountability Act of 1996 (HIPAA)** is a federal law that impacts many areas of healthcare, including insurance portability, code sets, privacy, security, electronic data interchange (EDI), and national identifier standards. HIPAA is divided into five titles, or sections. This chapter addresses Title II: Fraud and Abuse/Administrative Simplification.

The purpose of the **administrative simplification** title is to improve the efficiency and effectiveness of the business processes of healthcare by standardizing the EDI of administrative and financial transactions. This title was also designed to protect the privacy and security of **protected health information (PHI)** that is transmitted from one point to another. PHI includes health information in any format including paper, fax, and electronic. PHI is individually identifiable health information that is transmitted or maintained in any form or format by an organization subject to HIPAA. A third purpose is to reduce the cost of doing business in healthcare because of antiquated paper systems, nonstandard formats, and lack of accessibility to health records due to loss (45 CFR 160, 162, and 164 2013).

To be subject to HIPAA, an organization must meet the definition of a **covered entity (CE)** or be a business associate (defined later in this chapter). A CE is a health plan, healthcare clearinghouse, or healthcare provider that transmits any health information in electronic form for one of the covered transactions. A **health plan** pays for the healthcare provided to the individuals covered under the plan. These plans include medical, dental, vision, and other forms of health plans. Healthcare providers include hospitals, physician offices, long-term care facilities, ambulatory surgery centers, pharmacies, and other patient care providers. A **healthcare clearinghouse** collects billing data and processes it for the healthcare provider. The healthcare clearinghouse then submits the claim to the health plan for payment. The covered transactions that HIPAA addresses are:

- "Payment and remittance advice
- Claims status
- Eligibility
- Coordination of benefits
- Claims and encounter information
- Enrollment and disenrollment
- Referrals and authorizations
- Premium payment" (CMS 2020)

Health plans, healthcare clearinghouses, and healthcare providers that do not share patient information for one of these transactions are not CEs and, therefore, are not subject to HIPAA.

HIPAA has greatly impacted healthcare and the HIM profession as a result of changes in processes, emphasis on privacy and security, and patient rights. One of the sections in HIPAA is Administrative Simplification, which includes Transaction and Code Sets Rule, Privacy Rule, Enforcement Rule, Unique National Providers Identifiers, and the Security Rule. The Enforcement Rule and Unique National Providers Identifiers are outside the scope of this book. Although this chapter emphasizes security, as interrelated components of HIPAA, all three of the aforementioned rules are discussed.

Transaction and Code Sets Rule

The **Transaction and Code Sets Rule** was designed to standardize transactions performed by CEs. These standards apply to electronic transactions only, such as claim submission, eligibility queries, and many more insurance-related functions; however, paper submissions are similar. The Department of Health and Human Services (HHS) has assigned the responsibility of developing and maintaining standards for the Transaction and Code Sets rule to six organizations, called **designated standard maintenance organizations (DSMOs):**

- Accredited Standards Committee X12
- Dental Contact Committee of the American Dental Association
- Health Level 7 (HL7)
- National Council for Prescription Drug Programs

- National Uniform Billing Committee
- National Uniform Claim Committee (45 CFR 160, 162, and 164 2013)

Transaction and Code Sets standards cover the individual data elements and the format of the data for the claim submissions and other functions mentioned earlier in this chapter. The standards enable the use of **electronic data interchange (EDI)**, the transfer of data from one point to another without human intervention, which can significantly improve the efficiency of healthcare. The HIPAA transactions and code sets requirements use ASC X12 standards. These ASC X12 standards mandate the data to be submitted, formatting, and other attributes of the healthcare claims and other financial transactions.

CEs may follow the transaction requirements themselves and send formatted data to the clearinghouse for submission to the third-party payers. The CE also may send unformatted data to a clearinghouse or health plan and have the data converted into the appropriate transaction format.

Designated **code sets** are also a part of the HIPAA Transactions and Code Set rule. HIPAA defines a **code set** as a set of codes used to encode data elements (45 CFR 160, 162, and 164 2013). These codes record medical diagnoses, procedures, drugs, dental procedures, and other data elements. A code replaces larger pieces of data. For example, the ICD-10-CM code I10 means essential (primary) hypertension. HIPAA mandates the use of certain coding systems in the reporting of diagnoses, procedures, drugs, and more on medical and dental claims. These standards are:

- *International Classification of Diseases, Tenth Revision, Clinical Modification* (ICD-10-CM)
- *International Classification of Diseases, Tenth Revision, Procedural Coding System* (ICD-10-PCS)
- Current Procedural Terminology, Fourth Edition (CPT-4)
- Healthcare Financing Administration Common Procedure Coding System (HCPCS)
- Code on Dental Procedures and Nomenclature, Second Edition (CDT-2)
- National Drug Codes (NDC)

There are also nonmedical codes that can define medical specialties, claim adjustment reasons, reject reason codes, state abbreviations, remittance remarks, and more.

Privacy Rule

The HIPAA **Privacy Rule** controls how CEs, defined earlier in the chapter, may use PHI. **Business associates** are individuals or organizations that perform work on behalf of the CE and that require access to PHI. Examples of functions that business associates may perform are coding, release of information, and billing. Business associates are subject to HIPAA. HIPAA lists the specific data elements that determine whether or not information is PHI. If the information includes any of the data elements in figure 12.1, it is considered PHI and is therefore subject to the HIPAA Privacy Rule.

Figure 12.1. PHI identifiers

Names	Account numbers	Device identifiers and serial numbers
Dates, except year	Health plan beneficiary numbers	Internet protocol addresses
Telephone numbers	Certificate/license numbers	Full face photos and comparable images
Geographic data	Vehicle identifiers and serial numbers including license plates	Biometric identifiers (i.e. retinal scan, fingerprint)
FAX numbers		
Social Security numbers		
Email addresses		
Medical record numbers	Web URLs	

Source: HIPAA Journal 2017.

The Privacy Rule also lists the following PHI-related patient rights:

- Patient must be provided a notice of privacy practices that defines how PHI is used in the CE
- Patient has the right to inspect, copy, and receive a copy of the medical record
- Patient has the right to request an amendment to the health information
- Patient has the right to request communications from the CE through alternative means such as a post office box rather than the home address
- Patient has the right to report violations of the HIPAA Privacy Rule
- Patient has the right to request restrictions on how his or her PHI is utilized by the CE (Rinehart-Thompson 2018, 83-86)

The CE must have policies in place to allow a patient to claim these rights. Policies and procedures are important to the Privacy Rule compliance program since the rule focuses on processes and the people who develop and follow them rather than on technology. The need for policies and procedures to document security processes is mentioned throughout this chapter. These policies and procedures should be in writing and may be updated at any time. Once the policy and procedure or other required document is updated, replaced, or deleted, the document must be retained for six years from the date it was last in effect. This documentation must be available to members of the workforce responsible for implementing the procedures referred to in the documentation.

Security Rule

Security has two definitions that focus on different aspects of security:

1. The means to control access and protect information from accidental or intentional disclosure to unauthorized persons and from unauthorized alteration, destruction, or loss
2. The physical protection of facilities and equipment from theft, damage, or unauthorized access; collectively, the policies, procedures, and safeguards designed to protect the confidentiality of information, maintain the integrity and availability of information systems, and control access to the content of these systems.

A CE must address all of the aspects included in these definitions as they are all included in the Security Rule. The **Security Rule** defines the minimum that a CE must do to protect **electronic protected health information (ePHI)**, which is PHI that is "created, received, or transmitted" electronically by CEs (45 CFR 160, 162, and 164 2013). The Security Rule does not apply to PHI in other media such as paper, oral communication, and microfilm. ePHI can be communicated over the Internet or it can be stored electronically, such as on a magnetic drive. Voicemail, fax, and copy machines (unless the copy machine stores data) are not considered to be ePHI.

The Security Rule was developed to be technology neutral and scalable. Technology changes so fast that the Security Rule would need constant revision if specific technologies were mandated; therefore, the rule mandates what needs to be done but not how to do it. For example, the HIPAA Security Rule mandates that physical access to electronic information systems is limited to authorized staff. The rule does not tell the CE how that limitation is to be implemented, so the CE may use card keys, personal identification numbers, keys, biometrics, or other means (described later in this chapter) to control access. Scalable means that the HHS allows CEs to consider the size, complexity, and capabilities of the CE when developing the compliance strategy. The CE can also consider the infrastructure of the CE regarding technology, software, and hardware, as well as the costs of the security measures and the risks to the ePHI (AMA n.d.). Because of scalability, the HHS would expect more rigorous security measures from a 1,000-bed hospital than from a 60-bed hospital or a two-physician practice.

American Recovery and Reinvestment Act of 2009

The American Recovery and Reinvestment Act of 2009 (ARRA) introduced new requirements related to security: *Office of National Coordinators*

- Certification of EHRs
- Mandated HIPAA audits
- Increased severity of penalties
- Business associates subject to privacy and security regulations
- Breach notification

In order to become a certified EHR, the software must meet specified security standards. Vendors apply to have their EHR applications reviewed by one of the Office of the National Coordinator for Health Information Technology–Authorized Certification Bodies and Accredited Testing Laboratories. The benefit to becoming certified is that qualified healthcare providers are able to obtain incentive funds for using the certified EHR in a meaningful way. Refer to chapter 9 for additional information on the Promoting Interoperability program.

The increased penalties include prison as well as financial penalties and are discussed later in this chapter. Business associates and their responsibilities related to security are also covered later in this chapter. The breech notification requirements mandated that patients, the Security of the Department of Health and Human Services and in some cases the media must be notified when there is a privacy or security breach. Refer to chapter 9 for more information about EHRs.

CHECK YOUR UNDERSTANDING 12.1

1. To be subject to HIPAA, an organization must meet the definition of business associate or a(n) _____.
   a. Covered entity
   b. Accredited organization
   c. Administrative simplification
   d. Designated standard organization

2. One of the purposes of Title II: Fraud and Abuse/Administrative Simplification is to _____.
   a. Prevent security incidents from ever occurring in a healthcare organization
   b. Create socialized medicine in the United States
   c. Improve efficiency and effectiveness of healthcare business processes
   d. Establish a prospective payment system

3. Identify a HIPAA granted patient right.
   a. Amend their health record
   b. Access their health record
   c. To be notified that Medicare may not pay for healthcare services.
   d. Delete information that the patient disagrees with

4. Dr Smith is a solo practitioner. Hospital X is a 500 bed hospital. The concept that allows them consider to their size and resources when complying with the Security Rule is known as _____.

CHECK YOUR UNDERSTANDING 12.1 (*Continued*)

a. Technology neutral
b. Scalable
c. Business associate
d. Covered entity

5. Billing Plus is a company that will prepare and submit bill for the hospital. It is a _____.

a. DSMO
b. Business associate
c. Privacy Rule
d. Code set

Security Threats and Safeguards

Threats are the potential for a vulnerability to be exploited. **Vulnerabilities** are weaknesses that could be exploited, thus creating a breach of security. Threats come from internal and external sources. Internal threats come from employees, hardware factors (e.g. failure and stolen), and the environment (water leak, for example). Human threats, such as those performed by employees, can be intentional such as sabotage or they can be unintentional such as deleting the wrong data.

Threats due to human error are not intentional and result from mistakes or misunderstandings. Examples of human errors are cutting electricity to a building when digging, destroying the wrong disk, loading data on an Internet server by accident, and entering the wrong configuration setting. Conversely, some threats are classified as intentional activity, including intentional deletion or alteration of data, infecting the information system with viruses, and using data to steal a patient's identity. External threats can be caused by people outside the CE who attempt to gain unauthorized access. External threats also include natural disasters such as floods, tornadoes, and hurricanes, which may cause damage to the CE that destroys the information system or temporarily disables access to the information system.

The goals of the HIPAA Security Rule are to ensure the confidentiality, integrity, and availability of the ePHI – commonly known as the **CIA Triad**. Confidentiality means providing access to ePHI to only those who need it. **Integrity** is ensuring that data are not altered, either during transmission across a network or during storage. Integrity is discussed later in this chapter. ePHI must be available when needed for patient care and other uses when needed.

The Security Rule is designed to ensure that ePHI remains confidential and is protected from unauthorized disclosure, alteration, or destruction. The Security Rule utilizes administrative, physical, and technical safeguards to protect ePHI. Administrative safeguards are people-focused and include requirements such as training, policies, and assignment of an individual responsible for security. Physical safeguards are mechanisms in place to protect hardware, software, and data. The physical safeguards should protect ePHI from fire, flooding, unauthorized access to hardware, theft, and other hazards. Technical safeguards use technology to protect data and to control access to the data.

Administrative, physical, and technical safeguards are broken down into implementation specifications and standards. The standards tell the CE what must be done, whereas implementation specifications provide direction to help the CE comply with the standards. Each standard is identified as required or addressable. **Required standards** must be implemented by all CEs to protect the ePHI. **Addressable standards** must be evaluated by the entity to determine whether or not the standard is reasonable and appropriate. If the standard is reasonable and appropriate, then the CE must implement the standard. If it is not, then the CE has the flexibility to identify an equivalent method of accomplishing the same objective. For example, encryption is an addressable standard, but although the CE does not have to encrypt data, there has to be a method to protect the data from unauthorized use. The CE cannot determine that a standard is not reasonable and appropriate simply because it is expensive. There is no requirement for a standard to be deemed not reasonable and appropriate, but the CE must document the rationale (in case of audit) and what is being done to implement an equivalent method. Each type of safeguard will be discussed later in this chapter.

Administrative Safeguards and the Security Management Process

The Security Rule defines **administrative safeguards** as

> administrative actions, and policies and procedures, to manage the selection, development, implementation, and maintenance of security measure to protect electronic-protected health information and to manage the conduct of the covered entity's workforce in relation to the protection of that information (45 CFR 160, 162, and 164 2013).

A listing of the administrative safeguards required by the HIPAA Security Rule can be found in table 12.1.

Table 12.1. Administrative safeguards

Standards	Implementation Specifications
Security management	• Risk analysis • Risk management • Sanction policy • Information system activity review
Assigned security responsibility	• None
Workforce security	• Authorization and supervision • Workforce clearance procedures • Termination procedures
Information access management	• Isolating healthcare clearinghouse functions • Access authorization • Access establishment and modification
Security awareness and training	• Security reminders • Protection from malicious software • Log-in monitoring • Password management
Security incident procedures	• Response and reporting
Contingency plan	• Data backup plan • Disaster recovery plan • Emergency mode operation plan • Testing and revision procedures • Applications and data criticality analysis
Evaluation	None
Business associate contract and other arrangements	Written contract or other arrangement

Source: Adapted from 45 CFR 160, 162, and 164 2013.

Many of the security rule requirements require the development and implementation of policies to meet the administrative requirements. Some of the topics that must be addressed are risk analysis, risk management, sanction policy, and information system activity review.

Risk Analysis

Risk analysis is the process of identifying possible security threats to the CE's data and identifying which risks should be promptly addressed and which are lower in priority. The risk analysis process requires the CE to bring staff from across the CE together to identify the data that must be protected. The risk analysis includes estimating the potential costs associated with security breaches and how much it would cost to develop safeguards to prevent these incidents. The Department of Health and Human Services (HHS) has identified nine elements of risk analysis. These elements are shown in Table 12.2.

Table 12.2. Nine elements of risk analysis

Element	Description
Scope of the analysis	The risk analysis should cover all ePHI under the responsibility of the CE.
Data collection	The risk analysis should cover all ePHI no matter where it is stored, managed, and how it is used.
Identify and document possible threats and vulnerabilities	The risk analysis should identify all possible threats and vulnerabilities that apply to the specific CE based on location, situation, and more.
Assess current security practices	Assess current security practices to determine if they are appropriate and whether or not additional security practices are required.
Identify the likelihood that threat occurs	Determine which threats are more likely to occur than others given your location and situation.
Identify potential impacts	All potential impacts that could result from a threat should be identified so that the organization can be prepared for them.
Identify seriousness of risk	The seriousness of the risk is based on both the likelihood that something will occur and the impact that the risk would have on the CE.
Documentation of risk analysis	The CE should document the steps taken as well as their findings.
Periodic review and update	The risk assessment should be updated and revised periodically to ensure that it still meets the needs of the CE.

Source: Adapted from HHS 2010.

This risk analysis must include the risks to data confidentiality and integrity and the availability of the ePHI it controls. To accomplish this, the team has to identify the threats to and vulnerabilities of the CE. Vulnerabilities may be technical or nontechnical. A technical vulnerability are flaws in the computers, software and other equipment used. These flaw can be in the development of the technology, in the configurations or something else. Nontechnical vulnerabilities are administrative which would include lack of or poorly written policies (Shutters nd). Other examples of vulnerabilities would be connection to ePHI through the Internet and lack of detailed security policies, and procedures. The CE also must identify existing security controls such as firewalls, employee termination procedures, and virus protection software. In addition, the team must determine the impact of losing one or more information systems because of malware, sabotage, hardware failure, breach of privacy, or other failure. The risk analysis must also look for threats such as floods, fire, errors in data entry, viruses, and unauthorized access to ePHI. The Security Rule does not define the steps to be taken for risk analysis. It is left to each CE to develop and maintain its own plan for compliance.

Addressing the threats and vulnerabilities identified during the risk analysis helps prevent failure of information systems. While all information system failures are serious, some have a greater impact on the CE than others. For example, failure of the patient satisfaction database will not be as critical as the failure of the EHR. If the patient satisfaction system is not working for a week, the data entry will be backlogged and the reports may be delayed, but patient care goes on unimpeded. With the EHR, the patient's test results, allergies, past medical history, and other information may not be available, which severely impacts patient care. Not all risks are created equal so data criticality analysis is required to determine the risk for each information system. Each risk must be evaluated for the likelihood of the event happening. For example, if the CE is located in Alabama, the risk of an earthquake is low, but the risk of a tornado or hurricane will be high. The CE could categorize risks into high, medium, and low based on the impact that the threat would have on the CE. The CE would then need to address the threats—especially the ones deemed to be a high risk. If a vulnerability is exploited, the outcome resulting from the vulnerability could take a number of forms. According to the Centers for Medicare and Medicaid Services (CMS), potential impacts include destruction of ePHI, inappropriate access to ePHI, and more.

Based on the likelihood of risk, the impact on the CE, and other findings, the team must recommend controls to reduce the risk to the CE. Examples of controls are sanction policies, firewalls, encryption, and biometrics. These controls will be discussed later in this chapter. These proposals must be in compliance with the HIPAA security rule and be designed to reduce the risk and vulnerabilities to ePHI. The process, findings, and recommendations of the risk analysis process must be documented and retained.

Risk Management

Risk management is a comprehensive program of activities intended to minimize the potential for injuries to occur in a CE and to anticipate and respond to ensuring liabilities for those injuries that do occur. There must be processes in place to identify, evaluate, and control risk. The first step in risk management is the development of a risk management plan. This plan sets the priority for the implementation of the security measure identified in the security assessment. The plan should address the risk analysis plan as well as a mitigation plan. The mitigation plan will address each risk identified in the risk analysis and what the CE will do to reduce the probability that the risk will occur as well as the impact it would have on the organization (Compliancy Group nd). Risk assessment and risk management are not one-time events but rather ongoing processes. Although HIPAA does not mandate the frequency of reviews or updates, it does mandate that they must occur as necessary. This time period could be from one to three years, based on the needs of the CE.

In the security management process, the CE must manage security policies. The policies covered under this **security management plan** must include the policies required to prevent, identify, control, and resolve security incidents (45 CFR 160, 162, and 164 2013). The security management plan should be updated periodically to address changes in law, changes in the CE, and other issues.

Sanction Policy

Each CE must develop a sanction policy that addresses how employees will be penalized for failing to follow security policies and procedures. HIPAA does not require specific employee penalties, but requires the CE to determine how breaches and other violations should be handled. Employees should be notified of the policies and procedures and the penalties that come with violations. Sanctions should be based on the CE's policies as well as the severity of the violation (HIPAA Journal 2018). For example, an employee who fails to log off of a computer during a medical emergency should not be penalized in the same way as an employee who sells a celebrity's PHI to the tabloids.

Information System Activity Review

CEs are required to conduct an **information system activity review**, which monitors for the inappropriate use or disclosure of ePHI. HIPAA does not mandate the frequency of this review nor the way this review is to be conducted. These reviews should include logs, access, and incident reporting. The CE should monitor audit logs, the incident log, and other internal and external documentation to identify all successful and unsuccessful attempts to access ePHI (Amatayakul 2017, 377–378). For additional information on monitoring compliance, refer to chapter 13.

Assigned Security Responsibility

The Security Rule mandates an individual to be in charge of the security program for the CE. HIPAA calls this individual a **security official**; however, this position is frequently called chief security officer (CSO) by the CEs. The CSO is responsible for:

- Developing the security goals and objectives for the CE
- Determining how the goals and objectives will be met
- Advising administration regarding information security
- Determining reporting procedures
- Conducting adequate risk assessment and determining the appropriate level of risk acceptance
- Developing and monitoring the overall security program

The CSO works with others who assist in managing the CE's security program. This individual must have a strong understanding of both technology and the business practices of the CE. HIPAA gives little direction as to the role of the CSO, just that the responsibility should be given to a specific individual who is responsible for the overall security program. The CSO may have additional employees assisting. The CSO's role may be a full-time or part-time role, and the CSO may be the same or a different individual from the chief privacy official (CPO). The CPO is in charge of the privacy program for the CE.

Workforce Security

Policies and procedures should be in place to ensure that members of the workforce have the appropriate access to ePHI for their job. **Information access management** involves implementing policies and procedures to determine which employees have access to what information. One of the ways a healthcare clearinghouse can accomplish this is to isolate PHI from the rest of the clearinghouse's information. Some healthcare clearinghouses are owned and operated by large corporations that conduct business in many different industries. To protect the ePHI, it must be completely separated from the non-health clearinghouse segments of the business. For example, the data can be stored in a separate database and a separate network.

Additionally, each CE workforce member must be given access to data and system functionality, such as accessing the EHR, and then it must be specified what the user can do in the EHR, such as accessing whether or not a patient has an allergy. The CE must have a workforce clearance procedure. The **workforce clearance procedure** ensures that each member of the workforce's level of access is appropriate. The workforce includes all employees, students, volunteers, members of the board of directors, and others, paid or unpaid, who perform services for the CE. The access determination should be based on risk analysis and each employee's job description. This would require the CE to evaluate each user and their need for data and functionality. Authentication is covered later in this chapter. There must be a **termination process** to eliminate access to the information systems by a member of the workforce when that person's employment with the CE ends—either through resignation or through termination (firing). The **termination process** should also include review for job-appropriate access levels, to include more or less access to ePHI, as the individual's role in the CE changes. Termination in this context does not mean that the employee was fired but rather is leaving the CE for any reason. This termination should be performed immediately. For example, if an employee resigns and his or her last day ends at 5:00 p.m., then the access should be cancelled at or before 5:00 p.m.

All workforce members, including administration, board of directors, custodial staff, students, and volunteers, must receive **security awareness and training**, which educates CE employees about the CE's security policies and procedures. Basic training should cover general security policies, physical and workstation security, password management, importance of logging out, and other issues. Many workforce members will require additional security training appropriate to their job functions. For example, management staff will need training on monitoring procedures and security system assessment. HIPAA does not mandate the format that the training takes, but a recommendation is to include it in new employee orientation. Face-to-face training classes should be supported with periodic security reminders, which could take many formats, including:

- Screen savers
- Periodic e-mails
- Articles or statements in an employee newsletter
- Notices posted in public areas

HIPAA requires that documentation of the training, including the following, must be retained for six years:

- Sign-in sheets
- Handouts
- E-mail messages
- Training database identifying training and actions taken (Hjort 2003)

Training should be ongoing and provided whenever there are changes to policies and procedures or to areas related to security.

Managing a Security Incident

No matter how hard a CE strives to eliminate security incidents, they will still occur. The Security Rule defines a **security incident** as "the attempted or successful unauthorized access, use, disclosure, modification, or destruction of information or interference with system operations in an information system" (45 CFR 160, 162, and 164 2013). Because this definition is broad, the CE should define a security incident for itself. The security incidents should include both information technology incidents and physical security incidents. Examples of security incidents include: theft of password, virus or other malware, theft of media, and failure to delete account of former employee (Compliancy Group 2020).

ARRA requires CEs to actively identify and report security incidents. The security incident policies and procedures should identify how the incidents will be identified and to whom they should be reported. Employees have the responsibility to report security incidents as the incidents can result in fines, damage to the CE's reputation in the community, as well as lost revenue (MediaPRO 2019). Policies and procedures informed by the severity of the security incident should define how the CE will respond. If the incident suggests criminal activity or compromises the safety of an individual, the local law enforcement agency should be contacted.

Forensics is "used or applied in the investigation and establishment of facts or evidence in a court of law" (Vocabulary nd) is the process that should be used to gather evidence of the security incident. The steps in forensics investigation include:

- Policy and procedure development (including strict guidelines)
- Evidence assessment (determining what should be looked for)
- Evidence acquisition (how evidence will be captured)
- Evidence examination (analyzing data obtained)
- Documenting and reporting (documenting all activities performed) (Norwich University Online 2017)

The investigation may require hardware to be confiscated and stored in a secured location, network logs to be printed, data to be backed up, and other investigative steps. Failure to protect data may result in the intentional or unintentional destruction of evidence. "Spoliation is the destruction or alteration of a document that destroys its value as evidence in a legal proceeding" (US Legal 2019). During the course of the investigation, a number of steps may be taken such as:

- Recovering deleted files
- Recovering passwords
- Analyzing file access, creation, and modification times
- Analyzing system and application logs
- Determining user and application activity on a system (Derhak 2003)

Once a security incident (defined later in this chapter) is identified, the CE must mitigate its harmful effects and document both the incident and the outcome. **Mitigation** is the process of attempting to reduce or eliminate harmful effects of the breach (45 CFR 160, 162, and 164 2013). Harmful effects of a breach varies widely and can include public embarrassment, inability to obtain insurance, identity theft, loss of child custody, and much more. Even though it may not be possible to completely mitigate the effects, the CE must do everything possible to protect patients. The mitigation steps taken vary based on the situation. For example, if a patient's social security number is inappropriately disclosed, the CE may pay for the patient to monitor his or her credit report for a specified period of time.

Security events are anything security related that can impact the CE (Spacey 2016). The security event does not have to result in a breach of ePHI. Security events include noncompliance with security policies, errors made by employees, leaving computer without logging out, writing down passwords, and so forth.

Security events do not lead to harm however; steps should be taken to prevent the event from occurring again as harm could result in the future. Employees who are involved in a security event may need individual counselling or additional training.

The CSO should monitor trends in the types of security incidents and security events that occur. The identification of patterns from this trending yields valuable information regarding threats and vulnerabilities of the CE. Identifying the threats and vulnerabilities helps the CE determine where the problems are and what changes in security practices are needed. Security incidents may result in penalties, as discussed later in this chapter.

Ongoing Security Procedure Evaluation

Implementation of the security safeguards is not enough to comply with HIPAA security regulations. CEs must also critique its security program through ongoing monitoring and evaluation to identify areas for improvement. The evaluation must include both technical and nontechnical processes. Technical processes are those that use technology, such as encryption, access controls, firewalls, audit trails, and other technical tools. Nontechnical processes are the security measures that do not require technology, including policies and procedures, training, evaluations, monitoring, and other administrative responsibilities. The evaluation should address whether or not the CE is meeting the HIPAA security regulations and whether or not the program is still appropriate for the current status of the CE. CEs change over time because of growth (services, employees, and so forth), changes in policies, changes in technologies used, and changes in laws and regulations. The security program must keep up with these changes to ensure that the program is still meeting all HIPAA security regulations.

Contingency and Business Continuity Planning

When information systems are down, CEs must have a plan in place to continue business despite being unavailable to retrieve information, place orders, or perform other key tasks. This plan is called a business continuity plan (BCP). The BCP is a program that incorporates policies and procedures for continuing business operations during an information system shutdown. This shut down could be for upgrade of software, upgrade of hardware, hardware failure, and other reasons. The BCP should include when the plan should be implemented, who initiates the plan, which manual processes are to be used, what forms are needed, how to update the database once the system is again operational, and more.

A **contingency plan** is made up of policies and procedures that identify how a CE will react in the event of an information system emergency, such as power failure, natural disaster, a hacker, malware, or an information system failure. HIPAA calls this an emergency mode operation plan. A CE can take steps to reduce the risk of the EHR or other critical patient care information systems from being down or failing, but it cannot eliminate the possibility. Therefore, it is important to back up data so that if the information system fails, the data can be recreated from the backups. The CE must also update the information systems with data created during the downtime. The contingency plan should include a data-backup plan. The backup plan should address frequency of backups, where the backed-up data are stored, testing the backups, and more. The data-backup plan should include all critical sources of information, such as the EHR and clinical information systems. CEs may have a back-up data on site and a copy at a remote site that would not be impacted by the same natural disaster or other failure.

The contingency plan (emergency mode operation plan) must include manual processes to be implemented during the downtime. Examples of these manual processes include paper laboratory slips, microfilm of the master patient index, and health record forms, and much more. The forms, microfilm, and so forth must be immediately available in the event that the information system is down. The contingency plan must be tested periodically and revised as areas needing improvement are identified. Not all information systems are equivalent. Some information systems, like the EHR, cause turmoil in a healthcare organization if they are offline. Other information systems, such as a strategic decision-support system, have less impact on the healthcare organization because there is no direct impact on patient care. Each information system should be evaluated to determine how critical it is, and a plan of action should be implemented. The plan should also include a prioritized list of applications and data used to determine which information system should be addressed first if multiple information systems are down simultaneously. In a healthcare CE, the EHR and other patient care information systems would be the top priority, with nonpatient, nonfinancial systems, such as patient satisfaction and chart deficiencies, at the bottom. The priorities would be different for healthcare clearinghouses and health plans.

To help prevent failures due to hardware failure, redundancy is needed. **Redundancy** is duplication of data, hardware, cables, or other hardware components of the information system. As data are entered, it is also saved onto a second computer server, creating a way to access an operational information system with little to no downtime. It can also be used for networks, computers, and other hardware. For example, a large urban hospital may have multiple network cables that connect buildings by using cables that are buried under the street. If one cable fails, another cable takes its place in transmitting data.

Data Recovery

When the information systems are again functional, data recovery must occur. **Data recovery** is the process of recouping any data that has been lost from the information system crash as well as the data that was obtained during the downtime. Data backups may be used to bring the information system back to its original state. Data captured during downtime must be entered into the information system to bring it up to date. Lost data should be recoverable from backup servers or other storage media. Depending on the time since the last backup, little or no data may be lost. The CE must have current backups of the database to be able to re-create the data. Information systems should have a utility to restore data from the backup server or other storage media onto the database. This process should be tested periodically to ensure that the utility is working appropriately.

The CE may want to consider establishing a hot site. A hot site is a remote location that is set-up with an exact duplicate of the information systems and data. With a hot site, a healthcare organization can switch from its local information systems to the hot site automatically preventing downtime and data loss (Dooling et al. 2016, 9).

CHECK YOUR UNDERSTANDING 12.2

1. Identify a security incident.

   a. Monitor is turned toward the public.
   b. Computer is not logged out but it is located in a private office.
   c. Employee wrote down their password.
   d. Hacker attempted, but did not succeed, in accessing e-PHI

2. The process of developing policies used in determining what employees have access to is

   a. Information access management
   b. Workforce clearinghouse
   c. Termination process
   d. Business associate

3. The CE needs to determine the facts behind a security issue before going to court. This is known as:

   a. Workforce clearance procedure
   b. Forensics
   c. Spoliation
   d. Mitigation

4. Ensuring that data are not altered either during transmission across a network or during storage is _____.

   a. Integrity
   b. Accessibility
   c. Confidentiality
   d. Privacy

5. The CE is in the process of identifying possible security threats. This process is known as _____.

   a. Integrity
   b. Emergency mode operation
   c. Risk analysis
   d. Redundancy

Business Associate Contracts or Other Arrangements

Business associates (BA) are organizations that conduct business on behalf of the CE. Examples of BAs are contract coders, application service providers, transcription services, and billing services. These associates require access to PHI (45 CFR 160, 162, and 164 2013) in order to do their jobs. Therefore, BAs are subject to the HIPAA Security Rule. In order for the business associates to gain access to the ePHI, they must assure the CE that they will protect the ePHI and will notify the CE of any failures to do so that result in a breach. There must be a business associate agreement (BAA) between the CE and the BA that meets the requirements established in HIPAA. BAs are liable for noncompliance with the HIPAA privacy and security rules just as if they are a CE.

The BAA spells out the BA's responsibilities and how it should protect PHI. The BAA should also allow the CE to terminate the contract if the BA fails to meet the responsibilities in the BAA. The BAA must address certain required elements. Some of these required elements are found in Table 12.3.

Contract - Not valid if not signed [handwritten]

Table 12.3. Required elements of business associate agreement

Required Elements of Business Associate Agreement
Explains the permitted or required uses of PHI by the business associate.
Business associate is prohibited from using or disclosing PHI except as permitted.
Business associate is required to utilize safeguards to protect PHI.
Business associate is required to take appropriate actions to resolve breaches and violations.
The BAA can be terminated if the business associate does not protect the PHI.

Source: Adapted from HHS 2019.

Technical Safeguards

Technical safeguards are defined by the security rule as "the technology and the policy and procedures for its use that protect electronic protected health information and control access to it" (45 CFR 160, 162, and 164 2013). Technical safeguards use technology, policies, and procedures to protect ePHI from unauthorized access, destruction, or alteration. The policies, procedures, and documentation standards set by the CE define the requirements for the documentation required to show compliance with the technical safeguards. In this section access control systems and authentication, audit controls, and integrity are covered.

Access Control Systems and Authentication

Access controls are a computer software program designed to prevent unauthorized use of an information resource. CEs must define in their policies and procedures who can view, create, and modify data in an information system containing ePHI and use access controls to grant or limit those rights to employees who need them.

Types of Authentication

In **role-based authentication**, the functions and data available to the user are based on the role of the user. For example, a coder in the HIM department needs to review ePHI to properly code the health record; however, the coder would not need to add clinical information to the health record, and access controls would restrict the user from doing so. In role-based authentication, all coders have the same access, and all nurses have the same access. The nurses' functions and data will be different from those of the coders but will be the same for nurses in emergency department, medical-surgery nursing units, labor and delivery units and other departments. Appropriate rights are granted based on an employee's role in the organization. As the coder's (or other employee's) role in the CE changes, there must be a process in place to amend his or her rights. In this methodology, the user may have access to data and functionality that is not needed as the role of the users may vary slightly.

In **user-based authentication**, the functions and data available are based on the needs of the individual user, not all users with the same job title. For example, some HIM technicians may have the authority to combine duplicate health record numbers, but others would not have access to this function because there is not a need. This method is more specific to the user's needs than role-based authentication as the user gains the data and functionality that they need but no more. Evaluating each user individual is very time consuming.

Context-based authentication is an access control system that limits users to accessing information not only in accordance with their identity and role, but to the location and time in which they are accessing the information . This is helpful when there are employees, such as nurses, who work in various units or have different roles at different times. For example, a nurse who works full-time in the quality improvement department may work at a nursing unit to earn some extra money for Christmas. As the ePHI and functions needed to perform these roles differ, the access that she has depends on her role at the time.

There may be times when users need to have access to data they are not normally allowed. This is called **emergency access procedure**, or "break the glass." This access usually occurs during a medical emergency and may require a second password or a reason for access. Even in an emergency situation, there must be a way to identify who activated the emergency access and why. The emergency access control system should require a brief note from the user "breaking the glass" to justify why the data were needed. For example, "the patient 'crashed' while his nurse was at lunch." The use of the emergency access procedure must be audited to ensure that the emergency access procedures are only used when appropriate (Primeau 2017).

User Authentication Methods

Each user must have unique user identification that tracks that user's actions, although the specific identification technology is not mandated by HIPAA. Some CEs assign a **username**, a type of assigned user identification that may be based on the individual's name and is unique to that individual. For example, a username for Jane Doe could be jdoe or jane.doe. Many organizations utilize the same format for all users. If there are two users with the same name, the organization may add a 2, an additional or other means of distinguishing between the two users. For example, if two individuals are named jane.doe, then the second user may have an user name of jane.doe2. Other organizations assign a number or other identification information to each user. Social security numbers should never be used for user identification because of concerns about identity theft.

Methods of access control—commonly categorized as something you know, something you have, or something you are—can be used alone or in combination. See Table 12.4 for the differences in these methods of access controls. **One-factor authentication** utilizes one level of access control such as a username and password. There may be two requirements but they are both something you know. A one-factor authentication method could be something you have such as a token (described later in this section) as long as it is not used with another method (something you know or something you are). **Two-factor authentication** combines two different categories of access control, such as something you know and something you have. Common methods of access control—passwords, tokens and biometrics —are discussed in the following sections.

Table 12.4. Methods of access controls

Method	Explanation	Examples
Something you know	The user gains access to an information system based on something that they know.	User name Password Security questions
Something you have	This method gives users access to an information based on something that is in his or her possession.	Card key Token
Something you are	This method utilizes biometrics to uniquely identify the user.	Retinal scan Fingerprint scan Facial recognition Voice recognition

Source: ©AHIMA.

Passwords are a series of characters that must be entered to authenticate user identity; they are commonly used in conjunction with a username or identifier. Passwords, something you know, are an example of one-factor authentication.

Strong passwords should not be easily guessed. Passwords based on commonly known personal information, such as the user's name, child's name, dog's name, or favorite sports team are examples of passwords that may be easy to crack. Information systems vary in their password requirements. Some require the password to have a minimum number of characters such as seven or eight characters. The information systems frequently require two or more types of characters such as uppercase letters, lowercase letters, numbers, and symbols such as Gsge$26Y. Ideally, passwords should not contain a common word and should not be reused. Many information systems force the user to change the password periodically, such as every 30 days or once a year. The CE should establish strict rules for the use of passwords, including the format of the password, the frequency of change, and privacy of the password.

Policies should state that the password is confidential and cannot be shared with anyone else. Some users might write passwords down near the computer so they do not have to remember them. Users might also share their password with other users. For example, if a user forgot her password, she might ask another user to share his password, perhaps even out loud so that it is audible to others in the department and passers-by. Because audit trails, discussed in the next section, record not only what was done but also who did it, the user is responsible for every action under his or her username. This means that if an employee allows another user to user his or her access, then that user is responsible for anything that the other user does. Employees who violate policies related to passwords should be disciplined according to the policies of the CE.

One problem with passwords is that users often have too many of them to remember. Information systems throughout a CE frequently require different passwords, thus making it almost impossible for users to remember all of them. One way to overcome this issue is the use of single sign-on systems, which are designed so the user logs in one time. The user is then able to move from one application to another without entering another password. However, this single sign-on makes it even more important to protect the password so that the information system is not at risk of unauthorized access.

Completely Automated Public Turning Test to tell Computers and Humans Apart (CAPTCHA) may be used in conjunction with user names and passwords to help prevent computerized attempts to break into an information system. There are several methods of CAPTCHA. For example, there may be a series of images and the user has to identify the images with a traffic light, a store front, crosswalk, or something else. It may also ask the user to click a checkbox to indicate that the user is human. Another method is to type the word that is displayed in wavy fonts. The user has to not only use the correct user name and password but meet the CAPTCHA requirements in order to access the information.

A token used for security is usually a physical device that an authorized user of computer services is given to aid in authentication. **Tokens** may be used in conjunction with a password to provide **two-factor authentication** because a token and a password are two different types of authentications—something you know and something you have. Tokens used by themselves would be a one-factor authentication. Tokens are about the size of a credit card and contain a magnetic strip or chip that identifies the user. An algorithm displays a sequence of numbers in a liquid-crystal display (LCD) window. The characters in the LCD window change at specified intervals, for example, every minute. The user must enter the code on the token in order to access the information system. The problem with the use of tokens is that the token may be lost, which will result in the user being unable to access the information system and potential unauthorized access.

Biometric identifiers are based on a physical characteristic and are used to access the secure areas such as the data center or an information system. They are categorized as something you have. Retinal scans, fingerprints, facial recognition, and voice prints are biometric identifiers. National Institute of Standards and Technology (NIST)(2020) recommends that biometric identifiers should be used in conjunction as part of multi-factor authentication. For example, latex gloves may alter an individual's fingerprint enough to make it unrecognizable, preventing access to the information system.

One of the requirements in the HIPAA Security Rule's technical safeguards is the automatic log-off, which automatically logs the user off when a workstation is inactive for a specified period of time, such as five minutes. The amount of time should be a balance between the need for privacy and security and the need to give the user time to review the data. This automatic log-off helps prevent unauthorized users from accessing ePHI when an authorized user walks away from the computer without logging out of the information system. Prior to this log-off, a screen saver that blanks out the screen after a brief period of inactivity should be activated so that passing individuals would not see e-PHI.

Audit Controls

The CE must monitor the security program once it is implemented. One monitoring component required by HIPAA is implementing **audit controls,** the mechanisms that record and examine activity in information systems. Audit controls serve four purposes:

- Hold individual users personally responsible for their actions
- Use an investigation tool to identify cause of problem, the extent of the problem, and the way to restore the system back to normal operations
- Use real-time monitoring to identify breaches, technical problems, and other security issues quickly
- Watch for intrusions into the system so that the intrusion can be stopped before a breach occurs (Amatayakul 2004)

Audit trails are the record of these system activities, such as log-in, log-out, unsuccessful log-ins, print, query, and other actions. It also records user-identification information and the date and time of the activity. System-level controls monitor log-on and log-off activity and applications accessed by the user. Application-level controls track what information systems were used, what the user saw, and what he or she did. User-level controls record what actions the user initiated, such as resources accessed (Amatayakul 2004). Review of the audit trail can identify potential security incidents. For example, the audit trail may show that User A accessed a celebrity's health record when there was not a "need to know".

Audit trails are being subpoenaed to court as part of e-Discovery. e-Discovery is the revisions to the Federal Rules of Civil Procedure and Uniform Rules Relating to Discovery of Electronically Stored Information; wherein audit trails, the source code of the program, metadata, and any other electronic information that is not typically considered the legal health record is subject to motion for compulsory discovery. The court uses audit trails to prove or disprove access, alterations, review, documentation or other use of the information system.

Audits should be scheduled periodically but can also be performed when a problem is suspected, such as when a patient complains that his or her PHI has been released or in response to a newspaper article or other suspected incidents. For more on auditing, refer to chapter 13.

The security audit process should include **triggers** that identify the need for a closer inspection. A trigger is a flag that notifies the CE of a possible security issue that needs investigation. These trigger events cannot be used as the sole basis of the review, but they can significantly reduce the amount of reviews performed. Examples of triggers include user has same name as the patient and the patient is a well-known individual (celebrity, professional athlete, politician).

Just because a trigger is activated does not mean that there has been a breach. For instance, with common surnames, such as Smith and Jones, it would be easy for an employee named Smith to care for a patient named Smith who was not related; however, it should be investigated. The patient may or may not be related to the employee—after all, there are many Smiths, and the practice will not catch all relatives, but it is a way to identify something that should be investigated.

The security rule does not mandate a specific number of audits, but the CE should base the volume on the size and complexity of the CE, so the larger the CE, the more auditing would be performed. The findings of these audits should be reported all the way up the organizational chart to the board of directors. HIPAA requires that documentation of the audit activities be retained for six years.

Audit trails are not without their problems. Audit trails must be protected from alteration and deletion. One way to do this is to limit access to the audit log to only those who require access.

Audit-reduction tools are used to review the audit trail and compare it to facility-specific criteria and eliminate routine entries such as the periodic backups. This means that backups and other routine maintenance would be removed from the reports from which audits are conducted. The audit-reduction tools can also look for trends and behavior outside the norm. For example, if a nurse works only on the weekend and suddenly logs in on Tuesday, this would be cause for review. There may be a legitimate reason, such as the nurse changed shifts with another nurse, but the nurse could also have been snooping in a neighbor's ePHI. Another example is that a coder may be working late because he or she is taking a college class during the day. Finally, there are attack signature-detection tools that look for a specific sequence of events that may indicate a security problem, such as multiple failed attempts to log in to the information system or an employee who normally accesses the information from within the CE is accessing e-PHI remotely.

A review of the audit trail is not the only auditing that should be performed. Another means of auditing is touring the CE to ensure that security policies and procedures are being followed. This would be done by the CSO or a designee. Examples of actions that can be monitored in this way include ensuring that monitors are turned away from public areas, users log out of the information system when stepping away from the computer, fax machines with PHI are not in public areas, and no signs of passwords being written down or shared. More on auditing in chapter 13.

Integrity

Technology has advanced to a point at which an unauthorized user can capture data in transit and alter it. Therefore, CEs must confirm the integrity of data passed across a network. **Integrity** is the security principle that protects data from inappropriate modification or corruption. This includes both unintentional and intentional modifications and destructions. Unintentional modifications and destruction could occur if the wrong data are destroyed, the wrong backup is used to restore data, or an electrical fire destroys the computer. Examples of intentional modification and destruction include intentional deletion of data, induction of virus software, and changing the amount that the employee owes the healthcare organization for treatment provided. **Data integrity** is preserved when the message received is confirmed as identical to the one sent. Integrity can be validated with checksum validation, defined as a "sum derived from the bits of a segment of computer data that is calculated before and after transmission or storage to assure that the data is free from errors or tampering" (Merriam-Webster 2020a).

Transmission security involves mechanisms designed to protect ePHI while the data are being transmitted between two points. These points can be internal or external to the CE. Encryption is frequently used to protect data as it moves across networks by preventing ePHI from being read by anyone with access to data during transmission. **Encryption** converts data from a readable form to unintelligible text. This is done with the science of cryptography, using mathematics to convert data into unintelligible data and back again. If encrypted data are intercepted during transmission, the health information is protected because the individual who intercepted the data cannot view it. Only authorized users are able to convert the data back into a readable format.

There are two categories of encryption: symmetric and asymmetric. Symmetric encryption uses a secret key to data. The computer sending the data uses the key to turn the message into the unintelligible format. The receiving computer uses the same key to revert the data back into its original format. In asymmetric encryption, an extremely popular method also known as public key infrastructure, two keys are used. The sending computer uses a private key to convert the data. The public key is provided, in the form of a signed certificate by a recipient-trusted certificate authority. to the computer with whom the sender is communicating. This public key converts the data into a readable format. A licensing agency called a certificate authority confirms the receiver's identity and relationship to the public key. In doing this, the certification authority issues a digital certificate to the receiver. This digital certificate is part of the integrity process because it ensures that plaintext messages are received without any alterations. Other components of public key infrastructure are It encompasses the policies, hardware, and software needed for the creation, revocation, management, distribution, and use of digital certificates and public key cryptography.

This encryption and decryption occurs instantaneously in the background. A public key infrastructure familiar to most people is the transport layer security (TLS), which is used to transmit protected information when conducting business transactions over the Internet. It prevents eavesdropping and tampering with the data being transferred (IETF 2018). In public key encryption, the public key allows the holder of the certificate to verify the message.

CEs rely heavily on networks to share information. These networks frequently allow users across the CE's campus and beyond to access ePHI. HIPAA mandates the use of network security methods to protect the ePHI as it travels across the network. **Network security** uses technology to protect the data transmitted across the network including firewalls and encryption. The CE should regularly perform penetration testing. Penetration testing is performed by a cyber security professional. This individual attempts to locate and take advantage of vulnerabilities in the CE's information system. The intent is to find and resolve the vulnerabilities before they can be used by a hacker (Cloudflare 2020).

A **firewall** is a computer system or a combination of systems that provide a security barrier or support an access control policy between two networks or between a network and any other traffic outside the network. This gatekeeper is physically located between the routes of a public network like the Internet and those of a private network. All data entering and leaving the CE must pass through the firewall. The firewall evaluates each packet of data to determine whether or not to let it through. This process is known as packet filtering. There are other types of firewalls too. The rules that determine what is let in and what is not are established by the healthcare organization. The data must meet those requirements or it is automatically blocked. For example, there may be a limit in the size of the file being transmitted. If the data passes the evaluation, the data are allowed in or out of the network. The firewall can be implemented in many ways. It can attach confidentiality messages to all e-mails that leave the CE, limit the size or type of file entering the CE's network, and can limit access to specific websites. The firewall may even scan the data to determine if a virus is attached to prevent a virus from being brought into the CE and spreading.

Another way to protect data as it is transmitting is a virtual private network (VPN). A VPN creates an encrypted tunnel through the Internet that allows data to be shared securely. It allows ePHI to be shared over a public network like the Internet and still be protected.

Intrusion detection systems (IDS) monitor networks and information systems to catch hackers and other intruders along with other security issues. The IDS notifies the information technology staff of the issue (Dill et al. 2016). The intrusion detection system assists the information system staff in monitoring the traffic on the Internet to ensure that it is legitimate and does not contain anything that will harm the ePHI or other data stored in the databases such as malware (addressed later in this chapter). Once a potential threat is identified, then the appropriate steps must be taken to not only protect the data but also keep a similar threat from happening again.

Intrusion prevention systems (IPS) monitor networks to identify possible malware threats. When identified, the IPS notifies the network administration and takes steps to stop the threat. This can take the form of shutting down access and altering firewall settings. The difference between an IDS and an IPS is how they handle an incident. The IDS simply notify the network administrator whereas the IPS will take steps to protect the network (Forcepoint 2020).

Data loss prevention (DLP) is a set of tools used to protect data. When a breach of policy is identified, the software notifies the organization and takes actions to prevent the unauthorized sharing of data. DLP is able to protect data at rest, data in motion as well as data in use. It also provides reports that can be used as part of the auditing and compliance required by HIPAA. These reports also identify the weaknesses in the organization's data security (Zhang 2020).

CHECK YOUR UNDERSTANDING 12.3

1. An audit-reduction tool will remove _____.
   a. invalid data
   b. routine maintenance events
   c. user's access
   d. outdated data

2. Converting data into unintelligible text is known as _____.
   a. Firewall
   b. Encryption
   c. Mitigation
   d. Intrusion detection system

3. Identify the type of authentication used when all coders have the same access to ePHI and functionality.
   a. User-based
   b. Role-based
   c. Context-based
   d. Both user-based and role-based

4. The access control used in the EHR requires a password and biometrics. This is an example of _____.

CHECK YOUR UNDERSTANDING 12.3 (*Continued*)

    a. Single-factor authentication
    b. Biometrics
    c. Two-factor authentication
    d. Tokens

5. Our information system just notified us that Mary Burchfield has just looked up another patient with the same last name. This notification is called a(n) _____.

    a. Trigger
    b. Audit reduction tool
    c. Integrity
    d. Audit control

Malicious Software

Malicious software, also known as malware, is designed to harm a computer. Some malware is more of a nuisance, whereas others destroy data or other files that may prevent the computer from operating or can steal data. HIPAA mandates that CEs take steps to protect data and information systems from malware. If malware is introduced into computers in the HIM department, it spreads and can ultimately mean that most, if not all, of the computers in the department are affected. If the computers are unusable, then most of the work in the department would be at a standstill. In this event, the contingency plan discussed earlier would be implemented. HIM professionals can help protect their computers by being cautious when opening attachments to e-mails or when using links within e-mails, by going to a company's website and logging in rather than using links in e-mail, and by otherwise being careful in what e-mails are opened, what software is downloaded, webpages that are visited, and so forth. Malware can also harm medical devices. **A medical device,** is "an article, instrument, apparatus or machine that is used in the prevention, diagnosis or treatment of illness or disease, or for detecting, measuring, restoring, correcting or modifying the structure or function of the body for some health purpose" (WHO 2020). Examples of medical devices are pacemakers and fetal monitoring systems. Medical devices often transport medical information via the internet. They pose a significant security risk as they typically do not have anti-virus software, encryption and have outdated operating software (Blacketer 2019). One of the benefits of telehealth is the ability of medical devices to report results to the healthcare provider via the internet. However, this technology also enables device vulnerabilities to be exploited by hackers. Medical devices are discussed in chapter 10.

Anti-malware and other software packages are designed to identify and stop or clean up malicious software, which includes viruses, worms, Trojans, bots, spyware, phishing, and ransomware.

Virus

A **virus** "propagates by inserting a copy of itself into and becoming part of another program. It spreads from one computer to another" (Cisco n.d.). The term "virus" is commonly used to indicate malware, but it is technically a specific type of malware. Viruses are designed to do a variety of destructive behaviors. For example, viruses can destroy data or damage the software that starts the computer. Viruses are frequently spread through e-mail through an attachment that is activated when opened. They can spread through the e-mail server and even the user's contact list in e-mail.

Worms

A **worm** is "standalone software and does not require a host program or human help to propagate" (Cisco n.d.). The worm is programmed to install itself onto a computer attached to a computer network and then moves to all computers on the network. It may harm the system or initiate a denial of service (DDoS). A distributed denial of service attack occurs when so much activity is sent to the website from multiple sources that the website crashes. The worm frequently spreads through e-mail attachments as well as files downloaded from the internet. The worm spreads to the e-mail server and then to all of the users listed in the contact list in e-mail.

Trojans

A **Trojan** is a type of malware that gives the appearance that it is perfectly legitimate software. This tricks the user into accessing it. Once accessed, the Trojan can perform a variety of actions, including pop-ups, deleting data, creating back doors, or other actions (Cisco n.d.). A back door is a way into the information system without going through the normal log-in process.

Bots

Bots perform automated tasks, such as gathering information and instant messaging, thus relieving a person the responsibility of doing it. These actions can be good or bad, depending on who initiates the bots and for what purposes (Cisco n.d.). Robotic process automation (RPA) bots perform tasks much quick and efficiently than humans. An example of a RPA bot is to automatically fill in forms (NICE nd). A malicious bot can be used to locate and access information stored on the computer such as passwords, usernames, credit card numbers, and other information. It can also be used to record keystrokes, send spam and participate in botnet attacks (computers controlled by malicious software without user's knowledge). The bot can be introduced into the computer by e-mail or social media. The computer can be protected from bots in many ways including the use of firewalls, keeping software up to date, and using anti-malware software (Norton n.d.a.).

Spyware

Spyware may be used to track keystrokes and passwords, monitor websites visited, or other actions and report these actions to the designated person or organization. Spyware is often classified as system monitors, adware, or tracking cookies. Computers are frequently infected with spyware through e-mail and downloaded files. The spyware may slow down the information system because of its increased activity. It contributes to identity theft and other breaches of privacy by sharing information. Essentially, spyware records computer usage without the user's knowledge and then provides this information to someone with whom the user may not want to share the information. Antimalware software would find and delete the spyware.

Ransomware

Ransomware is a type of malicious software that prohibits access to information systems in an organization. The ransomware programmer may demand money before they will deactivate the ransomware. Unfortunately, this type of malware is being used with more frequency. Use of ransomware rose by 350 percent in the fourth quarter of 2019 as compared to fourth quarter of 2018 (Corvus 2020). There are two main types of ransomware – locker and crypto. Locker ransomware shuts down or locks the hardware such as a computer or tablet. For example, it may prevent access or encrypt files. Crypto ransomware prevents access to the data itself (Rubens 2017).

This can have a major impact on a healthcare provider if it is unable to access the information needed in order to care for its patients. For example, DCH Health System was hit by ransomware. The CE decided to pay the required ransom to regain access to their information system. During the time that the information system was locked, the hospitals in the DCH Health System turned patients away and cancelled surgery (Srinivas 2019). Other ways of protecting a healthcare organization's computers from ransomware include:

- Back up computer
- Keep computer software current
- Be careful when opening email attachments
- Use technical tools such as antivirus software and firewalls.
- Ensure website addresses are correct (Department of Homeland Security 2019)

Social Engineering

Social engineering is the process of tricking someone into revealing information or doing something that will enable others to take advantage of them (Norton n.d.b.). There are six types of social engineering that users need to be aware of: baiting, phishing, email hacking, pretexting, quid pro quo, and vishing.

Baiting

Baiting works much like using a lure to catch a fish. The offender dangles something in front of the potential victim hoping that he or she will take the bait. Baiting takes many forms including downloading music or video; a price that is too good to be true, or something else (Webroot nd). It can also be leaving a thumbdrive in a public location hoping someone will access it and then be infected with sometime of malware (Norton n.d.b.).

Phishing

Phishing is "a scam by which an e-mail user is duped into revealing personal or confidential information which the scammer can use illicitly" (Merriam-Webster 2020b). The e-mail received may look official, but it is not. Its intent is to capture usernames, passwords, account numbers, and any other personal information. Users should be cautious in giving out confidential information such as passwords, credit card numbers, and social security numbers as many requests for this information received via e-mail is a phishing scam. Phishing can also install other malware such as ransomware.

Email Hacking and Contacts

With email hacking, the hacker takes over a user's email account. From there, the hacker is able to use the email address and contacts to trick others. The people in the contacts would trust the email as they know the sender or so they are tricked into believing. The hacker is then able to spread malware or trick the user in other ways (Norton ndb).

Pretexting

Pretexting is a type of social engineering that attempts to capture the user's attention so that they can be drawn in. The criminal then requests information from the recipient in order for the recipient to gain an inheritance, claim lottery winnings, or something else (Norton ndb).

Quid pro quo

Quid pro quo is a type of social engineering that proposes an exchange of some service with the victim being duped out of something. On the surface, it is a fair exchange but the victim always comes away losing in the exchange (Norton ndb). For example, someone may call claiming that they will pay the victim $100 for providing access to an information as part of a research study.

Vishing

Vishing is phishing that is verbally performed. The villain would use the phone to scam the individual out of personal information such as their social security number, bank account information, password, and more (Norton ndb).

Physical Safeguards

Physical safeguards are an important part of security. The Security Rule defines **physical safeguards** as "physical measures, policies, and procedures to protect a CE's electronic information systems, and related buildings and equipment, from natural and environmental hazards and unauthorized intrusion" (45 CFR 160, 162, and 164 2013).

Physical safeguards protect the hardware and software related to the ePHI. The physical plant and equipment must be protected from intentional and unintentional tampering or destruction.

The hardware must be protected from natural disasters such as tornadoes and floods. It must also be protected from fire, theft, and intentional tampering. The policies and procedures should also document how the CE is protecting the equipment from unauthorized access, tampering, and theft. Physical safeguards should include not only the computers and other hardware but also backup tapes. The required physical safeguards and their implementation specifications are listed in table 12.5.

Table 12.5. Implementation specifications for HIPAA physical standards

Standards	Implementation Specifications
Facility access controls	• Contingency operations • Facility security plan • Access control and validation procedures • Maintenance records
Workstation use	• None
Workstation security	• None
Device and media controls	• Disposal • Media re-use • Accountability • Data backup and storage

Source: Adapted from 45 CFR 160, 162, and 164 2013.

Facility Access Controls

The CE must implement **facility access controls**, which limit physical access to the data center and software to only authorized information system staff. Facility access controls must be documented in the policies and procedures. Access to the data center can be controlled by card keys, access codes, or other control methods. The fact that an individual is a member of the CE's workforce does not automatically authorize him or her to be in the data center. Access to the data center should be limited to individuals with a business need, such computer technicians and employees who work in the data center. There must also be policies and procedures regarding the handling of contractors and service technicians. In the event of a system outage, the appropriate staff and contractors must be able to access the information system so that the information system can be operational as quickly as possible. Individuals with authorized access should wear a picture identification tag at all times. Visitors to the area, such as computer vendors, consultants, and computer technicians, frequently are required to sign in and be escorted while in the data center.

Cameras may be used to record individuals going into the data center and other areas where hardware is located. The video can be used to determine who had access to the data center or other critical areas in the event of a security incident.

Some of the physical safeguards are as simple as locking doors, using an alarm system, bolting the equipment to a desk, and using surge suppressors. Other safeguards include monitoring the temperature of the room so that the computers do not become too hot or too cold because extreme temperatures can damage the computers. There should also be a system in place to extinguish fires.

These physical safeguards will need to be maintained and updated as appropriate to ensure that they continue to protect the ePHI. Examples of this maintenance include installing new security cameras, changing locks, or knocking down walls to expand the size of the data center. The CE must maintain documentation of the preventive maintenance and repairs made. This documentation can be as simple as a logbook or as complicated as a specialized database, depending on the size and complexity of the CE.

Workstation Use and Security

Workstations include not only desktop computers but also handheld devices, laptops, and other pieces of equipment that manage ePHI. Workstations must be protected from unauthorized access, physical access and tampering. This can be accomplished in a number of ways, such as placing the workstations behind closed doors or other types of barriers. Black-out screens can be used to prevent unauthorized users from seeing the content on the screen when walking by the computer or looking at it over the shoulder of the user. Policies and procedures should be in place to protect the workstations from theft and other threats. Workstations—including computers, tablets, and laptops that access ePHI—should be used appropriately by the workforce members. It is up to the CE to define what is appropriate.

It is easy for thieves to pick up computers or other pieces of hardware and walk off with them. Someone might also insert flash drive to download malware or steal data. To protect hardware, security measures can include bolting hardware to desks and locking doors. Security of mobile devices is discussed later in this chapter.

Device and Media Controls

Media, which includes computer hard drives and removable digital storage, must also be protected from loss and destruction. Examples of removable digital storage are external hard drives, thumb drives, CDs, and optical disks. Media that store ePHI must have policies and procedures that control its movement and storage. Because media is small and easily portable, it is easy for employees to move the media and for it to get lost. It is also easily stolen. The CE could create a log to track receipt or removal of the media so that an individual is responsible for the media.

With the advent of portable devices such as tablets and mobile phones, tracking media is becoming more and more difficult because the devices are moved around for use in patient care. The actions, and not the location, of the workstation matter, so the policies should apply to computers at employee's workstations and other locations. It is easy to lose CDs and other media that store ePHI, so CEs must have a policy in place to protect them from loss or destruction. The media must be tracked throughout the CE. This can be done by creating a log that requires staff to check out the media, much like checking a book out of the library or tracking a health record.

Once the media is no longer needed, there should be a formal process for its disposal. Workstations and other media cannot just be thrown away or sold. If ePHI is disposed of improperly, these computers could be found at garage sales and thrift shops still containing this confidential information. Deletion of the ePHI stored on the media does not render it inaccessible; there are utilities, or software programs, that can undelete files. Because of this capability, the media itself needs to be destroyed, or the media should be degaussed. **Degaussing** is application of a magnetic field to the media to render the data on it useless. Degaussing renders data impossible to recover and is not reversible. Unfortunately, this does not work on Solid State Drives. Another method for sanitizing the traditional hard drive of a computer is overwriting (writing data over the existing data) the data stored on the hard drive. The data may have to be overwritten multiple times in order to prevent recovery. CDs, USB drives, and other media may also be pulverized.

There may be times that the CE wishes to reuse media on which ePHI is stored. For example, workstations frequently may be moved from one location to another to make way for more powerful workstations. The security rule allows this reuse if the ePHI is removed according to policy. Electronic media, computers, and other hardware may be moved within the CE, but there must be a record of where all of the workstations and media are at any given time and who is responsible for the equipment. When a computer has ePHI stored on it, the data should be backed up before the computer is moved. Another method of protecting ePHI when computers are moved is to store the data on a network so that the ePHI is not at risk. If ePHI is stored on the workstation, that data must be removed before the computer is transferred from one location to another or before it is scrapped or sold.

Mobile Security

Mobile devices take many forms, including tablets, smartphones, and thumb drives, and are easily stolen, lost, or misplaced. They are used in healthcare to facilitate communications both between staff and patients as well as accessing information systems. The mobile devices can be used for dictation, photos, and accessing health records. Due to their small size, they are easy to lose and easy to steal. This is why protecting the mobile device is critical.

Every item should have a property control tag attached so that the hardware can be tracked as it moves throughout the CE. This property control tag assigns a unique identifier to the hardware, allowing it to be inventoried. For example, the healthcare organization would know that hardware 12345 is a personal computer that is assigned to Mary Smith in the HIM department. The CE may also want to investigate security options for portable devices such as those that monitor the location of devices. When an inventory is performed, the CE knows exactly where pieces of hardware should be located and what has been moved. Best practices for the use of mobile devices in a CE include:

- Use authentication methods to control access
- Utilize encryption
- Install remote wiping and remote disabling software
- Do not allow use of data sharing applications on device (for example Dropbox)
- Update software frequently
- Use official sources of software (such as Google Play)
- Protect data when using public Wi-Fi (Becker's Health IT 2020)

Staff members who use mobile devices should be trained on the associated privacy and security responsibilities, including physical security, logging off, and other operations.

Some CEs allow healthcare providers to access ePHI on their personal tablet or phone. This practice is known as bring your own device (BYOD). If BYOD is used, there must be policies and procedures in place to address security issues such as encryption and remote wipe.

Appropriate steps should be taken to investigate all lost and stolen devices. If the device is not located, then a remote wipe should be initiated. **Remote wipe** is used when data must be deleted from the mobile device remotely because it has been lost or stolen. This prevents data stored on the remote device from being accessed by unauthorized users. The remote wipe is also used when the mobile device is transition from one employee to another (TechTarget n.d.). Mobile Device Management (MDM) software is used to determine what mobile devices are authorized to access the CE's network, what applications can be installed on the devices, locating devices when misplaced, and protecting devices in the event they are stolen (ManageEngine nd). The protection of devices does include remote wiping.

Fire and Natural Disasters

As discussed earlier, media can be destroyed by natural disaster or fire. CEs should have contracts with restoration companies in place in advance of a natural disaster so that efforts to repair the damage from water, fire, mold, chemical spills, and more can occur quickly. These types of events support the need for backups as described earlier. One CE that implemented a document management system created a backup file of their scanned health records. The problem was because this CE stored the backup file about 15 feet from the original disk. The HIM department, where the original and backup media were stored, was located in the basement, so if there had been a flood or other disaster both copies would have been lost. Backup files should be stored on an off-site server that would not be at risk for the same disaster. For example, a CE in Georgia could have its data backed up on an information system in Montana. This eliminates the possibility of the same event damaging both the original and the backup databases.

Penalties

The oversight of the HIPAA Security Rule has been given to the Office of Civil Rights, which has the right to award civil and criminal penalties. These penalties are awarded when the individual knowingly and willfully violates the security rules. There are four tiers of civil penalties, which are shown in table 12.6.

Table 12.6. Civil penalties for security rule violations

Violation Category	Each Violation	Annual Cap
Did Not Know	$119 – $59,522	$1,785,651
Reasonable Cause	$1,191 – $59,522	$1,785,651
Willful Neglect—Corrected	$11,904 – $59,522	$1,785,651
Willful Neglect—Not Corrected	$59,522 – $1,785,651	$1,785,651

Source: HHS 2020.

Certifications

There are three privacy or security certifications: Certified in Healthcare Privacy and Security (CHPS), Certified Information Security Manager (CISM), and Certified Information Systems Security Professional (CISSP). The CHPS is designed specifically for healthcare, whereas the CISSP and CISM are general security certifications.

Certified in Healthcare Privacy and Security

The **Certified in Healthcare Privacy and Security (CHPS)** credential demonstrates advanced privacy and security skills. These advanced privacy and security skills exceed those in the Registered Health Information Administrator or Registered Health Information Technician examinations. It is sponsored by the American Health Information Management Association (AHIMA). The CHPS examination includes both technical and managerial issues, including a number of topics related to privacy and security. Figure 12.2 shows AHIMA's CHPS competency domains.

Figure 12.2. CHPS domains

Domain 1: Ethical, Legal, and Regulatory Issues/External Environmental Assessment (23–27%)
Domain 2: Program Management and Administration (23–27%)
Domain 3: Information Technology/Physical and Technical Safeguards (23–27%)
Domain 4: Investigation, Compliance, and Enforcement (23–27%)

Source: AHIMA 2019.

Certified Information Systems Security Professional

The **Certified Information Systems Security Professional (CISSP)** certification is sponsored by the International Information Systems Security Certification Consortium [(ISC)²]. It is a generic security certification and therefore is not healthcare specific [(ISC)² n.d.].

Certified Information Security Manager

The **Certified Information Security Manager (CISM)** is sponsored by ISACA. It is an international security examination covering a number of security related topics such as information security governance and incident management (ISACA 2020).

CHECK YOUR UNDERSTANDING 12.4

1. Identify the type of malware that can capture keystrokes.

   a. Spyware
   b. Trojan
   c. Virus
   d. Worm

2. Identify the type of malicious software that denies an organization access to its own information system.

   a. Ransomware
   b. Phishing
   c. Denial of service
   d. Worm

3. Identify a facility access control.

   a. Contingency plan
   b. Backup
   c. Card key
   d. Media controls

4. Remote wipe is used to _____.

   a. Routinely delete ePHI when using BYOD.
   b. Delete ePHI in mobile devices when they are stolen.
   c. Eliminate malicious software.
   d. Prepare an information system for reinstalling data from a backup.

5. A pacemaker is an example of a(n) _____.

   a. Medical device
   b. Mobile device
   c. Media control
   d. Remote wipe

Real-World Case 12.1

Fountain View Hospice is an inpatient hospice that has an EHR. Because of a hurricane, the town, including the hospice, was flooded. Patients had to be evacuated and the data center was underwater. The hospice backs up its files daily and the files are stored at a vendor site across town. The vendor's office was unaffected by the flood, so the backup files are safe however the vendor does not have a copy of the Hospice's EHR application as a hot site. The flood waters have receded and the building is undergoing renovations. The vendor has stated that there is no way to recreate their application and so a full implementation of the EHR will be necessary and could take a year or more. In the meantime, the hospice will have to operate using paper health records. The hospice will have to pay to select and implement the new information system as well as manage the paper health record.

Real-World Case 12.2

Anywhere Hospital was attacked by WannaCry, a type of malware, and is unable to access the EHR. The hospital is routing patients to other emergency rooms, cancelling elective surgeries, and is struggling to treat patients. They are not able to identify allergies, past medical history, and other critical health information. A ransom of $20,000 was requested. The chief security officer and the chief executive officer conferred and decided to pay the ransom since they could easily come up with the amount requested. They felt it would be cheaper to pay the ransom than lose patient revenue. They were also concerned with the possibility of providing poor quality of care during this time and were afraid that the hospital could lose the respect of the community. They paid the ransom using bitcoin and were given the key to access the data.

REVIEW QUESTIONS

1. Identify where ePHI is stored.

   a. Voicemail
   b. Paper health record
   c. Fax machines and EHR
   d. EHR

2. Amanda has resigned from her position in the HIM department. She finishes her last shift at 5:00 p.m. today. Identify the activity that must be implemented.

   a. Termination procedure
   b. Workforce clearance process
   c. Information access management
   d. Addressable standard

3. Identify the type of encryption used when both the sending and receiving computers use the same key.

   a. Public key
   b. Asymmetric
   c. Symmetric
   d. Private key

4. HIPAA security standards whereby the CE can determine if the standard is reasonable and appropriate is known as _____.

   a. Addressable
   b. Optional
   c. Noncompulsory
   d. Voluntary

5. Identify an example of administrative safeguards.

   a. Emergency access procedure
   b. Mechanism to authenticate ePHI
   c. Security awareness and training
   d. Audit controls

6. Access controls are classified as something you know, something you have, and something you _____.

(Continued)

REVIEW QUESTIONS (*Continued*)

   a. Are
   b. Choose
   c. Design
   d. Develop

7. Caring Healthcare has two different healthcare facilities. They need to share e-PHI between the two organization. Recommend a method for sharing it securely.

   a. Firewall
   b. Mitigation
   c. Virtual private network
   d. Emergency access procedure

8. One of the nurses in the quality management department has decided to work a few shifts on the nursing units in order to earn some extra money. When she logs in with her normal sign-in, she has certain functionality; when she logs in differently to work on the nursing unit, she has different functionality. This is known as _____.

   a. Role-based authentication
   b. User-based authentication
   c. Context-based authentication
   d. Emergency access procedure

9. Identify the true statement about audit logs.

   a. Audit logs should be protected
   b. Audit logs only capture actions that are outside the norm.
   c. Audit logs monitor only user actions.
   d. Audit logs should be available to a wide range of employees to facilitate audits.

10. Identify the type of social engineering that proposes an exchange with the victim.

   a. Quid pro quo
   b. Phishing
   c. Vishing
   d. Pretexting

References

45 CFR 160, 162, and 164. HIPAA administrative simplification regulation text. 2013 (unofficial version, as amended through March 26). https://www.hhs.gov/sites/default/files/hipaa-simplification-201303.pdf.

Amatayakul, M. 2004. Kick starting the security risk analysis. *Journal of AHIMA* 75(7):46–47.

Amatayakul, M. 2017. *Health IT and EHRs: Principles and Practice*. Chicago: AHIMA.

American Health Information Management Association (AHIMA). 2019. Commission on Certification for Health Informatics and Information Management (CCHIIM) Candidate Guide. https://www.ahima.org/media/mhjapwhx/revised-candidate-guide-8-6-2020.pdf.

American Health Information Management Association. 2017. *Pocket Glossary of Health Information Management and Technology,* 5th ed. Chicago: AHIMA.

American Medical Association. n.d. HIPAA Security Rule & Risk Analysis. https://www.ama-assn.org/practice-management/hipaa/hipaa-security-rule-risk-analysis.

Becker's Health IT. 2020. 7 Best Practices for HIPAA Mobile Device Security. https://www.beckershospitalreview.com/healthcare-information-technology/7-best-practices-for-hipaa-mobile-device-security.html.

Blacketer, C. 2019. Managing Medical Device Security Risk: It takes a Village. https://medcitynews.com/2019/08/managing-medical-device-security-risk-it-takes-a-village/.

Centers for Medicare and Medicaid Services. 2020. Transactions Overview. https://www.cms.gov/Regulations-and-Guidance/Administrative-Simplification/Transactions/TransactionsOverview.

Cisco. n.d. What Is the Difference: Viruses, Worms, Trojans, and Bots? Accessed January 7, 2018. http://www.cisco.com/web/about/security/intelligence/virus-worm-diffs.html.

Compliance Group. nd. What is HIPAA Risk Management? https://compliancy-group.com/what-is-hipaa-risk-management/.

Compliancy Group. 2020. What is a "Security Incident" under the HIPAA Security Rule? https://compliancy-group.com/what-is-a-security-incident-under-hipaa-security-rule/.

Corvus. n.d. Security Report: Health Care – Hospitals, Providers and More. https://info.corvusinsurance.com/hubfs/Security%20Report%202.2%20-%20Health%20Care%20.pdf.

Davis, J. B. 2003. *HIPAA Compliance Manual: A Comprehensive Guide to the Administrative Simplification Provisions for Health Care Professionals*. Los Angeles: PMIC.

Department of Health and Human Services. 2020. *Federal Register*. Annual Civil Monetary Penalties Inflation Adjustment. https://www.govinfo.gov/content/pkg/FR-2020-01-17/pdf/2020-00738.pdf.

Department of Health and Human Services. 2019. Business Associates. https://www.hhs.gov/hipaa/for-professionals/privacy/guidance/business-associates/index.html.

Department of Health and Human Services. 2010. Guidance on Ris Analysis Requirements Under the HIPAA Security Rule. https://www.hhs.gov/sites/default/files/ocr/privacy/hipaa/administrative/securityrule/rafinalguidancepdf.pdf

Department of Homeland Security. 2019. Security Tip: Protecting Against Ransomware. https://www.us-cert.gov/ncas/tips/ST19-001.

Derhak, M. 2003. Uncovering the enemy within: Utilizing incident response, forensics. *In Confidence* 11(9):1–2. http://library.ahima.org/doc?oid=59731#.WoN3deRy5jo.

Dill, M. W., S. Lucci, and T. Walsh. 2016. Understanding cybersecurity: A primer for HIM professionals. *Journal of AHIMA* 87(4). http://bok.ahima.org/doc?oid=301408.

Dooling, J. A., T. Rihanek, D. Warner, and L. A. Wiedemann. 2016. Disaster Planning and Recovery Toolkit. http://bok.ahima.org/PdfView?oid=301964.

Forcepoint. 2020. What is an Intrusion Prevention System (IPS)? https://www.forcepoint.com/cyber-edu/intrusion-prevention-system-ips.

HIPAA Journal. N.d. Is HIPAA Violation Grounds for Termination. https://www.hipaajournal.com/hipaa-violation-grounds-for-termination/.

HIPAA Journal. 2017. What is Considered PHI Under HIPAA? https://www.hipaajournal.com/considered-phi-hipaa/.

Hjort, B. 2003. Practice brief: HIPAA privacy and security training (updated). http://library.ahima.org/xpedio/groups/public/documents/ahima/bok1_048509.hcsp?dDocName=bok1_048509.

Internet Engineering Task Force. 2018. The Transport Layer Security (TLS) Protocol Version 1.3. https://tools.ietf.org/html/rfc8446.

International Information Systems Security Certification Consortium [(ISC)²]. n.d. CISSP®—Certified Information Systems Security Professional. https://www.isc2.org/cissp/default.aspx.

ISACA. 2020. Certified Information Security Manager (CISM). https://www.isaca.org/credentialing/cism.

ManageEngine. nd. What is Mobile Device Management (MDM)? https://www.manageengine.com/mobile-device-management/what-is-mdm.html.

MediaPRO. 2019. Why Every Employee is a Vital Part of Security Incident Response. https://www.mediapro.com/blog/every-employee-vital-part-security-incident-response/.

Merriam-Webster. 2020a. Checksum. https://www.merriam-webster.com/dictionary/checksum.

Merriam-Webster. 2020b. Phishing. https://www.merriam-webster.com/dictionary/phishing.

National Institute of Standards and Technology. 2020 Digital Identity Guidelines. https://pages .nist.gov/800-63-3/sp800-63b.html#biometric_use.

NICE. nd. What is a bot in RPA? https://www.nice.com/rpa/rpa-guide/what-is-a-bot-in-rpa/.

Norton. n.d.a. What are Bots? https://us.norton.com/internetsecurity-malware-what-are-bots .html.

Norton. n.d.b. What is Social Engineering? Tips to Help Avoid Becoming a Victim. https:// us.norton.com/internetsecurity-emerging-threats-what-is-social-engineering.html.

Norwich University Online. 2017. 5 Steps for Conducting Computer Forensics Investigations. https://online.norwich.edu/academic-programs/resources/5-steps-for-conducting-computer -forensics-investigations.

Primeau, D. 2017. How Small Organizations Handle HIPAA Compliance. http://library.ahima .org/doc?oid=302074#.WlgMFeRy5jo.

Rubens, P. 2017. Common Types of Ransomware. https://www.esecurityplanet.com/malware /types-of-ransomware.html.

Shutters, K. n.d. HIPAA Vulnerabilities, Threats and Risks. http://www.hipaaalli.com/2018/04 /hipaa-vulnerabilities-threats-and-risks/.

Srinivas, R. 2019. 7 Times Ransomware Became a Major Healthcare Hazard. https://www .cisomag.com/7-times-ransomware-became-a-major-healthcare-hazard/.

TechTarget. n.d. Remote Wipe. https://searchmobilecomputing.techtarget.com/definition /remote-wipe.

University of Alabama at Birmingham (UAB). 2020. UAB Data Classification Rule. https://www .uab.edu/it/home/policies/data-classification/classification-rule.

USLegal 2019. Spoliation Law and Legal Definition. https://definitions.uslegal.com/s/spoliation/

Vocabulary. n.d. Forensic. https://www.vocabulary.com/dictionary/forensic.

Webroot. n.d. What is Social Engineering? Examples & Prevention Tips. https://www.webroot .com/ie/en/resources/tips-articles/what-is-social-engineering.

World Health Organization (WHO). 2020. Medical Devices. http://www.who.int/medical _devices/definitions/en/.

Zhang, E. 2020. What is Data Loss Prevention (DLP)? A Definition of Data Loss Prevention. https://digitalguardian.com/blog/what-data-loss-prevention-dlp-definition-data-loss -prevention.

Security Compliance and Monitoring

Learning Objectives

- Differentiate between auditing and monitoring.
- Assist in the auditing and monitoring of HIPAA security rule compliance activities.
- Document audit process and findings.

Key Words

Auditing
Benchmark
Compliance
Compliance plan
Corrective action
  plan
Dashboard
Data analysis
Data display

Department of Health and
  Human Services Office
  of Civil Rights (OCR)
Evidence
External audit
Field work
Internal audit
Metric
Monitoring

Objective evidence
Process audit
Product audit
Resolution agreement
Standard
System audit
Threshold
Visual observation

Covered entities (CEs) and business associates (BA) are mandated to prove their compliance with the Health Insurance Portability and Accountability Act of 1996's (HIPAA) security rule standards. Compliance is the process of establishing an organizational culture that promotes the prevention, detection, and resolution of instances of conduct that do not conform to federal, state, or private payer healthcare program requirements or the healthcare organization's ethical and business policies. In other words, the CE (defined in chapter 12) proves that it is following the requirements of the security rules. The OIG, who is responsible for enforcement of the security rule, published some tips for the development of a culture of compliance in a CE. These tips include:

- Make compliance a priority: Compliance cannot be put off or conducted when it is convenient. It must be an ongoing process. There must be resources provided for compliance which include staff and money as well as other resources.

- Identify areas of risk: These risks for the CE would be identified during the risk assessment described in chapter 12. These risks can be hackers, natural disasters, and much more. Each of these risks must be addressed as part of the compliance plan described later in this chapter. The CE must take steps to avoid or reduce the amount of risk for each. For example, the CE would utilize fire suppression systems, take steps to block hackers such as a firewall, plan for power outages, and so forth.

- Know what you can and cannot do: All employees at a CE must be trained on what they can and cannot do related to the HIPAA Security Rule. This would include ongoing education of security awareness, policies and procedures, privacy, saving electronic protected health information (ePHI) on personal devices, and much more.

- Ask for assistance: Asking for assistance applies to both the CE and the workforce members. If a member of the workforce is unclear on a policy, how to download data, how to delete data appropriately, and so forth, then they should ask for help rather than risk being accused of a security violation in case something goes wrong such as uploading ePHI to the internet. There are many ways that a CE can ask for help if they are unsure of how to comply with the security rule. A few include contacting other CEs to learn how they are complying with a specific standard, contacting the Department of Health and Human Services (HHS), and hiring a consultant (OIG n.d.).

Parts of this chapter are about compliance in general and can therefore be used for monitoring compliance with anything; however, the focus of the chapter will be the HIPAA security rule as discussed in chapter 12. This chapter will address the importance of compliance, auditing and monitoring, the Office of Civil Rights, what to audit, and training as well as compliance monitoring and information systems.

Importance of Compliance

As mentioned earlier, compliance is mandated by HIPAA. Failure of the CE to meet the HIPAA security rule requirements will result in penalties which may be financial and/or prison. Because of the severity of these penalties, it is critical that a CE prove that they are complying with the HIPAA security rule as discussed in chapter 12. Another importance reason for compliance is that the CE does not want to make the evening news with the headline due to a security breach. Bad press can damage the image of a CE and make it hard for it to regain the public's trust. For example, if a hospital makes the evening news because of a privacy or security breach, patients may choose to receive their care at another hospital.

Each CE will need to develop a compliance plan. A compliance plan is a process that identifies how a healthcare organization CE will operate ethically to accomplish its goal of providing high-quality medical care and efficiently operating a business under various laws and regulations (MedProGroup 2018).

Covered Entity Compliance Plan

The OIG recommends that each CE create a compliance plan that included seven fundamental elements. The elements are:

- Written policies, procedures as well as standards of conduct
- Compliance officer
- Training and education
- Effective communication
- Enforcement
- Prompt response to noncompliance (OIG nd)

Before, each of these elements are discussed, an introduction to auditing and monitoring will be discussed.

Introduction to Auditing and Monitoring

Auditing and monitoring may sound the same, however there is a distinct difference between the two concepts. Auditing has two definitions:

- A function that allows retrospective reconstruction of events, including who executed the events in question, why, and what changes were made as a result.

- To conduct an independent review of electronic system records and activities in order to test the adequacy and effectiveness of data security and data integrity procedures and to ensure compliance with established policies and procedures.

Audits are performed by the compliance officer to make sure that auditing and monitoring is both being done and is effective in its design (Kusserow 2017). This compliance official is generally the chief security official. This role was discussed generally in chapter 12. The role specific to compliance will be covered later in this chapter. Auditing would review the monitoring program to ensure that it is effective at getting the CE to accomplish the anticipated outcome.

Monitoring is keeping a watchful eye on compliance activities to detect any issues that need to be addressed by management (Aleixo 2018). Monitoring includes keeping current on regulations and laws, establishing standards, developing policies and procedures, and training. Monitoring should be conducted throughout the healthcare organization depending on what is being monitored. For example, someone in information technology would monitor issues identified by the intrusion detection system (discussed in chapter) and someone in the training department might monitor participation in security training. The monitoring also looks for policy violations and errors, as well as other issues. Reviews are conducted by department managers to determine if the standards are being met (Kusserow 2017).

Auditing and monitoring are not a one-time task but should be ongoing. Auditing and monitoring work together to ensure that the CE is meeting the requirements of the HIPAA security rule. Monitoring is actually part of the auditing process. When an area of noncompliance is found, the CE must take immediate action to correct the issue. All auditing and monitoring activities must be documented and retained as evidence that the CE is complying with the HIPAA security rule. More on this process later in this chapter.

Internal vs. External Audits

Both internal and external audits should be used in any compliance program. Internal audits are performed by the CE's staff to determine whether or not the CE is in compliance with HIPAA, policies and procedures, laws, regulations, or other requirements. Depending on the compliance plan and policies and procedures, these audits may be performed daily, weekly, monthly, or at other intervals.

External audits are performed by consultants or others who do not work for the CE. The purpose of an external audit is to confirm that the internal audits are identifying the risks and issues that it should. These external audits may be performed annually.

There are consultants who specialize in compliance auditing. These consultants are hired to perform the external audits. The contract between the CE and the consulting firm would spell out deliverables (reports, data, recommendations), areas to be audited, purpose of audit as well as normal contract clauses such as a termination.

There are three types of audits that a CE may perform: process, product, and system. The process audit confirms that the CE's performance of tasks is meeting established standards. For example, are 100% of triggers reviewed (see chapter 12). The product audit is evaluating a product or services to ensure that is meets expected requirements. For example, confirming that the network firewall is working to block spam, malware, and more. The system audit reviews activities to ensure that the system used is appropriate and effective (American Society for Quality 2020).

For example, investigating the training program will determine how effective it is, if the required documentation is present and so forth.

Written Policies, Procedures, and Standards of Conduct

Written policies and procedures are an important part of the security rule's administrative standards. The policies and procedures should include a variety of topics including sanctions, access authorization, and work station use. These policies and procedures must be retained for six years from the date it was created or from when it was phased out. The CE must have a method in place for the storage and destruction of the policies and procedures as appropriate once the retention period has passed. For example, the policies and procedures will be shredded or deleted.

These policies and procedures must be available to employees at the CE so that they can refer to them at any time. Posting these policies and procedures on an intranet allows members of the workforce to access them quickly and easily as well as requiring updates to be posted in one and only one location.

A code of conduct is a description of how a CE's employees are expected to behave. The code of conduct varies from organization to organization but address operations, the organization's core values and the organizational culture (Munim 2017). For example, employees are expected to report privacy and security concerns.

Chief Security Official (Compliance Officer)

The chief security official (CSO) is an executive level position that is in charge of the security program including compliance. This person does not manage the security program alone but should have an advisory committee to assist in the process. This committee would be made up of information technology staff, health information management staff, risk managers, legal counsel, and others involved in security. The committee would advise the CSO, examine results of the auditing and monitoring, review the compliance plan, and more. The CSO works with staff who implement the compliance plan, conduct the audits, and more. This staff includes employees throughout the program and varies by CE. For example, the HIM director might monitor the audit trail of his or her staff in one CE and in another it might be performed by the CSO's staff.

Training and Education

As stated in chapter 12, all members of the workforce must undergo continuous training related to security. All members of the workforce must have security awareness training. Additional training will be held for employees based on the role they have in the organization. For example, workforce members in the information technology would be trained on access to the data center, terminating workforce member's access to information systems, monitoring the intrusion detection system, and more. This may be controlled by the CSO or it may be the responsibility of a training department. Regardless of who is in change, the two must work together to ensure the employees are receiving the training that is need.

There must be a plan in place to schedule and develop the training that will be performed. The CE must prove to the OIG that there is a plan to ensure ongoing training on security awareness, employee's role in security, security policies related to the employee's role, and other security related topics.

Training must be ongoing and can take many forms. There needs to be a plan in place to ensure this occurs as well as documentation of the training. Example of documentation required include:

- Sign-in sheets
- Handouts
- Training materials
- Fliers
- Emails
- Newsletters
- Quizzes

The documentation can be housed in the CSO's office, the training department, human resources, or the employee's department according to the CE's policy.

There must be a schedule of the training as well as a mechanism in place to track employees who have completed training and when training is needed. This tracking can be a part of a spreadsheet, a database, or an information system devoted to tracking training. Department directors would need to be notified when their employees are behind in the training so that he or she can ensure that the employee gets caught up on the training. Failure to participate in the training should lead to disciplinary actions and could result in termination.

Effective Communication

Effective communication is defined as "communication between two or more persons with the purpose of delivering, receiving, and understanding the message successfully" (Kashyap 2019). In other words, it is getting your point across to the listener. Workforce members must be kept in the loop on upcoming changes in policies, upcoming training and other information related to security. The communications should be retained for proof that information was communicated to employees. This documentation would be part of the compliance plan. There are four skills that help encourage effective communication. These are:

- Engaged listener: Being an engaged listener is more than just understanding what is being said; it is also understanding what the speaker does not say. Understanding the other individual's emotions and where they are coming from is an important part of engaged listening as this understanding would shape what the speaker communicates and how they communicate it.

- Nonverbal communications: The listener's nonverbal communication such as facial expressions, body language, eye contact, and more lets the speaker know that the listener is engaged or unengaged. For example, if the listener checking their phone, reading a report, or are otherwise distracted, then the speaker feels that the listener does not care what is being said.

- Stress: Some communications can be stressful. For example, if a manager is counseling an employee responsible for a security violation, it can be stressful to both the manager and the employee if the individual is not comfortable with confrontation. The manager to minimize the stress by taking time to think about what he or she wants to say, communicating clearly, and summarizing what is said.

- Assertive: Being assertive in communication is the speaker being open and honest as well as respecting others rather than forcing his or her beliefs on the listener (Robinson et al. 2019). For example, an employee needs to understand why the security policies and monitoring is in place and why the employee can or cannot do something. The employee will be more open to following the policy rather than a "thou shall not" mandate.

Enforcement

The security rule mandates a sanction policy that defines what penalties will be given if a workforce member fails to follow the appropriate security measures (45 CFR 164.308(a)(1) (ii)(C)). Not all violations are created equal. There is a big difference between a careless error and selling protected health information to a tabloid. Because of this, there should be tiers of penalties or sanctions so that the penalty is equal to the action. These tiers are establishing by the CE. For example, if a workforce member does not log out of the EHR and walks away, a verbal or written warning might be all that is needed. On the other hand, if a workforce member uses protected health information to open a credit card in that patient's name, then termination of employment would be appropriate. In this case, law enforcement would need to be informed. Any security breach would need to reported to the OIG. Spelling out the penalties in the policy not only lets the members of the workforce know what to expect but it also helps apply penalties uniformly across the CE. The CSO and the advisory committee would be key to the development of the enforcement process.

Prompt response to noncompliance

Violations must be addressed promptly to not only prevent further violations from occurring but to protect the CE in the event of an OIG security audit. These audits can be performed when a complaint is received, but the CE can also be identified for an audit randomly or due to their past performance (past breaches).

Once a violation is identified, the CE must resolve the problem. As stated earlier, any security breach must be reported to the Secretary of Health and Human Services (HHS). When a security breach is identified, then the patients, the media, and HHS must be notified as per the breach notification rule. A breach is defined by CMS as "an impermissible use or disclosure under the Privacy Rule that compromises the security or privacy of the protected health information" (45 CFR § 164.400-414). For example, if an employee leaves a laptop in his or her car and that laptop is stolen, it is a security breach if the laptop contained unsecured ePHI (not encrypted).

The patient is always notified when there is a breach of his or her electronic protected health information (ePHI). The media is notified if the number of patients impacted by the breach is more than 500. The Secretary of HHS is notified as soon as possible not to exceed 60 days if the number of patients exceed 500. If the number of patients is less than the 500, then the Secretary of HHS is notified electronically.

A pattern of breaches or a significant breach can trigger an audit as it raises a red flag that the CE may not be complying with the security rule. It is better for the CE to identify the issue and resolve it before the OIG identifies the problem for the CE. This does not mean that no penalties will be awarded but the penalties should be reduced.

The resolution of the violation would vary according to the problem and according to policy. Examples of resolutions include, but are not limited to, the following: change in policy and procedure, training, employee sanctions, and so forth.

When a breach has occurred the CE must take immediate steps to mitigate (limit) the impact that the breach has on a patient. Mitigation can take many forms depending on the breach. It can be writing letters to employers, or others, credit monitoring, providing information to courts, and much more.

Standards

A standard is a scientifically based statement of expected behavior against which structures, processes, and outcomes can be measured. Standard is also the term used by HIPAA to spell out the requirements of the regulation. The term *standard* in both contexts give the CE something that they can measure themselves against. For example, the HIPAA Security rule mandates protecting the physical hardware that stores ePHI. These standards should be the basis upon which the compliance program is based with regards to what is audited and monitored. For example, 99 percent of the members of the workforce participate in security training. Each CE will establish their own standards for compliance with HIPAA and HITECH.

Benchmarking

Benchmarking is the systematic comparison of the products, services, and outcomes of one organization with those of a similar organization, or the systematic comparison of one organization's outcomes with regional or national standards (Oachs and Watters 2020). This means that a 900-bed teaching hospital would compare itself to another large teaching hospital, not a physician practice or a small community hospital. Benchmarking is a key part of any compliance program as it helps the CE understand how they compare to other comparable CEs. If the CE's standards are lower than the comparable CEs, operations related to that standard would need to be reviewed in depth to identify why the standard is lower than it should be.

CHECK YOUR UNDERSTANDING 13.1

1. The CE conducts audits and takes steps to ensure that they meet the requirements of the HIPAA security rule. This process is known as:

   a. Auditing and monitoring
   b. Security program
   c. Organizational culture
   d. Compliance

2. Security training should be based on the:

   a. Length of time the workforce member has worked at the CE
   b. Education of the workforce member
   c. Department in which the employee work
   d. Role workforce member has in the CE

3. Penalties for non-compliance with the HIPAA security rule is (are):

   a. Financial only
   b. Prison only
   c. Financial and prison
   d. Exclusion from the Medicare program

4. The Secretary of HHS should be notified of any security breaches that impact more than _____ patients.

   a. 250
   b. 500
   c. 750
   d. 1,000

5. The CE hired a consultant to come review their security program. This is known as a(n)

   a. External audit
   b. Internal audit
   c. Process audit
   d. System audit

Department of Health and Human Services

The Department of Health and Human Services' Office of Civil Rights (OCR) is in charge of oversight for the HIPAA Security Rule. Initially, CEs were only audited if there was a complaint or other reason to suspect a violation of the HIPAA security rule. With the passage of HITECH, the OCR HIPAA security audit, known as a compliance review, can occur at any time for both CE and business associates. This is only one of the ways that HITECH increased the emphasis on compliance. The other components were through education and making BA subject to HIPAA. This section will address the OCR's audit program, resolution agreements, and the results of their audit program.

The OCR identifies a random sample of CEs and business associates who are selected for an audit. The selected CE and business associates may be reviewed remotely at the OCR's office which is known as a desk audit or it may be an onsite audit at the CE. The CEs and business associates are notified of the audit and required to submit specified documents. Much of the audits will focus on the CE's policies and procedures to ensure that it supports the CE's security program. The CE and business associates will be notified of the OCR's initial findings and will be able to respond to the findings. If issues are identified through the desk audit then a compliance review onsite may be conducted to investigate the issues further (HHS 2016). The audit process for a security rule complaint is shown in Figure 13.1.

Figure 13.1. HIPAA privacy & security rule compliant process

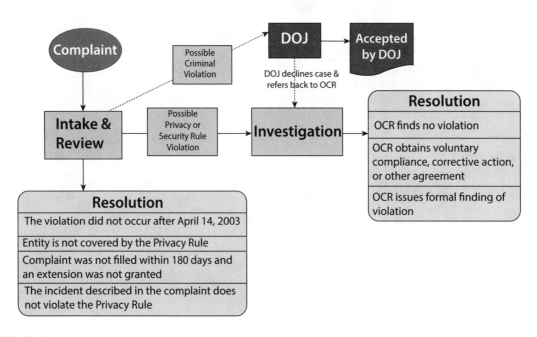

Source: HHS 2017a.

When the OCR investigates security complaints, it reviews the complaint in a process known as intake & review. During this process, OCR confirms that the alleged behavior occurred after HIPAA went into effect; that it was done by a CE; that, if true, it would be a violation of the privacy or security rule; and that the complaint was filed within 180 days of when the issue was identified or should have been identified (HHS 2017b).

After the intake & review, the OCR can take one of five actions:

- Close the investigation after review when there is obviously no compliance issue. For example, the organization in question is not subject to the HIPAA security rule or ePHI is not involved.

- Provide technical assistance to the CE or business associate. Technical assistance would include education of the CE or business associate.

- Investigation indicates that there was not a violation and therefore, no action is required.

- Corrective Action Obtained occurs when the OCR investigate and provides technical assistance, which generally results in mandated changes made in their compliance program. A resolution agreement is made between OCR and the CE or Business Associate.

- OCR may opt to not investigate further for some reason such as a natural disaster or is being addressed by the Department of Justice (HHS 2019a).

Results of the OCR Audit Program

OCR's enforcement in 2018 (the most recent year available at the time this chapter was written) exceeded $28 million. This enforcement came about through settlements and judgements. When a CE or BA have been found to be noncompliance with the security rule, the decision on civil monetary penalties can be awarded in two ways – through settlements or negotiations. In a settlement, the CE or BA negotiate with the OCR to establish the civil monetary penalties. Judgements are awarded to CE or BA when the case goes to court. The 2018 penalties were awarded to a number of different types of organizations including hospitals, a physician office, a health record storage company, and an insurer. Table 13.1 shows number of cases processed by the OCR. These figures show that OCR has continued to increase the number of cases reviewed of cases.

Table 13.1. Total cases

	Complaints	Compliance Reviews	Technical Assistance	Total Cases	Of Those, Settlements or CMPs	% of Total Cases
2015	17620	176	4008	21904	6	0.0275%
2016	23900	335	6458	30692	13	0.0424%
2017	23717	396	7559	37672	10	0.0316%
2018	23717	438	7243	32771	10	0.0305%
2019	29853	338	9060	39251	10	0.0255%

Source: HHS 2020.

Resolution Agreement

A resolution agreement is an agreement between the OCR and either a CE or business associate (BA). The resolution agreement describes the failure of the CE to meet the HIPAA requirements, any civil monetary penalties, a corrective action plan, and more. The corrective action plan (CAP) portion outlines the CE or BA's responsibilities over a designated period (HHS 2019b). During the CAP period, the CE or BA would have to periodically report to the OCR their progress towards compliance. Civil money penalties are described in chapter 12.

Audit Program

Every CE and BA should have an audit program. It should begin at the top with the chief executive officer and the chief security officer as their focus on the program will ensure that employees understand the importance of the audits. There are a number of benefits to a strong audit program. These include:

- Presence of policies and procedures
- Oversight of ethical and moral values
- Education of employees
- Monitoring activities related to security
- Consistent disciplinary actions
- Feedback that result in improved actions (Reachout 2016)
- Identify what is going on in the organization

- Resolve issues before they become serious
- Determine where resources should be focused (Cochran 2017, 7)

The HIPAA security rule has many standards that must be audited or monitored. The audits and monitors can take a number of formats based on the HIPAA standard. Sometimes it is as simple as ensuring that a policy and procedure is in place and is updated periodically. Sometimes it is more complicated such as conducting a periodic risk analysis.

There are five stages of an audit. These stages are selection, planning, fieldwork, reporting, and follow-up (University of Oregon n.d.).

Selection

Selection identifies what needs to be audited. The areas chosen would be based on the risk to the CE (University of Oregon n.d.). In this case, the areas chosen would be based on the HIPAA security rule requirements. For example, the risk assessment should not only be performed periodically but it should identify significant risks to ePHI.

HIPAA is divided into administrative, physical, and technical safeguards which are discussed in chapter 12. All of these must be audited/monitored on an ongoing basis. Refer to Tables 13.2 – 13.4 provides examples of administrative, physical and technical safeguards that should be audited and/ or documented.

Table 13.2. Examples of administration safeguards and proof of compliance

Sample Administrative Safeguards	Sample Proof of Compliance
Policies and procedures	• Presence of policies and procedures • Documentation that policies and procedures are followed • Retention of policies and procedures for required period.
Business associate agreements	• Business associate agreement with every business associate • Business associate agreement has mandated content
Risk analysis	Documentation of periodic risk analysis and its findings
Sanction policy	Presence of sanction policy and compliance with that policy
Audit trail	Documentation of ongoing review of audit trail
Chief security officer	Appointment of a chief security officer that is in charge of the security program.
Workforce security	Process to determine access needs of users
Termination procedures	Employees are immediately removed from information systems when they leave the CE

Source: Adapted from 45 CFR §§164.308.

There are also many physical standards that must be audited/monitored. See Table 13.3 for a list of some of the physical safeguards that should be included.

Table 13.3. Examples of physical safeguards and proof of compliance

Sample of Physical Safeguards	Sample Proof of Compliance
Contingency operations	Contingency plan
Access controls	Use of access controls such as passwords
Workstation security	Monitors turned away from public
Device and media controls	• Policies on protecting devices • Data center with card key • Computers locked to desk • Mobile devices tracked • Log vendor and others who access data center • Inventory of devices

Source: Adapted from 45 CFR §§164.310.

There are also many technical safeguard standards that must be audited/monitored. See Table 13.4 for a list of some of the physical safeguards that should be included.

Table 13.4. Examples of technical safeguards and proof of compliance

Sample of Technical Safeguards	Sample Proof of Compliance
Transmission security	Is encryption used? If not, document alternative transmission security
Access controls	Each user has a unique identifier Use of password or other access control
Emergency access procedure	• Existence of "break the glass" access • Documentation of use of "break the glass" access with monitoring
Integrity	Technology used to protect the integrity of ePHI
Encryption	Use of encryption to transmit ePHI

Source: Adapted from 45 CFR §§164.312.

Planning

Planning audits begin at a high level by identifying the scope of the audits and the objectives of the audits to be conducted (University of Oregon n.d.). In other words, what the CE wants to accomplish with the audits. The plan should include the frequencies of audits, monitoring to be performed, mitigation to be enacted, and so forth. The planning would include the scheduling of the major activities of the audit. The schedule keeps the auditors on track so that the audits do not get behind. It should also include developing metrics.

Metrics

A metric is "a standard of measurement" (Merriam-Webster 2020). The CE should establish metrics for many of the HIPAA security measures. Examples of metrics include number of breaches, number of employees going through training, number of audit trail audits, number of triggers investigated, date policies reviewed, and so much more.

Each metric should have a threshold attached to it. The threshold is the desired level of performance for that metric. The goal is to meet or exceed the threshold. If the threshold is not met, then the CE needs to determine what should be done in order to improve performance. The threshold will vary based by metric. For example, 98% of visitors to the data center are logged as they enter and leave the data center. The threshold should be reasonable as employees get frustrated if they are unable to meet the too high standard.

Fieldwork

Fieldwork is the process of completing the audit. This includes data collection and data analysis. Depending on what is being audited, fieldwork could include interviews, reviewing laws, regulations and policies, review of policies and procedures, and so forth. It could also be monitoring actions taken by employees (for example, monitoring audit trails) and much more (University of Oregon n.d.). The evidence collected not only identifies areas for improvement but also identifies areas where the CE is doing well.

To have a successful audit, the auditors must have accurate and objective evidence. Evidence is the data collected in order to determine the compliance or noncompliance with the standards. The objective evidence should be unbiased, factual (real), first hand (observed by auditor), traceable (able to go back and look at data), and impersonal (focused on the process rather than the person or persons performing the process) (Cochran 2017, 56).

Visual observation is also a way to gather evidence through watching what occurs (Cochran 2017, 58). For example, security monitoring can be conducted by walking around to ensure computer monitors are turned away from the public, mobile devices are protected, and so forth. Visual observation not only looks for compliance, but it can also confirm what the auditor has been told.

Audit

CEs do not have enough staff in order to do 100% compliance auditing. For example, the staff cannot monitor 100% of all the activities recorded in the audit trail as this indicates every view, every piece of data entered, every deletion, and so forth. There is just too much data for this to be feasible. This is why sampling of data is utilized. For example, with the audit trail, a single unit for the day shift might be reviewed, specific individuals may be audited, or simply a random sample. A full discussion of sampling is beyond the scope of this textbook.

The scope of the audit is the first step in performing the audit as it outlines what is audited. The next step is to create the audit plan. The audit plan guides the auditors as it explains what will happen, when it will happen, and how it will happen. The audit plan is used by both the auditors and auditee in order to prepare for audits (Cochran 2017, 87, 88, 91, 92). The data is then collected and data analysis is performed. A report is then created. Reports will be covered later in this chapter.

Data Collection

Data collection is an important part of any audit. The data collected should support the purpose of the audit. For example, if an audit is being performed on access controls then data collected should include policy and procedures for assigning access controls, type of access controls used, termination of access, appropriateness of access, and more. However, there is no need to collect data on encryption or other transmission security methods as you just have to show that they are in place and operational. The data collected during an audit can come from information systems, interviews, surveys, review of documents, and more. The data collected can be either quantitative (numerical) or qualitative (non-numeric) depending on the audit being conducted. An example of quantitative data that might be collected is the number of security breaches for the month of December. An example of qualitative data is a policy that covers how workforce clearances will be performed.

Some data, like the audit trail, is automatically captured while other data will have to be captured manually. Unfortunately, not all audit trails are adequate which may cause a compliance issue. Manual data collection includes employees participating in training, mitigation taken, when policies and procedures are reviewed, and more. The CE can utilize databases, spreadsheets, dashboards, or other data collection tools. Regardless of how the data is collected, steps must be taken to ensure data quality since "garbage in, garbage out". In other words, if the quality of the data is not adequate, the resulting information will have little to no value. For more on data quality, refer to chapter 2. See figure 13.2 for an example of a data collection tool.

Data Analysis

A full discussion of data analysis is outside the scope of this textbook; however, it is important to have a basic understanding of data analysis as part of the compliance program. Data analysis is a body of methods that help describe facts, detect patterns, develop explanations, and test hypotheses. Data analysis can include descriptive statistics, inferential statistics, data display, and more. This analysis enables the CE to determine what is working well and what needs improvement.

Documentation of Compliance Activities

The HIPAA security rule requires the retention of certain documents for a period of six years from the date of creation or the last time that it was in force. This includes policies and procedures, training documentation, audit reports, and more. The CE must be able to retrieve the policies and procedures and other documents when required by an OCR investigation or other reason. At the end of the security rule mandated period, the document can be destroyed unless prohibited by state law or another requirement to retain longer.

Corrective Action Plan

A corrective action plan (CAP) is a written plan of action to be taken in response to identified issues. The CAP document outlines the issues and the steps needed to meet the desired thresholds. Examples include workforce training, new technologies, change in policies, and so forth. The content will be based on the issue, such as outdated risk analysis, and what needs to be done, such as complete a new risk analysis. The CAP should be specific, given deadlines, and hold the CE accountable.

Reporting

It is often said about health record documentation "if it's not documented, you didn't do it." This could be said about auditing and monitoring as well. This phrase illustrates the importance of documenting compliance efforts. For example, a physician may perform a diabetic foot exam, as is required by quality metric, but fail to document the exam. This lack of documentation means that when the data is collected, the evidence of the diabetic foot exam is not present.

Reporting the findings of an audit can be oral and/or written; however, any oral reporting should be documented as evidence of the report. One purpose of the report is to notify management of the findings as well as the recommendations for improvement. It is also an important defense in case of an OCR audit.

There are certain components that should be included in any report. These include:

- Title of report
- Date of report
- Date that the report covers
- Content of report

The report may contain the process followed or it may simply present the findings. Frequently data display tools are used. Data display is a method for presenting or viewing data. The data display tools include tables, graphs, infographics, and other displays utilized. These tools are beyond the scope of this course.

Figure 13.2. Data collection tool

Training Log

Employee ID	Employee Last Name	Employee First Name	Initial Security Awareness Training	2020 Annual Training	2021 Annual Training	2020 1st Qtr Refresher	2020 2nd Qtr Refresher	2020 3rd Qtr Refresher	2021 1st Qtr Refresher	2021 2nd Qtr Refresher	2021 3rd Qtr Refresher	2021 4th Qtr Refresher
223588	Johnson	Jared	☑ Yes	☑ Yes	☑ Yes	☑ Yes	☑ Yes	☑ Yes	☑ Yes	☐ Yes	☑ Yes	☐ Yes
223598	Smith	Susanna	☑ Yes	☑ Yes	☑ Yes	☑ Yes	☑ Yes	☑ Yes	☑ Yes	☑ Yes	☑ Yes	☐ Yes
223602	Jones	Elizabeth	☑ Yes	☑ Yes	☑ Yes	☑ Yes	☑ Yes	☑ Yes	☑ Yes	☑ Yes	☐ Yes	☐ Yes
223603	Bain	Grant	☑ Yes	☑ Yes	☑ Yes	☑ Yes	☑ Yes	☑ Yes	☑ Yes	☑ Yes	☑ Yes	☐ Yes
223064	Richards	Phyllis	☑ Yes	☑ Yes	☑ Yes	☑ Yes	☑ Yes	☑ Yes	☑ Yes	☑ Yes	☑ Yes	☐ Yes
223112	Flynn	Alyssa	☑ Yes	☑ Yes	☑ Yes	☑ Yes	☑ Yes	☑ Yes	☑ Yes	☑ Yes	☐ Yes	☐ Yes
223145	Michaels	Alaina	☑ Yes	☑ Yes	☑ Yes	☑ Yes	☑ Yes	☑ Yes	☑ Yes	☑ Yes	☑ Yes	☐ Yes
223147	Abbott	Robert	☑ Yes	☑ Yes	☑ Yes	☑ Yes	☑ Yes	☑ Yes	☑ Yes	☑ Yes	☑ Yes	☐ Yes
223153	Terrill	Thomas	☑ Yes	☑ Yes	☑ Yes	☑ Yes	☑ Yes	☑ Yes	☑ Yes	☑ Yes	☑ Yes	☑ Yes

Source: ©AHIMA.

Reports should be created monthly, quarterly, and annually. This enables managers to not only look at current data however look at trends over time. An example of a table showing the annual audit trail monitoring activities is shown in Figure 13.3.

Figure 13.3. Example of report

Audit Trail Report			
January 1 - December 31, 20XX			
Month	Number of Audit Trail Entries Audited	Potential Security Breach Investigated	Security Breaches Confirmed
January	589	6	1
February	1,255	10	2
March	1,022	7	1
April	1,159	4	0
May	845	3	0
June	789	3	1
July	981	2	0
August	897	4	0
September	1,157	4	0
October	1,066	7	2
November	1,074	4	1
December	542	5	1
Total	11,376	59	9

Date of Report 1/2/20XX

Source: ©AHIMA.

Follow-up

These findings of the audit/monitoring should be shared with the chief security officer and the compliance committee as it is their responsibility to monitor the compliance or lack of compliance with the security rule. The workforce that is responsible for the metric(s) audited/monitored should be notified of the results as well.

When issues are identified, the topic should be rereviewed after corrective action plans have been enacted in order to confirm that the changes were effective. For example, if a change in policy was enacted, then the metric needs to be reassessed to determine if the expected change occurred and if additional alterations in the policy are needed to reach the desired threshold. If the desired threshold is met, that does not mean that the metric no longer needs to be audited/monitored. It would continue to be monitored as per the compliance program schedule.

Training

The HIPAA security rule mandates ongoing security training. This means that the CE not only has to train new employees but existing employees as well. There is no mandate for a specific schedule so the CE has flexibility. The CE must prove that the training was performed. This proof is shown through the documentation. As stated in earlier in this chapter, the documentation includes sign-in sheets, training materials, and more. The security rule does not mandate a particular format such as paper or electronic – just that the materials are retained for six years. Auditing would be required not only to confirm presences of the documentation but that all members of the workforce are included in the training. The documentation would also need to prove that the CE ensured that the workforce gets the appropriate level of training. All members of the workforce would need security awareness training but some would need more in-depth training. The in-depth training would be developed based on the role that the workforce member has in the CE. For more on training, refer to chapter 12.

Compliance Monitoring and Information Systems

Technology can be a valuable tool in compliance audits and monitoring as well as investigations of breaches. It can be used to track compliance efforts, investigate issues, create reports, and much more. The technology utilized can include computer forensics, databases, and dashboards.

Computer Forensics

Computer forensics is the "application of investigation and analysis techniques to gather and preserve evidence from a particular computing device in a way that is suitable for presentation in a court of law" (Techtarget n.d.). In computer forensics, steps are taken in order to isolate the computer's storage media so that it cannot be destroyed or altered, either accidently or on purpose. The hard drive is then copied so that investigators can research what happened by using the copy, not the original. This prevents changes from being made in the original so that it can be used in court or for other purposes (Techtarget n.d.). Review of the hard drive may identify unauthorized deletions, evidence of hacking, alteration of data, and much more.

Databases

A database is an organized collection of data, text, references, or pictures in a standardized format, typically stored in a computer system for multiple applications. A database can be created to store compliance activities and the results. The database could track training, audits, actions, and so forth. The database can be used to create reports, download into spreadsheets, trending, and more. As with all databases, data quality is always critical. Refer to chapter 3 for more on data quality.

Dashboard

A dashboard is a display of process measures to help leaders follow progress to assist with strategic planning. The dashboard will display the metrics established by the CE so that the chief security officer will know where the CE stands with regards to compliance with the HIPAA security rule. The dashboard might include the number of security breaches, number of patients impacted by security breaches, percentage of employees who are current on training, the number of members of the workforce current on their training, number of patients impacted by security breach, number of triggers reviewed, and more.

CHECK YOUR UNDERSTANDING 13.2

1. Identify the entity with oversight of the HIPAA security rule.

   a. Office of the Inspector General
   b. Office of Civil Rights
   c. Centers for Medicare and Medicaid Services
   d. Office of the National Coordinator of Health Information Technology

2. The document issued by OCR that outlines the failures of the CE and what their responsibilities are is known as:

   a. Policy and procedure
   b. Resolution agreement
   c. Audit
   d. Report

3. Identity the correct statement regarding auditing the security rule.

   a. The audit program is only required for the technical safeguards.
   b. The audit program is based solely on risks.
   c. The audit program includes administrative, physical, and technical safeguards.
   d. The audit program utilizes only automatically captured data.

4. A body of methods that help describe facts, detect patterns, develop explanations, and test hypotheses is known as:

   a. Data analysis
   b. Monitoring
   c. Auditing
   d. Data collection

5. The CE has a suspected security breach. They need to review data on the hard drive. The first step is to:

   a. Check the database
   b. Isolate storage media
   c. Review the audit trail
   d. Copy the hard drive

Real World Case 13.1

In 2019, the University of Rochester Medical Center (URMC) was penalized $3,000,000 for failure to meet the HIPAA security rule requirements. The personal laptop of a resident was stolen. This laptop contained unencrypted ePHI. Investigation of the incident by HHS resulted in a number of violations:

- Disclosure of 43 patient's ePHI due to the stolen laptop
- Failure to conduct comprehensive risk analysis
- Failure to implement appropriate policies and procedures to protect hardware and other electronic media, share policies and procedures with workforce
- Failure to encrypt and decrypt ePHI or to implement an equivalent measure

HHS developed a corrective action plan which would last for two years. During this time URMC had to conduct a risk analysis, develop and implement a risk management plan, implement HHS's recommendations, develop policies and procedures related to risk analysis and risk management, report failures and more, URMC had to submit a report within 120 days and submit annual reports.

Source: HHS 2019b.

Real World Case 13.2

Tuscaloosa Medical Center has just been notified via letter that they have been selected for a security audit by the OCR. This review is not due to a compliant but rather a random review. The letter states that they will receive additional information and instructions within the next month. Tuscaloosa Medical Center is a 400-bed hospital with a wide range of services. They frantically begin reviewing their security plan and all of the actions they have taken over the past few years as they wait for the additional information.

REVIEW QUESTIONS

1. An engaged listener

   a. Understands only the words.
   b. Understands what is said and not said
   c. Interprets nonverbal communications
   d. Is stressed by the message received

2. An audit is conducted to determine if the security compliance program is working. This type of audit is known as:

   a. Product audit
   b. Process audit
   c. System audit
   d. Monitoring

3. Security complaints are reviewed in a process known as:

   a. Intake & review
   b. Resolution agreement
   c. Investigation
   d. Compliance

4. The goal to meet or exceed is known as:

   a. Metric
   b. Threshold
   c. Selection
   d. Resolution agreement

5. Field work would include:

   a. Developing thresholds
   b. Observations
   c. Data analysis
   d. Planning

REVIEW QUESTIONS (*Continued*)

6. Unbiased, factual, first hand, traceable, and impersonal evidence is known as _____ evidence.

   a. Fact-based
   b. Impartial
   c. Independent
   d. Objective

7. The data collected for an audit should

   a. Address what happened today
   b. Support the purpose of the audit
   c. Be easy to collect
   d. All be electronically captured

8. The audit step that requires the CE to determine if a change in policy worked is known as:

   a. Follow-up
   b. Planning
   c. Field work
   d. Reporting

9. Training documentation must be retained for _____ years.

   a. 4
   b. 6
   c. 8
   d. 10

10. The tool used to display current status of metrics is known as:

    a. Database
    b. Report
    c. Dashboard
    d. Computer forensics

References

45 CFR §§164.30—164.312. 2013. Security and Privacy. https://www.hhs.gov/sites/default/files/ocr/privacy/hipaa/administrative/combined/hipaa-simplification-201303.pdf.

45 CFR 164.308(a)(1)(ii)(C). 2013. Administrative Safeguards. https://www.govregs.com/regulations/expand/title45_chapterA_part164_subpartC_section164.308#title45_chapterA_part164_subpartC_section164.308.

45 CFR §§ 164.400-414. 2013. Breach Notification Rule. https://www.hhs.gov/hipaa/for-professionals/breach-notification/index.html.

Aleixo, J. 2018. Healthcare Compliance Auditing and Monitoring. https://emptech.com/healthcare-compliance-auditing-monitoring/.

American Health Information Management Association. 2017. *Pocket Glossary of Health Information Management and Technology,* 5th ed. Chicago: AHIMA.

American Society for Quality. 2020. What is Auditing? https://asq.org/quality-resources/auditing#ThreeTypes.

Cochran, C. 2017. Internal Auditing in Plain English. Patton Professional: Chico, CA.

Department of Health and Human services. 2020. Enforcement Results by Year. https://www.hhs.gov/hipaa/for-professionals/compliance-enforcement/data/enforcement-results-by-year/index.html

Department of Health and Human Services. 2019a. Enforcement Data. https://www.hhs.gov/hipaa/for-professionals/compliance-enforcement/data/index.html.

Department of Health and Human Services. 2019b. Resolution Agreement. https://www.hhs.gov/sites/default/files/urmc-ra-cap-508.pdf.

Department of Health and Human Services. 2017a. Enforcement Process. https://www.hhs.gov/hipaa/for-professionals/compliance-enforcement/enforcement-process/index.html.

Department of Health and Human Services. 2017b. What OCR Considers During Intake Review. https://www.hhs.gov/hipaa/for-professionals/compliance-enforcement/examples/what-ocr-considers-during-intake-and-review/index.html.

Department of Health and Human Services. 2016. HIPAA Privacy, Security, and Beach Notification Audit Program. https://www.hhs.gov/hipaa/for-professionals/compliance-enforcement/audit/index.html#who.

Kashyap, D. 2019. Here's How Effective Communication is in the Hands of 73% of Professionals. https://www.proofhub.com/articles/effective-communication.

MedProGroup. 2018. Developing an Effective Compliance Plan: A Guide for Healthcare Practices. https://www.medpro.com/documents/10502/2837997/Guideline_Developing+an+Effective+Compliance+Program.pdf.

Merriam-Webster. 2020. Metric. https://www.merriam-webster.com/dictionary/metric.

Munim, A. 2017. 18 of the Best Code of Conduct Examples. https://i-sight.com/resources/18-of-the-best-code-of-conduct-examples/.

Oachs, P. K. and M. L. Watters. 2020. Health Information Management: Concepts, Principles, and Practice. AHIMA Press: Chicago.

Office of the Inspector General. nd. Health Care Compliance Program Tips. https://oig.hhs.gov/compliance/provider-compliance-training/files/Compliance101tips508.pdf.

Reachout. 2016. How to Put Together an Effective Audit Program. https://www.reachoutsuite.com/put-together-effective-audit-program/.

Robinson, L., J. Segal, & M. Smith. 2019. Effective Communication. https://www.helpguide.org/articles/relationships-communication/effective-communication.htm.

Techtarget. n.d. Computer Forensics. https://searchsecurity.techtarget.com/definition/computer-forensics.

University of Oregon. n.d. Audit Process. https://internalaudit.uoregon.edu/report/audit-process.

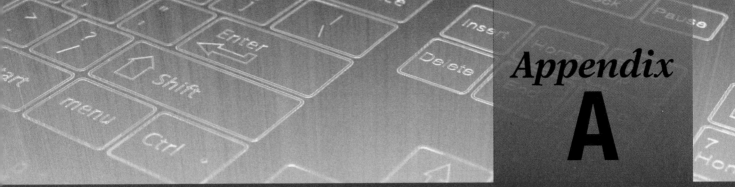

Source: American Health Information Management Association. 2010. RFI/RFP template (Updated). http://library.ahima.org/xpedio/groups/public/documents/ahima/bok1_047959 .hcsp?dDocName=bok1_047959.

The request for information/request for proposal (RFI/RFP) process is vital to procuring a system that meets organizational and user needs. Because of this, it is imperative that adequate time be allotted for the process.

This template is provided as a sample tool to assist healthcare providers as they issue an RFI or an RFP for electronic health record (EHR) or component systems. It is meant to be used in conjunction with the practice brief titled "The RFP Process for EHR Systems."

Healthcare providers should customize this sample template by using the components that are applicable for their needs, adding components as necessary, and deleting those that are not.

Sections 1 and 2 should be completed by the facility.

1. Introduction (introducing the facility to the vendor)
   a. Brief Description of the Facility
   b. Facility Information
      i. Complete Address
      ii. Market (acute, ambulatory, long-term care, home health)
      iii. Enterprise Information. The organizations should provide all relevant information including whether the facility is a part of a healthcare delivery system, the facilities that are included in the project, and their locations.
      iv. Size. The organization should provide any information that will be relevant to the product such as the number of discharges, visits, beds, etc.
      v. General Description of Current Systems Environment. The organization should provide general information regarding current information systems structure (i.e., hardware and operating systems).
   c. Scope
      The organization should provide a brief narrative description of the project that the RFP covers and the environment sought (e.g., phased approach, hybrid support).

2. Statement of Purpose
   a. Overall Business Objectives/Drivers
      The organization should list high-level business goals it is looking to achieve by implementing the software.

b. Key Desired Functionality
When requesting information for the facility-wide solution (e.g., EHR), the organization should list the various features and functions of the system desired, as well as any pertinent details.

   i. Clinical Repository

   ii. Clinical Documentation

   iii. Computerized Physician Order Entry (CPOE)

   iv. Ancillary Support (e.g., laboratory, radiology, pharmacy, etc.)

   v. Picture Archiving Communication System (PACS)

   vi. Electronic Document Management/Document Imaging

   vii. Customizable Workflow Management

   viii. Interoperability (e.g., for health information exchange)

   ix. Patient Portals

   x. Other

c. HIM Department Operations
When requesting information for the HIM solution, the organization should list the various processes and functions of the system it is looking for, as well as any pertinent details.

   i. Chart Analysis/Deficiency Management

   ii. Coding/Abstracting

   iii. Patient Identity Management/Electronic Master Patient Index (e-MPI)

   iv. Health Record Output and Disclosure Management

   v. Release of Information

   vi. Screen Input Design

   vii. Support for Mandated Reportable Data Sets

   viii. Other

d. System Administration—Records Management and Evidentiary Support
This functionality is applicable to or used for all components or modules of an application. Facility requirements for this functionality should be specified in the detailed system requirements.

   i. User Administration

   ii. Access Privilege Control Management

   iii. Logging/Auditing Function

   iv. Digital Signature Functions

   v. Records Management Function

   vi. Archiving Functions

   vii. Continuity of Operations (e.g., support for backup, recovery)

   viii. Maintenance of Standardized Vocabularies and Code Sets

e. Future Plans
General description of long-term plans, including identified future systems environment and projected timetables.

Sections 3 and 4 should be completed by the vendor.

3. Requirements
Vendors should provide availability and timelines for development of software to fulfill requirements not available at this time.

a. User Requirements

Each functional area is expected to have its own set of user requirements.

Sample questions related to HIM functional user requirements and features are provided below. This table is a sample only. Organizations must customize this RFP template to meet their needs.

Functional User Requirements/Features (Also refer to certification requirements and Health Level Seven (HL7) EHR System Functional Model (EHR-S FM) for other key requirements/features.)	Available	Custom Developed	Future Development	Not Available
Chart Completion/Deficiency Analysis				
Can the organization define the intervals for aging analysis (e.g., 7 days, 14 days, 21 days, etc.)?				
Does the system allow for standard and ad-hoc reporting for chart deficiency/delinquency analysis?				
Can delinquency reports be sent to physicians/clinicians in electronic (e.g., e-mail or fax) and paper formats (letters)?				
Does the system allow you to define or detail all deficiencies by provider, by area of deficiency, or other combinations (e.g., group practices, etc.)?				
Does the system allow the organization to list all records (charts) by the deficiency type?				
Can deficiency analysis be conducted at the time the patient is prepared for discharge from the facility?				
Does the system support most industry standard dictation systems to allow transcribed reports to be easily and efficiently completed?				
Does the system allow for end-user notification when information identified as incomplete/missing is completed?				
Coding Completion/Analysis				
Does the system support automation of coding work flow (e.g., computer-assisted coding)?				

(Continued)

Functional User Requirements/Features (Also refer to certification requirements and Health Level Seven (HL7) EHR System Functional Model (EHR-S FM) for other key requirements/features.)	Available	Custom Developed	Future Development	Not Available
Does the system support automated case assignment to work queues?				
Can the user assign cases based on special attributes (e.g., VIP, dollars, or case type such as cancer or trauma, etc.)?				
Does the system support online communication between employees and managers?				
Does the system support most industry standard encoders/groupers?				
Does the system support both on-site and remote coding activities?				
Does the system support assignment of high-risk coding to supervisory staff or allow coding verification as staff complete cases?				
Does the system contain tools for monitoring and evaluating the coding process?				
Does the system support electronic query capabilities?				
Coding/Transaction Standards (see also Section 4.k)				
Does the system support ICD-10-CM and/or ICD-10-PCS in addition to ICD-9-CM?				
Does the system use General Equivalence Mappings (GEMs), such as between ICD-10-CM/PCS and ICD-9-CM or SNOMED CT and ICD-9-CM?				
Is the system compliant with the Version 5010 transaction standard?				
Health Record Output and Disclosure				
Does the system allow a unified view of all component subsystems of the EHR at the individual patient level and at the date of service encounter level for purposes of disclosure management (including the ability to print and generate electronic output)?				

Does the system provide the ability to define the records or reports that are considered the formal health record for a specified disclosure or disclosure purposes?			
Does the system allow VIP patients to be flagged and listed confidentially on corresponding reports (i.e., census)?			
Does the system produce an accounting of disclosure, reporting at a minimum the date and time a disclosure took place, what was disclosed, to whom, by whom, and the reason for disclosure?			
Does the system provide the ability to create hard copy and electronic output of report summary information and to generate reports in both chronological and specified record elements order?			
Does the system provide the ability to include patient identifying information on each page of electronically generated reports and provide the ability to customize reports to match mandated formats?			
Does the system allow for redaction and recording the reason, in addition to the ability to redact patient information from larger reports?			

Release of Information (Note: Administrative release of information functionality may or may not be an integral component of an EHR system.)

Does the system support HIPAA management of non-TPO disclosures?			
Does the system track and report the date/time release of information requests are received and fulfilled?			
Does the system allow the ability to track whether the release of information consent/authorization was adequate, in addition to a corresponding disposition?			
Does the system generate invoices with user-defined pay scales?			

(Continued)

Functional User Requirements/Features (Also refer to certification requirements and Health Level Seven (HL7) EHR System Functional Model (EHR-S FM) for other key requirements/features.)	Available	Custom Developed	Future Development	Not Available
Does the system allow tracking of payments received?				
Does the system generate template letters for standard correspondence (e.g., patient not found, date of service not valid, etc.)?				
Does the system allow information to be released electronically?				
Authentication				
Does the system authenticate principals (i.e., users, entities, applications, devices, etc.) before accessing the system and prevent access to all nonauthenticated principals?				
Does the system require authentication mechanisms and can the system securely store authentication data/information?				
If user names and passwords are used, does the system require password strength rules that allow for a minimum				
number of characters and inclusion of alphanumeric complexity, while preventing the reuse of previous passwords, without being transported or viewable in plain text?				
Does the system have the ability to terminate or lock a session after a period of inactivity or after a series of invalid log-in attempts?				
Access Controls				
Does the system provide the ability to create and update sets of access-control permissions granted to principals (i.e., users, entities, applications, devices, etc.) based on the user's role and scope of practice?				
Does the system inactivate a user and remove the user's privileges without deleting the user's history?				

Does the system have the ability to record and report all authorization actions?				
Does the system allow only authorized users access to confidential information?				
Does the system prevent users with read and/or write privileges from printing or copying/writing to other media?				
Does the system define and enforce system and data access rules for all EHR system				
resources (at component, application, or user level, either local or remote)?				
Does the system restrict access to patient information based on location (e.g., nursing unit, clinic, etc.)?				
Does the system track restrictions?				
Does the system have the ability to track/audit viewed records without significant effect on system speed?				
Does the system allow for electronic access to specified patients/encounters for external reviewers?				

Emergency Access Controls

Does the system allow emergency access regardless of controls or established user levels, within a set time parameter?				
Does the system define the acceptable circumstances in which the user can override the controls for emergency access, as well as require the user to specify the circumstance?				
Does the system require a second level of validation before granting a user emergency access?				
Can a report be generated of all emergency access use?				
Does the system provide the ability to periodically review/renew a user's emergency access privileges?				

(Continued)

Functional User Requirements/Features (Also refer to certification requirements and Health Level Seven (HL7) EHR System Functional Model (EHR-S FM) for other key requirements/features.)	Available	Custom Developed	Future Development	Not Available
Does the system provide the ability to generate an after-action report to trigger follow-up of emergency access use?				
Information Attestation				
Does the system provide the ability for attestation (verification) of EHR content by properly authenticated and authorized users different from the author (e.g., countersignature) as allowed by users' scope of practice, organizational policy, or jurisdictional law?				
If more than one author contributed to the EHR content, does the system provide the ability to associate and maintain all authors/contributors with their content?				
If the EHR content was attested to by someone other than the author, does the system maintain all authors and contributors?				
Does the system provide the ability to present (e.g., view, report, display, access) the credentials and the name of the author(s) and the attester, as well as the date and time of attestation?				
Data Retention, Availability, and Destruction				
Does the system provide the ability to store and retrieve health record data and clinical				
documents for the legally prescribed time or according to organizational policy and to include unaltered inbound data?				
Does the system provide the ability to identify specific EHR data for destruction and allow for the review and confirmation of selected items before destruction occurs?				

Does the system provide the ability to destroy EHR data/records so that data are not retrievable in a reasonably accessible and usable format according to policy and legal retentions periods, and is a certificate of destruction generated?			

Record Preservation

Does the system provide the ability to identify records that must be preserved beyond normal retention practices and identify a reason for preserving the record?			
Does the system provide the ability to generate a legal hold notice identifying whom to contact for questions when a user attempts to alter a record on legal hold or an unauthorized user attempts to access a record on legal hold?			
Does the system provide the ability to secure data/records from unauditable alteration or unauthorized use for preservation purposes, such as a legal hold?			
Does the system provide the ability to merge and unmerge records?			
Does the system allow a record to be locked after a specified time so no more changes may be made?			

Minimum Metadata Set and Audit Capability for Record Actions

Does the system capture and retain the date, time stamp, and user for every object/ data creation, modification, view, deletion, or printing/export of any part of the medical record?			
Does the system retain a record of the viewer?			
Does the system retain a record of the author of a change?			
Does the system retain a record of the change history?			

(Continued)

Functional User Requirements/Features (Also refer to certification requirements and Health Level Seven (HL7) EHR System Functional Model (EHR-S FM) for other key requirements/features.)	Available	Custom Developed	Future Development	Not Available
Does the system retain a record of the source of nonoriginated data?				
Does the system retain the medical record metadata for the legally prescribed time frame in accordance with the organizational policy?				
Does the system include the minimum metadata set for a record exchanged or released?				
Pending State				
Does the system apply a date and time-stamp each time a note is updated (opened/signature event)?				
Does the system display and notify the author of pending notes?				
Does the system allow the ability to establish a time frame for pending documents before administrative closing?				
Does the system display pending notes in a way that clearly identifies them as pending?				
Does the system allow the author to complete, edit, or delete (if never viewed for patient care) the pending note?				
Amendments and Corrections				
Does the system allow the author to correct, amend, or augment a note or entry?				
Does the system allow the author to indicate whether the change was a correction, amendment, or augmentation?				
Does the system record and display the date and time stamp of the change?				
Does the system provide a clear indicator of a changed record?				
Does the system provide a link or clear direction to the original entry/note?				

Does the system retain all versions?				
Does the system disseminate updated information to providers that were initially autofaxed?				
Documentation Succession Management and Version Control				
Does the system manage the succession of documents?				
Does the system retain all versions when a change is made?				
Does the system provide an indicator that there are prior versions (when appropriate)?				
Does the system indicate the most recent version?				
Retracted State				
Does the system allow for removing a record or note from view?				
Does the system allow for access of a retracted note or record?				
Does the system allow the user to record the reason for retraction?				
Does the system allow for notification of the viewers of the data to present correct information (if applicable)?				
Data Collection and Reporting				
Does the system allow for real-time data collectionand progress measurement against preset targets?				
Does the system produce reports on turnaround days, dollars pending, costs per				
chart by process, days to billing, and so on, as related to AR?				
Does the system have the ability to track clinical decision-making alerts (e.g., when they were added to the system or discontinued, used, ignored, etc.)?				

(Continued)

Does the system comply with meaningful use reporting requirements?				
Patient Financial Support				
Is your proposed solution fully integrated (or able to interface with the patient financial system), offering users an electronic form of the business office?				
Can patient information be placed in folders to easily identify those details that refer to the patient (guarantor) account(s)?				
Can you electronically capture, store, and retrieve computer-generated documents and reports, such as the UB-04 or the CMS 1500, which are HIPAA transaction standard compliant?				
Patient Portals				
Does the system allow for electronic patient access (e.g., Web portal)?				
Health Information Exchange				
Does the system enable participation in local health information exchange initiatives?				

b. System Requirements

Organizations should provide a list to vendors of what current technology needs to be supported. Vendors should then provide information on their system's available requirements.

Sample questions related to system requirements and features are provided below. This table is a sample only. Organizations must customize this RFP template to meet their needs.

System Requirements/Features (*Also refer to certification requirements and Health Level Seven (HL7) EHR System Functional Model (EHR-S FM) for other key requirements/features.)	Available	Custom Developed	Future Development	Not Available
General System Requirements				
Is the system integrated or interfaced?				
Does the system provide the ability to archive via tape, CD, or DVD? Describe any other options.				
Are the COLD (computer output to laser disc) data streams available in ASCII (American Standard Code for Information Interchange)?				

Does the system support audit trails at the folder level for managing access, editing, and printing of documents?				
Does the system make audit trail logs available to the organization, including the date, time, user, and location?				
Does the system support an online help function/feature?				
Is the proposed solution scalable (e.g., can it support 50 to 800 workstations, concurrent users, etc.)?				
Does the system have the capability of recording change management logs related to platform upgrades and patches?				
Can the system identify or distinguish the facility location in a multi-entity environment?				
Can the system support a centralized database across multiple facilities?				
How compliant is your product with the HL7's EHR-S FM and EHR profiles? (Please provide us with your HL7 EHR-S FM and profile conformance statements.)				
System Security				
Does the system monitor security attempts for those without user rights and those logged in the audit trail/log?				
Does the system track all activity/functions, including where they change the database, and can they be managed through the audit trail/log?				
Does the system use encryption methods that render protected health information unreadable in compliance with the latest industry approaches and guidelines?				
Technical Requirements				
Do communication components include TCP/IP (transmission control protocol/ internet protocol)?				

(Continued)

System Requirements/Features (*Also refer to certification requirements and Health Level Seven (HL7) EHR System Functional Model (EHR-S FM) for other key requirements/features.)	Available	Custom Developed	Future Development	Not Available
Does the system use CCITT Group III, IV for compression schemes?				
Does the system support standard HL7 record formatting for all input and output?				
Does the system support SQL for communication?				
Does the system support thin client PCs?				
Is the system sized for capacity to allow for planning? Describe your recommendations.				
Does the system support disk shadowing and system redundancy provisions? Please describe.				
Can your solution be supported as an Application Service Provider (ASP) hosted model?				
Does the system support browser-based options?				
Integration of Narrative Notes				
Does the system support HL7's Clinical Document Architecture Release 2 (CDA-R2) standard for the encoding of narrative, text-based clinical information?				
Does the system receive, display, transform, and parse CDA-encoded clinical documents as described in the HL7 CDA-R2 Implementation Guides for document types, such as History and Physical Note, Consultation Note, Operative Note, and Diagnostic Imaging Report?				
Does the system receive, display, transform, and parse CDA-R2-compliant documents with encoded headers (Level 1 encoding)?				
Does the system process CDA-R2-compliant documents that include Level 2 encoding?				
Does the system process CDA-R2-compliant documents that include Level 3 encoding?				

c. Interfaces

Organizations should provide a list of existing interfaces that will need to be supported, as well as new interfaces that will have to be created and supported, including any pertinent interoperability information that exists and will be needed in the future. Vendors should provide information regarding their system's ability to meet the organization's interface requirements.

4. Vendor Questionnaire

The organization should request information about the vendor and the product to assist with decision making.

a. Vendor Background and Financial Information
   i. Company Name and Geography. The organization should request an address of a branch close to the facility, as well as the headquarters. Staff may want to visit both.
   ii. Company Goals
   iii. Year the Company Was Established, Significant Company Merges, Acquisitions, and Sell-offs
   iv. Whether the Vendor Is Public or Privately Owned
   v. Bankruptcy/Legal Issues (including under which name the bankruptcy was filed and when, or any pertinent lawsuits, closed or pending, filed against the company)
   vi. Research and Development Investment (expressed in a total amount or percentage of total sales)
   vii. Status of Certification

b. Statement of Key Differentiators

The vendor should provide a statement describing what differentiates its products and services from those of its competitors.

c. Customer Base and References
   i. Customer List (or total number of customers per feature or function, if a list of customers cannot be provided owing to confidentiality/privacy concerns)
   ii. References That Can Be Contacted. The vendor should provide references the facility can contact/visit based on product features and functions most suitable to the facility, as well as those using the latest versions of the software.

d. Qualifications
   i. The vendor should provide a list of qualifications and resume, including a sample list of similar projects and clients.

e. User Participation
   i. User Groups

   Organizations should provide a list of the user groups and ask whether it can attend a meeting or a call for review purposes.

   ii. Requirements Gathering

   The vendor should request information regarding customer participation in requirements-gathering stages of system development. How is customer feedback, such as requests for new requirements, handled?

f. Technology

The vendor should provide technology specifications that support the product (e.g., database, architecture, operating system, ASP versus in-house, etc.).

g. Services

The vendor should describe the services offered and corresponding fees (if applicable).

   i. Project Management

   ii. Consulting

   iii. MPI Cleanup

   iv. Integration

   v. Legal Health Record Definition

   vi. Process Reengineering

   vii. Other

h. Training

The vendor should outline the training provided during and after implementation.

i. Product Documentation. The vendor should specify the product documentation that is available and its formats.

j. Implementation/Migration. The vendor should provide detailed information about the implementation such as the timelines and resources required.

k. Data Conversion

   i. If the system is not currently ICD-10-CM/PCS or Version 5010 compliant, describe plans for becoming compliant by regulatory required dates.

   ii. How will the system handle both ICD-9-CM and ICD-10-CM/PCS data?

   iii. How long will the system support both ICD-9-CM and ICD-10-CM/PCS codes?

   iv. If the system uses General Equivalence Mappings (GEMs), such as between ICD-10-CM/PCS and ICD-9-CM, describe how the integrity of the maps is maintained.

   v. Describe other data conversions (e.g., document imaging, platform conversions).

l. Maintenance

   i. Updates/Upgrades

   The vendor should provide information on how the system is maintained, including how often the updates/upgrades are applied, methods used (e.g., remotely, on-site), and by whom.

   ii. Compliance with Meaningful Use Incentive Requirements

   The vendor should provide its plan for addressing meaningful use on an ongoing basis, including plans for achieving corresponding certification requirements.

   iii. Expected Product Lifetime

   The vendor should outline the expected time frame for the next version requiring a different platform or operating system upgrade

   iv. Customer Support

   The vendor should outline the types of customer support packages offered (e.g., 24/7, weekday only), methods of support (e.g., help desk or tickets), and the tools used (e.g., 800 number, e-mail, web-based, etc.).

   v. Expected Facility Support

   The vendor should outline the number of full-time employees expected to support the product at the facility.

m. Pricing Structure

    i. Product Software Pricing

        1. Price

        The vendor should provide the price of the proposed solution, broken down by application/module, including licensing fees.

        2. Cost of Ownership (breakdown over a certain number of proposed contract years)

        3. Other Costs (maintenance, upgrades, consultation and support fees, post-implementation training and services, travel, etc.)

        4. Discounts (available discounts such as those based on participating as a beta site)

    ii. Invoicing (fee schedule and terms)

    iii. Return on Investment

    iv. Acceptance Period

    The vendor should outline the terms for validating the product after implementation and the refund policy

n. Warranty

The organization should request a copy of the warranty, as well as how it is affected by maintenance and support agreements after the implementation period

Sections 5 and 6 are to be completed by the facility.

5. Vendor Requirements and Instructions

a. RFP Questions

The facility should provide the name and contact information of one person to whom all questions concerning the RFP should be directed. Generally, questions about the RFP must be submitted in writing within a given time frame, and the questions and answers are distributed to all vendors responding to the RFP. Provide the preferred method of contact, such as fax number or e-mail.

b. Response Format, Deadline, and Delivery

c. Contract Duration

The facility should request that the vendor to disclose how long the returned information will be considered valid.

6. Terms and Conditions

a. Confidentiality

State confidentiality rules in regard to the information the facility disclosed in the RFP as well as the rules pertaining to the information provided by the vendor).

b. Information Access

The facility should describe who will have access to the returned RFP and for what purpose.

c. Bid Evaluation and Negotiation

The facility should briefly describe the evaluation process and the deadlines and provide the appropriate information if vendors are allowed to negotiate after the evaluation is complete.

d. Formal Presentation

The facility should describe process and format requirements if the vendor is invited to present the software product suite.

e. Acceptance or Rejection

The facility should describe how the vendor will be notified regardless of whether the product is selected or not.

f. Contract Provisions

The facility should note the sections of the RFP response that can be included in the final contract.

g. Type of Contract

The facility should let the vendor know if this will be firm fixed price, cost plus fixed fee, a time and materials, or other type of contract.

Check Your Understanding Answer Key

Chapter 1

1.1.

1. **b.** Extranets are used to access the healthcare facility's systems by those outside of the organization.
2. **b.** Cloud computing is the delivery of computational services (e.g., analytics, storage, and application sharing) by a vendor over the Internet.
3. **a.** Documenting patient care at the bedside is known s point of care.
4. **a.** Financial applications were the first information systems used in healthcare organizations.
5. **b.** The intranet can be used to store policies, menus, forms, and more.

1.2.

1. **d.** While both the RHIA and RHIT certifications have some coding included, the only one of these certifications that is solely coding is the CCS.
2. **d.** Dashboards provide current status on key indicators.
3. **a.** Prescriptive analytics uses descriptive data to make recommendations for the future so it helps the healthcare organization decide their best options.
4. **b.** Many HIM professionals are able to work from home and some HIM departments are now virtual.
5. **d.** Clinical pathways are a tool designed to coordinate multidisciplinary care planning for specific diagnoses and treatments.

Chapter 2

2.1.

1. **d.** Data integrity tools include edit checks and required fields.
2. **c.** Hot spots provide additional information about the data element.
3. **c.** Radio buttons are good for a small number of entry choices such as with gender.

    4. b. Health records are a primary data source.

    5. a. Drop down boxes are good to limit entries but allows a number of options from which to choose.

2.2.

    1. d. Authorship is identifying who created an entry.

    2. c. Data cleansing is looking for and addressing duplication of data, missing data, and outliers.

    3. a. Documentation integrity issues include copy and paste, authorship, amendments, and more.

    4. a. Data relevancy is the extent to which healthcare-related data are useful for the purposes for which they were collected.

    5. b. Data consistency ensures that like data are the same on each document or computer screen

Chapter 3

3.1.

    1. c. Autonumbering provides a unique number that will never be assigned again.

    2. a. Normalization is breaking the data elements into the level of detail desired by the healthcare facility.

    3. b. A record is data collected on a single patient.

    4. a. Words such as "and," "or," and "not" are used to restrict queries.

    5. c. The data dictionary specifies the metadata including the length of a field.

    6. c. A mask allows the user to enter characters without the formatting. The information converts the data into the correct format.

    7. a. New question, need to provide rationale

    8. d. New question, need to provide rationale

    9. b. New question, need to provide rationale

    10. d. New question, need to provide rationale

    11. a. New question, need to provide rationale

3.2.

    1. a. An entity is a person, location, thing, or concept that is to be tracked in the database.

    2. c. A data flow diagram shows how data flows within an information system.

    3. b. An attribute is a fact about an entity.

    4. a. A relational database stores data in rows and columns—in other words, a table.

    5. b. A use case is used to show developers how users will use the information system.

Chapter 4

4.1.

    1. b. A project lasts for a finite period of time and has a specific outcome. Implementing an EHR is a project.

2. **c.** A feasibility study is conducted by the healthcare organization to determine if a proposed IS is an appropriate option to meet the objectives of the healthcare organization

3. **d.** The critical path shows the steps that must stay on track to prevent the implementation date from slipping.

4. **c.** The Gantt chart is a project management tool that records specific tasks, their start and end dates, the person responsible for the tasks, and any connections between tasks.

5. **a.** Scope creep occurs when the definition of the project expands during the project.

4.2.

1. **a.** Functional requirements are a list of functions or tasks that the IS must be able to perform.

2. **b.** Questionnaires allow for a large number of users to provide input about the needs of the IS as the results are easy to collect and analyze.

3. **a.** The RFI requests basic information on an information system.

4. **b.** The design stage is where the required functionality is identified.

5. **d.** Alpha sites partner with the IS vendor in order to design an IS.

4.3.

1. **b.** Spreadsheets can be used to compare responses to RFPs.

2. **c.** Escrow is a situation in which a third party holds a copy of the software in case the vendor goes bankrupt.

3. **c.** Contracts should always be a win-win.

4. **c.** : Creating a prototype is a way to quickly design and develop an IS.

5. **d.** A software license describes what the healthcare organization can do with the software.

Chapter 5

5.1.

1. **d.** Setting configurations populate tables, control when bills drop, and more.

2. **c.** Computer screens are read from left to right and top to bottom.

3. **a.** Site preparation is ensuring there is space, electrical sockets, and anything else needed to add computers to an area.

4. **a.** Data conversion is changing data from one format to another.

5. **d.** Reengineering is evaluating the way the healthcare organization does business in order to improve efficiency

5.2.

1. **b.** The testing plan should create a realistic test environment, which is an exact duplicate of the IS in use, excluding the live data. In this test environment, changes can be made to the IS and then tested to see what happens.

2. **d.** The parallel go-live model operates the old information system and the new information system to ensure the new information is working as expected.

3. a. Adults like to have a say in their education, and they have a need to see the relevance of what they are learning.

4. b. Rationale: Volume testing confirms that the IS and the network can handle the large volume of users and data.

5. c. Support and evaluation include day to day maintenance and determining what you could do better with the next implementation.

Chapter 6

6.1.

1. b. Health informatics is the scientific discipline that is concerned with the cognitive, information-processing, and communication tasks of healthcare practice, education, and research, including the information science and technology to support these tasks.

2. a. Data analytics is the science of examining raw data with the purpose of drawing conclusions about that information; it is a subset of informatics.

3. d. Mapping specialist must be an expert in both ICD-9-CM and ICD-10-CM systems so that they can correctly create the links between old and new diagnostic codes.

4. d. The chief security officer (CSO) is responsible for protecting data from unauthorized access, alteration, and destruction.

5. a. Hard skills include: informatics, data analytic, and data use..

6.2.

1. c. The encoder is specialty software used by coders to select the appropriate code for the diagnosis(es) and procedure(s) supported by the health record.

2. c. The automated codebook encoder is an encoder that lists diagnoses and procedures in alphabetic order much like the alphabetic index located in the International Classification of Diseases, Tenth Edition, Clinical Modification (ICD-10-CM) and Current Procedural Terminology (CPT) codebooks.

3. a. The grouper is a computer program that uses specific data elements to assign the diagnostic and procedural codes entered into the encoder into the appropriate Medicare severity diagnosis-related groups (MS-DRG) or other diagnosis-related group (DRG).

4. b. The ROI system is designed to manage the processing of requests for protected health information (PHI) received and processed by the HIM department. Use of the information system begins when a new request is entered into it. It continues to track the request as it is processed and acts as a historical database of all requests processed and ultimately used to generate reports.

5. c. A disclosure management system tracks the disclosures made throughout the healthcare facility for reporting purposes. This tracking is required by the Health Insurance Portability and Accountability Act (HIPAA). The covered entities must provide the patient with an accounting of disclosures upon request.

6.3.

1. d. One of the data elements unique to the cancer registry include ICD-O codes.

2. a. A registry is a collection of care information related to a specific disease, condition, or procedure that makes health record information available for analysis and comparison.

3. **b.** The chart locator system, also called chart tracking system, is designed to identify the current location the paper health record or information.

4. **d.** The cancer registry information system tracks information about the patient's cancer TNM (tumor, node, metastasis) stage.

5. **a.** Trauma registry software tracks patients with traumatic injuries from initial trauma treatment to death.

6.4.

1. **c.** CDI is the process a healthcare entity undertakes that will improve clinical specificity and documentation that will allow coders to assign more concise disease and procedural classification codes

2. **a.** The physician uses the dictation system to dictate, but the HIM department uses the system to transcribe the report.

3. **d.** The healthcare quality indicator system is an abstracting system that records information about the patient and the care provided to the patient.

4. **a.** Birth certificate software will capture the minimum data set established by the National Center for Health Statistics (NCHS) and any state-required data.

5. **c.** Expanders allow transcriptionists to type an acronym such as "CHF" and the full phrase "congestive heart failure" will automatically be spelled out, thus saving keystrokes and time.

Chapter 7

7.1.

1. **c.** The financial information system is critical to the fiscal health of the healthcare facility. The healthcare facility must receive accurate financial information in a timely manner to monitor and manage the finances of the healthcare facility.

2. **a.** The encoder is a specialty software that helps the coders determine the most appropriate diagnostics and procedural codes which in turn are used to determines reimbursement for the healthcare facility.

3. **c.** The human resources information system (HRIS) tracks employees within the organization. This tracking includes promotions, transfers, terminations, performance appraisal due dates, and absenteeism.

4. **a.** HIM professionals should be involved in the development and management of the chargemaster. The codes and charges must be updated at least annually.

5. **d.** Both ICD-10 and CPT classification codes are updated on a regular basis. These changes must be implemented and verified within the facility's chargemaster.

6. **c.** In addition to improving the coding process, CDI also improves and supports data quality, availability, and usability—all key aspects of data governance. The quality of this documentation is vital in order to properly evaluate patient care, meet all regulatory requirements, and obtain the appropriate amount of reimbursement

7.2.

1. **c.** It is a patient-identifying directory referencing all patients related to an organization and which also serves as a link to the patient record or information, facilitates patient identification, and assists in maintaining a longitudinal patient record from birth to death.

2. **d.** An EIS dashboard report gives administration-structured information to make intelligent decisions for the future.

3. **c.** Algorithms are used by organizations to determine the "probability of a duplicate in order to identify potential duplicate MPI entries."

4. **b.** Advantages of the EIS include assistance in making strategic decisions about the facility.

5. **a.** An IDS is an organizational arrangement of a network of health providers that may include hospitals, physicians, and health maintenance organizations (HMOs) that provide coordinated services along the continuum of care from ambulatory, acute, and long-term care and may extend across a geographical region.

7.3.

1. **d.** The scheduling system can assist with many management functions. The reporting capabilities of the scheduling system can track cancellations, resource utilization, patient volume, and other topics important to management.

2. **b.** The R-ADT system generates some key reports used by many departments within the facility. These include the daily admission list, discharge list, census report, transfer list, and bed utilization reports. The facility may also generate monthly, quarterly, yearly, and ad hoc reports to show type of patient treated, number of discharges, number of admissions, occupancy rates, and other information needed.

3. **a.** The scheduling system can help with this by scheduling tests, beds, operating rooms, staff, and other resources wisely.

4. **a.** With the focus by the Joint Commission on patient safety, the physical plant is focused on providing equipment and a healthcare environment that is vital to the well-being of the guests, staff, and ultimately the patients within the facility.

5. **d.** The R-ADT system issues the health record number assignment to the patient folder.

Chapter 8

8.1.

1. **c.** OCR is defined as a method of encoding text from analog paper into bitmapped images and translating the images into a form that is computer readable.

2. **a.** Target sheets are blank pages, except for a barcode, that will tell the scanner and ultimately the computer the content of the pages that follow.

3. **c.** Indexing is the abstracting of data that will be used to retrieve the image.

4. **c.** There must be an electronic or computerized print tracking log, similar to an audit log, that indicates who requested or submitted the print order, where the printing occurred (which printer was used and in what area of the healthcare facility), date and time of printing, what forms or reports were printed, and any other pertinent information the healthcare facility deems appropriate.

5. **a.** Annotation is the ability to alter the image in some way. The highlighting tool highlights important sections of text, much like a highlighter pen on paper.

6. **c.** Providers agree to contracts with fiscal intermediaries to receive payments when the patient's health is improved, their chronic disease(s) are more efficiently managed so that they suffer from less complications, and they live healthier lives based on established criteria

7. **d.** CDS encompasses a variety of tools to enhance decision-making in the clinical workflow.

8.2.

1. **d.** In a PACS, x-rays, MRIs, mammograms, and other radiological examinations are stored digitally, thus eliminating the need to store and manage the physical film.

2. **d.** A radiology information system (RIS) is used to collect, store, and provide information on radiological tests such as x-rays, ultrasound, magnetic resonance imaging (MRI), computerized tomography (CT), and positron emission tomography (PET).

3. **b.** The ability of these images to be viewed from any location by the radiologist and other users is called teleradiology.

4. **a.** Currently, LISs involve many interfaces since they are still typically stand-alone systems, separate from the EHR. It is important for these interfaces to work seamlessly with the specified EHR system to ensure integration with the clinical and communications needs of the healthcare facility (Biedermann and Dolezel 2017, 84).

5. **c.** Picture archival communication system (PACS) is an integrated computer system that obtains, stores, retrieves, and displays digital images.

6. **a.** The LIS can assist management in running the laboratory department through the management reporting capabilities. It should be able to generate reports such as the number of tests run per month, the tests ran, turnaround time, and productivity reports on individual laboratory technicians

8.3.

1. **c.** A nursing information system will document the nursing care provided to a patient. Clinical documentation is any manual or electronic notation or recording made by a physician or other healthcare clinician related to a patient's medical condition of treatment.

2. **b.** The PIS can be stand-alone or integrated with other systems in the healthcare facility such as CPOE.

3. **b.** Smart cards enable portable storage of health and insurance information.

4. **d.** Telehealth, also known as telemedicine, is the use of telecommunications and networks to share medical and nonclinical information between a patient and a healthcare provider located at different sites.

5. **d.** The HIM professional is typically not a direct user of the various CISs discussed throughout this chapter; however, the HIM professional accesses the information through either the CIS or the EHR.

Chapter 9

9.1.

1. **b.** With its seminal publication, *To Err Is Human: Building a Safer Health System*, the Institute of Medicine, now the National Academy of Medicine (NAM), advocated for the use of health information technology (HIT) to help prevent many of mistakes that regularly occur in the delivery of healthcare that lead to the injuries and deaths of tens or thousands of patients (NAM 2000, 1).

2. **b.** Reminders can notify physicians of screenings that should be performed based on the patient's age and gender.

3. **a.** The CCR is a core data set, which is the most relevant administrative, demographic, and clinical information about a patient's healthcare, covering one or more healthcare encounters.

4. **d.** A longitudinal health record is a permanent record of significant information listed in chronological order and maintained across time, ideally from birth to death.

5. **a.** An EHR is designed to not only be used by the originating healthcare entity but be able to be referred to and transmitted to authorized and authenticated users at other healthcare entities.

9.2.

1. **b.** The PHR contains health information that comes from both the physician and the patient, but the PHR is controlled by the patient.

2. **c.** The CPOE system notifies clinical departments, such as the laboratory, radiology, physical therapy, and dietary departments, of orders made by the physician.

3. **c.** As of 2015, approximately 97 percent of hospitals had certified EHR technology.

4. **c.** The Affordable Care Act (ACA) and the Healthy People 2020 campaign support monitoring population health to create social and physical environments that promote good health.

5. **b.** EMAR, also referred to a bar-code medication administration record (BC-MAR) automates many of the medication administration processes in a healthcare facility.

9.3.

1. **a.** One of the primary barriers to EHR implementation is cost.

2. **a.** The EHR enables quick access to patient records for more coordinated, efficient care.

3. **a.** HIT has a significant role in improving the health of not only a medical practice's population, but the population on the community level.

4. **a.** Interoperability is the ability of different information systems and software applications to communicate and exchange data.

5. **b.** The hybrid record is a combination of paper and electronic health records; a health record that includes both paper and electronic elements.

6. **d.** Natural language processing (NLP) is the conversion of unstructured data into structured data through the use of computer algorithms or statistical methods.

9.4.

1. **c.** Messaging standards may also be called interoperability standards or data exchange standards.

2. **b.** Diagnostic and Statistical Manual of Mental Disorders (DSM) is a classification system of mental disorders used by mental health providers

3. **a.** Semantics is a "branch of linguistics dealing with the study of meaning, including the ways meaning is structured in language and how changes in meanings and form occur over time

4. **d.** The National Council for Prescription Drug Programs (NCPDP) is an independent SDO and is ANSI-accredited. These standards were developed for and used by retail pharmacies and payers for claims, eligibility, and remittance advice. These e-prescription standards, called SCRIPT, control data to be shared for new prescriptions, refills, and other communications between physicians and pharmacies

Chapter 11

11.1.

1. **b.** HIE is defined as the formal agreed-upon process for the seamless exchange of health information electronically between providers and others with the same level of interoperability, according to nationally recognized standards, typically through a HIO that serves as an intermediary to facilitate access and retrieval of clinical data to provide safer, timelier, efficient, effective, equitable, patient-centered care.

2. **d.** Interoperability is defined as the capability of different information systems and software applications to communicate and exchange data.

3. **c.** The Office of the National Coordinator (ONC) for Health Information Technology (ONC) was established in 2004 as a result of an executive order by President George W. Bush calling for the healthcare industry to implement an electronic system for health records and to have an interoperable communication system between all HCOs by 2014.

4. **b.** Based on the hardware and equipment connectivity used in the exchange, this type of interoperability allows any computer or device to exchange data with another computer or device without corrupting the data or creating errors.

11.2.

1. **a.** LHIOs and RHIOs are groups of healthcare organizations in specific geographic areas that share electronic health information according to accepted standards.

2. **b.** Equity of treatment and services with improved health outcomes leading to a reduction of health disparities.

3. **a.** In 2016, follow-up research from Johns Hopkins University School of Medicine indicated that number may well be above 250,000 deaths per year, making medical mistakes the third leading cause of death in the United States.

4. **a.** The eHealth Exchange Sequoia Project is a group of "federal agencies and non-federal organizations that came together under a common mission and purpose to improve patient care, streamline disability benefit claims, and improve public health reporting through secure, trusted, and interoperable health information exchange."

5. **c.** BYOD (bring your own device) refers to healthcare providers using their personal smart phones and other devices and the increase in mobile technology.

11.3.

1. **d.** Must be used in a meaningful way such as e-prescribing (eRx) and computerized provider order entry (CPOE).

2. **b.** Meaningful use (MU) is a regulation that was issued by the Centers for Medicare and Medicaid (CMS) on July 28, 2010, outlining an incentive program for eligible professionals (EPs), eligible hospitals, and critical access hospitals (CAHs) participating in Medicare and Medicaid programs that adopt and successfully demonstrate meaningful use of certified EHR technology.

3. **a.** CEHRT must be evaluated independently of the vendor by the ONC or designee that the EHR in question must meet identified criteria and standards for functionality and interoperability in order to qualify for the MU incentive program.

4. **d.** They CQMs are criteria and tools to measure or quantify healthcare processes, outcomes, patient perceptions, and organizational structure and/or systems that

relate to one or more of the quality goals for health care: effective, safe, efficient, patient-centered, equitable, and timely.

5. **a.** Population health, or public health, focuses on preventing, diagnosing, and treating an entire group of people rather than one person at a time.

6. **d.** Query-based exchange is a find-and-seek request for information that is sent through the HIO to find any health information on a specified individual.

11.4.

1. **a.** Identity or patient matching is the process in which the HIO identifies the right person within the database to exchange information between HCOs.

2. **c.** Consent management has nothing to do with the consent for treatment but rather consent or approve the HIO to transmit health information between two or more authorized entities.

3. **b.** A biometric is a physical characteristic of the patient or users (such as fingerprints, voiceprints, retinal scans, iris traits) that systems store and use to authenticate identity of the patient or before allowing the user access to a system.

4. **b.** The *opt-out with exceptions* model sets the default for health information for patients to be included, but the patient can opt-out completely or allow only select data to be included.

5. **a.** Opt-in consent means that the patient must specifically agree to have the personal health information accessible for the HIE.

Chapter 12

12.1.

1. **a.** Only covered entities are subject to HIPAA.

2. **c.** One of the purposes of administrative simplification is to improve the efficiency and effectiveness of healthcare business processes such as claims submission.

3. **b.** One of the rights given to patients by HIPAA is the ability to access their health record. The answer cannot be amend their health record as the right is patients have the right to "request" an amendment not demand one.

4. **b.** The concept that allows CEs to consider the size, complexity, and capabilities of the CE when developing the compliance strategy is known as scalable.

5. **b.** Business associates do work on behalf of the CE that requires access to ePHI.

12.2.

1. **d.** The hacker attempted to access e-PHI. The attempt does not have to be successful in order to meet the definition of a security incident. The other options are all security events.

2. **a.** Information access management is establishing the process for determine what employees will have access to. Workforce clearance is applying those policies to give the employee the appropriate level of access.

3. **b.** Forensics is determining the facts for court.

4. **a.** Integrity is ensuring that data are not altered either during transmission across a network or during storage.

5. c. Risk analysis is the process of identifying possible security threats to the CE's data and identifying which risks should be promptly addressed and which are lower in priority.

12.3.

1. b. Audit-reduction tools are used to review the audit trail and compare it to facility-specific criteria and eliminate routine entries such as the periodic backups.

2. b. Encryption is turning data into unreadable text.

3. b. This methodology controls access to an information system based on the user's role in the organization. All individuals with that same role will have the same capabilities.

4. c. The user name and password is only a single factor authentication as it utilizes only the "what you know" methodology.

5. a. Triggers can be used to flag suspicious activities for further review.

12.4.

1. a. Both bots and spyware can capture keystrokes.

2. a. Ransomware is a type of malicious software that prohibits access to information systems in an organization. The ransomware pro-grammer may demand money before they will deactivate the ransomware.

3. c. Organizational access control is a physical safeguard that controls access to the data center and other resources.

4. b. Remote wipe removes data from a mobile device. While it can be used to delete data from a BYOD, it would not be used routinely.

5. a. Medical devices are used to treat patients.

Chapter 13

13.1.

1. a. Compliance is the process of establishing an organizational culture that promotes the prevention, detection, and resolution of instances of conduct that do not conform to federal, state, or private payer healthcare program requirements or the healthcare organization's ethical and business policies.

2. d. Training will be based on the role the employee has in the organization.

3. c. The penalties include financial penalties as well as prison time.

4. b.

5. a. External audits are performed by consultants or others who do not work for the CE. The purpose of an external audit is to confirm that the internal audits are identifying the risks and issues that it should.

13.2.

1. c. The Department of Health and Human Services' Office of Civil Rights (OCR) is in charge of oversight for the HIPAA Security Rule.

2. b. A resolution agreement is an agreement between the OCR and either a CE or business associate (BA). The resolution agreement describes the failure of the CE to meet the HIPAA requirements, any civil monetary penalties, a corrective action plan, and more.

3. **c.** HIPAA is divided into administrative, physical and technical safeguards All of these must be audited/monitored on an ongoing basis.

4. **a.** Data analysis is a body of methods that help describe facts, detect patterns, develop explanations, and test hypotheses.

5. **b.** In computer forensics, steps are taken in order to isolate the computer's storage media so that it cannot be destroyed or altered either accidently or on purpose. The hard drive is then copied so that investigators can research what happened by using the copy, not the original which prevents changes from being made in the original so that it can be used in court or for other purposes.